Mary Lindner
A Child's Mind Required!

Mary Lindner

A Child's Mind Required!
Evaluation Results on a Health Promoting
Initiative on AIDS and Sex Education for
Primary Schools

Budrich UniPress Ltd.
Opladen & Farmington Hills, MI 2010

All rights reserved. No part of this publication may be reproduced, stored in or introduced into a retrieval system, or transmitted, in any form, or by any means (electronic, mechanical, photocopying, recording or otherwise) without the prior written permission of Barbara Budrich Publishers. Any person who does any unauthorized act in relation to this publication may be liable to criminal prosecution and civil claims for damages.

You must not circulate this book in any other binding or cover and you must impose this same condition on any acquirer.

A CIP catalogue record for this book is available from
Die Deutsche Bibliothek (The German Library)

© 2010 by Budrich UniPress Ltd. Opladen & Farmington Hills
www.budrich-unipress.eu

ISBN   978-3-940755-30-8

Das Werk einschließlich aller seiner Teile ist urheberrechtlich geschützt. Jede Verwertung außerhalb der engen Grenzen des Urheberrechtsgesetzes ist ohne Zustimmung des Verlages unzulässig und strafbar. Das gilt insbesondere für Vervielfältigungen, Übersetzungen, Mikroverfilmungen und die Einspeicherung und Verarbeitung in elektronischen Systemen.

Die Deutsche Bibliothek – CIP-Einheitsaufnahme
Ein Titeldatensatz für die Publikation ist bei Der Deutschen Bibliothek erhältlich.

Budrich UniPress Ltd.
Stauffenbergstr. 7. D-51379 Leverkusen Opladen. Germany

28347 Ridgebrook. Farmington Hills, MI 48334. USA
www.budrich-unipress.eu

Jacket illustration by disegno, Wuppertal, Germany – www.disenjo.de
Printed in Europe on acid-free paper by paper & tinta, Warszaw, Poland.

TABLE OF CONTENTS

LIST OF FIGURES AND TABLES _____09
ABBREVIATIONS_____13
SUMMARY_____15
PROLOGUE _____16
ACKNOWLEDGEMENTS _____17
FOREWORD _____20

CHAPTER ONE　　　*Introduction* _____21

CHAPTER TWO　　　*Psychosocial Causes of Unsafe Health Behaviour of South African Children and Adolescents*
2.1　Introduction _____29
2.2　HIV/AIDS Epidemic and its Impacts on the South African Society _____30
2.3　Factors Contributing to the Transmission of HIV among Children and Adolescents in South Africa _____33
2.4　Learning Processes to Enhance Health – The Application of the Social Cognitive Theory by Bandura (1986) _____42
2.5　Conclusion _____55

CHAPTER THREE　　*Life Skills Interventions on HIV/AIDS in South Africa*
3.1　Introduction _____57
3.2　Sub-Saharan School-based Life Skills Initiatives on HIV/AIDS with Pre-Adolescents_____57
3.3　A Case of a School-based Life Skills Programme on HIV/AIDS in South Africa _____66
3.4　Factors Influencing the Implementation at School Level _____67
3.5　Conclusion _____71

CHAPTER FOUR　　　*A Needs Analysis for Health Interventions – Case Study of Kayamandi*
4.1　Introduction _____73
4.2　The History and Geographical Development of Kayamandi _____74
4.3　Socio-demographic Conditions _____78
4.4　Health Status of the Population _____83

4.5	Crime Rate	88
4.6	Educational Status of the Population	90
4.7	Existing Infrastructure	91
4.8	Conclusion	97

CHAPTER FIVE *Research in the Conditions of a Developing Country – Aims and Challenges*

5.1	Introduction	99
5.2	Psychosocial Research in the Conditions of a Developing World	100
5.3	Aims, Objectives, and Ethics of the Study	101
5.4	The Procedures of Selecting Communities and Primary Schools	104
5.5	Negotiation Access for Psychosocial Research in a Semi-urban Setting in South Africa	107
5.6	Unanticipated Events – Resulting Limitations	111
5.7	Conclusion	113

CHAPTER SIX *Methodology of the Study*

6.1	Introduction	115
6.2	Methods of the Needs Analysis	115
6.3	Methods of the Process Evaluation	120
6.4	Methods of the Outcome Evaluation	127
6.5	Conclusion	137

CHAPTER SEVEN *The Child Mind Project – Implementation Process*

7.1	Introduction	139
7.2	Background of the Study	140
7.3	Coordination Structures and Community-wide Implementation Procedures	141
7.4	The Learning Programme	145
7.5	Involvement of Health Promotion Trainers, the Class Teacher and Parents	157
7.6	Special Influences and Events during the Pilot Study	160
7.7	Conclusion	165

CHAPTER EIGHT *Assessment of the Programme by Health Promotion Trainers and Learners*

| 8.1 | Introduction | 167 |

8.2	Results of the HPTs' Reports	168
8.3	Results of Learners' Reports	178
8.4	Evaluating Social Behaviour of Four Children	183
8.5	Conclusion	192

CHAPTER NINE   *Results of the Outcome Evaluation*

9.1	Introduction	195
9.2	Effects of the Programme Regarding Individual Protective Variables	196
9.3.	A Descriptive Analysis of Particular Segments of the Learning Model and Outcomes Regarding HIV/AIDS	208
9.4	Results of the Opinion Poll	215
9.5	Conclusion	215

CHAPTER TEN   *Developing an Understanding of the Evaluation of the Proximal and Distal Context*

10.1	Introduction	219
10.2	Ethnic Diversity and Cultural Heritage	219
10.3	Physical Environment – Prevailing Risks to Health	220
10.4	Insights into Family Structures and Realities	225
10.5	The Existing Educational System	227
10.6	Conditions in Kayamandi – Strengths and Challenges	229
10.7	Children's Analysis of their Demands	235
10.8	Conclusion	236

CHAPTER ELEVEN   *Discussion of Research Findings*

11.1	Introduction	239
11.2	The Applicability of the Coordination Structure	240
11.3	The Main Columns – Incorporation of Parents, Class Teacher and Health Promotion Trainers	243
11.4	Applied Methods for Creating Emotional and Intellectual Safety	248
11.5	Research Gaps – Considerations Regarding Learning Outcomes on the Individual Level	252
11.6	Conclusion	255

EPILOGUE	257
REFERENCES	259

APPENDICES

Appendix A	Checklist for Casual Observation	277
Appendix B	Questionnaire for Field Interview	278
Appendix C	Health Promotion Trainers' Report	280
Appendix D	Checklist for Participant Observation	281
Appendix E	Revised Questionnaire	283
Appendix F	Commitments and Rules	291
Appendix G	Group Statistics (T-Test)	292
Appendix H	Correlation between Gender and the Evaluation Variables within the Intervention Group	293
Appendix I	Pearson Correlation Regarding Age of Samples – Intervention Group	296
Appendix J	Multiple Comparisons for Knowledge Scale 2 – Intervention Group	298

LIST OF FIGURES AND TABLES

FIGURES

Figure 1.1. Location of Kayamandi Settlement in Stellenbosch (Dennerlein & Adami, 2004).

Figure 2.1. HIV Prevalence among Respondents aged two Years and older by Sex and Age Group, South Africa 2005 (HSRC, 2005).

Figure 2.2. Bandura's Model of the Social Cognitive Theory (1998).

Figure 2.3. Research Model for Organizing the Relationship between psychological Competencies, interpersonal Conditions, and environmental Factors.

Figure 4.1. Kayamandi Structure in 1939 (Dennerlein & Adami, 2004).

Figure 4.2. Kayamandi Structure in 2004 (Dennerlein & Adami, 2004).

Figure 4.3. Formal Housing (Detached Houses) (Bicher, 2005).

Figure 4.4. Informal Housing (Shacks) (Bicher, 2005).

Figure 4.5. School Building – Ikaya Primary School (Bicher, 2005).

Figure 7.1. Project Structure of the Child Mind Project illustrating its six Levels.

Figure 7.2. Three Basic Components of the Presented Life Skills Programme on AIDS and Sex Education (see also PPASA, 1997).

Figure 8.1. Comparison between Results of Self-Assessment and Method by Health Promotion Trainer 1 (HPT1).

Figure 8.2. Comparison between Results of Self-Assessment and Method by Health Promotion Trainer 2 (HPT2).

Figure 8.3. Girls' General Attitude towards the Life Skills Programme during Intervention I.

Figure 8.4. Boys' General Attitude towards the Life Skills Programme during Intervention I.

Figure 8.5. Illustration of the Results on the Assessment of Like and Dislike towards Content and used Method by Girls of the Intervention Group.

Figure 8.6. Illustration of the Results on the Assessment of Like and Dislike towards Content and used Method by Boys of the Intervention Group.

Figure 9.1. Responses on – "Who do you live with at the Moment?" (Eleven Responses clustered in Six Categories) – Existing Family Units in the Intervention Group and Control Group at Pretest in March 2003.

Figure 9.2. Means of the Psychological and Social Variables for the Intervention Group (IG) over four Test Phases.

Figure 9.3. Means of the Psychological and Social Variables for the Control Group (CG) over four Test Phases.

Figure 9.4. Means for Knowledge Scale 1 for Intervention Group (IG) and Control Group (CG) over four Test Phases.

Figure 9.5. Means of Knowledge Scale 2 of the Intervention Group (IG) and Control Group (CG) over four Test Phases.

TABLES

Table 3.1. Characteristics of Sub-Saharan School-based Life Skills Initiatives on HIV/AIDS and Sex Education – Four Examples.

Table 3.2. Summary of Evaluation Methods on Sub-Saharan School-based Life Skills Initiatives on HIV/AIDS and Sex Education – Four Examples.

Table 3.3. Summary of Results on Knowledge, Attitudes, and Intentions on Sub-Saharan School-based Life Skills Initiatives on HIV/AIDS and Sex Education – Four Examples.

Table 3.4. Summary of Results on Communication and Behaviour on Sub-Saharan School-based Life Skills Initiatives on HIV/AIDS and Sex Education – Four Examples.

Table 5.1. Duration of Research from 2002 until 2004 and Content of Research.

Table 6.1. Design of Field Interviews illustrated with its Six Phases.

Table 6.2. Interobserver Reliability measured by Kendall's Tau B and Pearson Correlation and Interobserver Agreement measured by Kappa.

Table 6.3.	Factorial Analysis with repeated Testing with Intervention Group (IG) and Control Group (CG).
Table 6.4.	Data Analysis of Questionnaire by Cronbach Alpha, Number of Items, and Selectivity of Scales.
Table 7.1.	Organizational Structure of the Child Mind Project.
Table 7.2.	Topic One – Self-Esteem with Lesson Goal and applied Methods.
Table 7.3.	Topic Two – Relationships with Family and Friends with Lesson Goal and applied Methods.
Table 7.4.	Topic Three – Understanding my Body with Lesson Goal and applied Methods.
Table 7.5.	Topic Four – Health and Hygiene with Lesson Goal and applied Methods.
Table 7.6.	Topic Five – HIV/AIDS with Lesson Goal and applied Methods.
Table 7.7.	Topic Six – Sexual Abuse with Lesson Goal and applied Methods.
Table 7.8.	Topic Seven – Caring for an ill Person with Lesson Goal and applied Methods.
Table 7.9.	Topic Eight – Coping with Death with Lesson Goal and applied Methods.
Table 8.1.	Observation Results from Observation Phase I and II of the four Participants – Verification or Falsification of the applied Research Hypothesis.
Table 9.1.	Results of the Factorial ANOVA of Knowledge Scale 1 with Group Variable (A) and Repeated Measurement Variable (B).
Table 9.2.	Differences between Means with regard to Knowledge 1 between Intervention Group (IG) and Control Group (CG) over four Test Phases.
Table 9.3.	Results of the Factorial ANOVA of Knowledge Scale 2 with Group Variable (A) and Repeated Measurement Variable (B).
Table 9.4.	Differences between Means in Knowledge Scale 2 between Intervention Group (IG) and Control Group (CG) over four Test Phases.

Table 9.5. Percentage of Right Answers in Knowledge Scale 1 in the four Test Phases and Significant Changes in the Number of Right Answers compared to Pretest Results of the Intervention Group (IG).

Table 9.6. Percentage of Right Answers in Knowledge Scale 2 in the four Test Phases and Significant Changes in the Number of Right Answers compared to Pretest Results of the Intervention Group (IG).

ABBREVIATIONS

AIDS	Acquired Immune Deficiency Syndrome
Bzga	Bundeszentrale für gesundheitliche Aufklärung [Federal Centre for Health Education]
CADRE	Centre for AIDS Development Research and Evaluation
CG	Control Group
CIAC	Crime Information Analysis Centre
CMP	Child Mind Project
DAAD	Deutscher Akademischer Austauschdienst [German Academic Exchange Service]
DramAide	Drama Approach to AIDS Education
EU	European Union
HBM	Health Belief Model
HIV	Human Immunodeficiency Virus
HIVSP	HIV/AIDS/STD Strategic Plan for South Africa
HOD	Head of Department
HPT	Health Promotion Trainer
HSRC	Human Sciences Research Council
IG	Intervention Group
IPR	Index of Peer Relations
KTC	Kayamandi Town Council
MRC	Medical Research Council
NAMHC	National Advisory Mental Health Council
NBI	National Business Initiative
NDOE	National Department of Education
NDOH	National Department of Health
NFCS	National Food Consumption Survey
NGO	Non-governmental Organization
NIP	National Integrated Plan
NPPHCN	National Progressive Primary Health Care Network
OBE	Outcome Based Education
PAWC	Provincial Administration of the Western Cape
PGWC	Provincial Government of the Western Cape
PPASA	Planned Parenthood Association of South Africa
PSABH	Primary School Action for Better Health
PTT	Pilots Project in Southern Africa
RAPCAN	Resources Aimed at the Prevention of Child Abuse and Neglect

RDP	Reconstruction and Development Project
RLS	Rosa Luxemburg Stiftung [Rosa Luxemburg Foundation]
SA	South Africa
SAA	Stellenbosch AIDS Action
SAPS	South African Police Services
SATZ	South Africa and Tanzania Project
SCT	Social Cognitive Theory
SODI	Solidaritätsdienst-international e.V. [International Solidarity Service]
SPSS	Statistical Package for Social Sciences
STI	Sexually Transmitted Infections
STD	Sexually Transmitted Diseases
TB	Tuberculosis
UN	United Nations
UNAIDS	Joint United Nations AIDS Programme
UNICEF	United Nations Children's Fund
WC	Western Cape
WHO	World Health Organization

SUMMARY

Approximately two thirds (25.8 million) of the world's population infected with the Human Immunodeficiency Virus (HIV) are currently living in the sub-Saharan region. In South Africa, more than five million inhabitants are infected with the HIV-Virus. The South African group most vulnerable to HIV infection is young people between 20 and 34 years of age. It can thus be assumed that adolescents and children under the age of 15 are a less infected group and should therefore be *the major target of primary preventive approaches*. Consequently, this study is aimed at encouraging those skills and competencies required to cope with prevalent life tasks and to enhance the development of health behaviour to reduce the risk of HIV infection among pre-adolescent children (10-11 years of age) *before the onset of sexual activity*. This is done by means of a non-governmental and school-based *life skills programme on AIDS and sex education*, for socially disadvantaged children in the Western Cape Province of South Africa. The study, which is theoretically based on the *Social Cognitive Theory* (SCT) by Bandura (1986), used three types of evaluation to assess the personal, interpersonal and social context of the intervention undertaken. The *outcome evaluation* comprised a quasi-experimental research design with four test phases and was conducted by means of a self-administered questionnaire containing three psychological variables and two social variables. A *process evaluation* used the instruments of participant observation and reports to examine attitudes towards the intervention and other participating children as well as the health promotion trainers. A *needs analysis*, using the qualitative instrument of field interviews, examined risks and resources for child health within the environment of the case study. The results of the quantitative evaluation verify a significant increase in the participants' knowledge about HIV and the Acquired Immune Deficiency Syndrome (AIDS) from pretest to posttest phase. However, the follow-up tests show that *the effect of the programme is not sustainable* due to a relapse into a pretest knowledge level. Facing the insufficient sustainability of the evaluated programme, the results of the field interviews support the assumption that a magnitude of risk factors is evident in the environment of those children participating in the programme. These conditions assumingly not only negatively influence the mental, physical and social health from an early age on but *reduce the effect of the intervention* undertaken in this context. The thesis therefore concludes with recommendations for AIDS preventive and strengthening approaches for non-infected children living under these specific socio-economic and socio-cultural conditions, as they are most vulnerable to HIV infection.

PROLOGUE

How to Fight against a Snake

Once upon a time, a visitor from another world saw a wonderful place with purple flowers right in the middle of a sorrowful village. The beautiful and peaceful garden was surrounded by a high fence, making it inaccessible to everyone. The visitor lingered for a while in front of the main gate without entering. Meanwhile a woman stopped next to her and, with fear in her voice, she whispered: "Do not try to go in. Dangerous snakes live there." The visitor was surprised. There were no snakes to be seen, only wonderful, blooming and fragrant flowers. While the visitor was still deep in thought about the invisible snakes, other persons paused for a while next to her and told her stories about people who had seen snakes on this land. Now, the visitor became scared; if so many people were convinced of the existence of snakes, then they had to be there.

Weeks passed and the visitor could not forget that wonderful garden in the middle of such a sad town. She returned and to her surprise, this time, she found children playing in the forbidden area. While the children were building a fort underneath an old, wild tree, the visitor asked them: "What are you doing here? Didn't the people of this area tell you that you might get bitten by a snake when you enter this field?" And the children answered: "Yes, people tell many tales about the forbidden garden. We also know of one tale, which talks about snakes in the grass that might bite humans. But, this must be a myth because since we have been here we have not seen one snake." And then they carried on building their fort in this banned area, turning it into their own playground.

By Mary Lindner

ACKNOWLEDGEMENTS

The success of this study was undoubtedly ensured by the support of a lot of people, many of whom I would like to acknowledge in the following pages.

Special thanks go to my supervisors, Prof. Leslie Swartz from the University of Stellenbosch (US), who carefully secured the theoretical and ethical grounds for the study, and Prof. Dieter Kleiber from the Freie Universität in Berlin, who safeguarded the completion of this thesis. I would also like to express my gratitude to Prof. Gudrun Ehlert from the University of Applied Sciences in Mittweida and Prof. Sulina Green from the University of Stellenbosch, both of whom supported the purpose of my study right from the beginning. Dr Yalew Endawoke from the University of Addis Ababa and Dr Fred Mengering from the Technische Universität Berlin, who became valuable sources of fruitful discussions on the design of research instruments and statistical measurements, were instrumental in composing specific columns in this study.

I would also like to name some wonderful women working in the administration centres of foundations and universities who supported this study throughout its duration: Erika Thieme and Ursula Schlupeck from the University of Applied Sciences in Mittweida, Jane Moros and Helga Islam from the German Academic Exchange Service (DAAD), and the International Office team, specifically Dorothy Stevens, at the University of Stellenbosch. Special gratitude goes to the team of women from the Rosa Luxemburg Stiftung (RLS), who facilitated the financial basis of this study.

A person who expressed great trust in my skills and character was Dr Peter Stobinski, ret. Director of the Solidaritätsdienst-international e.V (SODI), which supported the project financially.

I would also like to thank the following people for their support, guidance and comments on my thesis during the long process of evaluating the programme in the field and writing up the results: Thuso Kewana Ceo, for his advice on African culture and community ethics; Songo Fipaza, for spending so much of his time doing the field trips with me; Yeki Mosomothane, for his work on community support and his often direct talks on ethics and the contents of such a programme; Ndudu Ndlebe, for her patience in discussing health purposes in the community with me and for carrying out a health workshop at the community clinic; and Mzwandile Mgabadeli, who always did his best to manage and resolve infrastructural barriers of the project within the school setting.

Then, I would like to name Brandon Ruth and Joy Wilson from Joy for Life, who were undoubtedly my greatest signposts in times of disorientation.

S. Gertrude Gedze, a Xhosa lady, and Anne Curnow, an Afrikaans lady, representing both the old and the new South Africa, supported me in a similar way and always had a warm welcome for me as a visitor to their loved country when I needed it most. People who have always been a tonic of humanism and have to be honoured in this acknowledgement are my friends Alexandra Baer, Heidi Lohmeier, Katrin Morgeneyer, Sebastian Dathe and Jacqueline Sidi-Boumedien. Vera Dittmar holds a special position in this group of people. She has always been the best critic of my work, but also the first emotional pillar when I stumbled, and therefore had a great impact on the success of this work.

During the course of the study the team members of the research and project team became much more than colleagues – they became the Child Mind 'feste'. First of all I would like to thank Christine Buchinger and Christina Otto, who volunteered as research assistants. They always kept in mind to be as objective as possible. The supporting teacher, Roselind Xhamela, was a welcome partner during the intervention phase. She often invested additional time in the project and dealt bravely with resistance against the project in the school setting more than once. In the same way I would like to name Zanele Kobus, the class teacher of the control group at the Nomlinganiselo Primary School, who was always able to incorporate my visits to the school without long pre-meetings and spent so much of her leisure time to meet for discussions on the project. It is difficult to find the right words to express what a great honour it was for me to work with two extremely courageous and open-minded young women, Patricia Mangena and Anneliesa Charmaine Mbena, the leading health promotion trainers in the Child Mind Project (CMP). They gave life to this project against all odds and despite the fears they had or which they experienced in their community.

Most importantly, I am very grateful to and impressed by the parents and children of the intervention and control group, who have always been a ray of hope and a fountain of new experiences and insights for the project, for the research part, and for me.

My final and affectionate acknowledgement is to my parents. Although my time in South Africa was not easy for them, they were always there to support me in my aims. Today I can say that what I really learned from all my experiences in the field is that I was in the privileged position of being able to grow up with loving and caring parents, who always put me first.

This book is dedicated to Anneliesa Charmaine Mbena,
a highly intelligent and courageous young woman
who died under unknown circumstances
after giving birth to her baby boy
in December 2003.

FOREWORD

Convinced that every chapter of this thesis undoubtedly constitutes a piece of the greater puzzle of this research work, I would like to give some advice to readers regarding possible points of interest, so as to simplify the reading process. Readers who have a research background might find it more interesting to focus on the chapters which explain the research model used (chapter 2), the methodology of the study (chapter 6), the research results (chapter 7 to 10) and the final discussion (chapter 11). The chapters listed above would perhaps be of less interest to readers who are actually working in the field of life skills education and AIDS prevention. These readers might be more interested in the chapters which describe the negotiation processes preceding the project (chapter 5) and explain the Child Mind Project with reference to its pedagogical approach and realisation of content (chapter 7). They might also find some useful recommendations for the implementation of similar projects in similar environments in chapter 11. Readers who are unfamiliar with practical research in a developing-world context should focus on the first five chapters in order to enhance their understanding of the difficulties faced by researchers striving to realise their aims and goals in this particular kind of research context.

CHAPTER ONE
Introduction

The United Nations Conventions on the Rights of the Child, the legal foundation for the rights of all children worldwide, pleads for a standard of living with adequate physical, mental, spiritual, moral and social development of children in the present and the future (Article 27). In accordance with the Convention, a 'healthy' child development is defined as one that strives for the *protection* (Article 19), *health and well-being* (Article 24), and *education* (Article 28/29) of the child (United Nations [UN], 1989). However, the reality always appears somehow different from legal ideals.

In 2004, the United Nations Children's Fund (UNICEF) reported that *poverty, conflict and AIDS* are denying more than one billion children worldwide a peaceful childhood. These three conditions create seven basic deprivations that children feel and which have a powerful impact on their futures, namely inadequate shelter, no access to sanitation or clean water, lack of access to information and education, no access to health care services, and food insecurity (UNICEF, 2004). Illustrated on the country South Africa, a positive and healthy child development can be tremendously effected if the chain of the three deprivations – poverty, conflict, and AIDS – is given.

The South African National Department of Health (NDOH) estimates that 14 million (approximately 30%) of the South African population experience food insecurity. Within this context, children, especially those in rural and semi-urban areas, are the most vulnerable to malnutrition which causes health implications ranging from growth failure, a reduced physical and mental capacity in childhood, to an increased risk of developing (diet-related) non-communicable diseases later in life (Mvulane, 2003).

A further problematic nature is the growing AIDS epidemic in South Africa. About a decade ago, the situation regarding the AIDS epidemic in South Africa was better than in some of its neighbouring countries. Today, HIV infection in South Africa is spreading at a rate of at least 1 700 new infections per day; one of the fastest-growing rates of HIV infection in the world. A study by the Human Sciences Research Council (HSRC) (2005) revealed that the highest HIV prevalence can be found in the 20- to 34-year-old age group, among which 24- to 29-year-olds are the worst infected (23.2%). This means, more than half of these new infections occur in young people (Skinner, 2000). Most infected people live in urban informal areas (25.8%) and are African and female (24.4%) (HSRC, 2005).

It has been estimated that by 2010, there will be more than two to three million orphans under the age of 16 who will be fending for themselves and their siblings in what is known as child-headed households (Padayachee, 2004). Thus, the loss of parents through AIDS, for example, puts especially children from socially-disadvantaged backgrounds in moreover unsafe living conditions and exposes them to a magnitude of insecure life situations, e.g. maltreatment and/or exploitation that most probably has negative effects on their physical health and mental well-being.

In other words, the described conditions above, widespread and growing poverty, an increasing intergenerational epidemic and high levels of violence in all its forms, cause especially great concern for those children who grew up in impoverished settings which prove their life more insecure. As it is stated in the United Nations Conventions on the Right of the Child (UN, 1989), interventions who shall improve the living situation for those children most in need must place the greatest emphasis to safeguard their basic needs on protection (Article 19 (1)), health and well-being (Article 24 (1/2), as well as education (Article 29a and b). Whereas *education,* as the third protective column, can be considered as extremely important for two main reasons. Education forms the foundation for the edification of a future society in long-term and in short-term, it can be regarded as the most significant resource to eliminate ignorance and illiteracy and to facilitate access to scientific and technical knowledge that conveys adequate information and skills for the protection and well-being of the individual (UN, 1989, Art. 28).

In regard to the United Nations (1989, Art. 29a), the development of the child's personality, talents and mental and physical abilities to their fullest potential should be in the centre of every educational process. A child needs to be prepared for a responsible life in a free society, in the spirit of understanding, peace, tolerance, equality of sexes, and friendship with all people, ethnic, national and religious groups and persons of indigenous origin (UN, 1989, Art. 29b). In other words, children and young people have to be considered important segments of the population as targets for any kind of educational purpose that strives to prepare them for present and future life demands. Health-promoting initiatives can be regarded as important and most effective pillars to close the gap between education, health and protection. Because their main goal is to train individuals' life-enhancing competencies and skills, they have an immediate and also a constant effect on the ability of the human to deal with present and future life tasks.

With this conviction in mind, the presented book describes the outcomes of a non-governmental and school-based life skills programme on AIDS and sex education targeting foremost the enhancement of adjusted coping strategies in terms of health, well-being and protective behavioural competencies for pre-adolescent children. Furthermore, the evaluated school-based life skills programme was characterised by a primary preventive approach, proposing that pre-adolescent children (10-11 years of age) should receive health and sex education before they develop a full value and behavioural system.

The consideration to target pre-adolescent children follows the assumption that pre-adolescents have neither developed health behaviour nor been sexually active, yet. Foremost, during the life stage of pre-adolescents, value and attitude systems only start to enlarge, behavioural patterns are in a permanent probation, bodily changes take place and the individual's social environment expands to no longer just include the family system but also the school and community. In this phase, they also start to formulate rational conclusions, enlarge their observational and testing spectrum, and consequently make decisions which result in concrete individual behavioural patterns. With this knowledge in mind, the conclusion can be drawn that a primary preventive approach can only have the greatest effect if within the participants does not exist an infection with HIV and they do not show risking-taking (sexual) health behaviour.

Chapter 2 opens the argumentation in which it formulates the above assertion into a scientific statement with the presentation of related results of recent studies on the psychosocial causes of unhealthy (sexual) behaviour among South African young people and children that contributes to HIV transmission. With regard to the development of health behaviour during different developmental stages from childhood to adolescence, three examples of risk factors for HIV infection of children and young people in South Africa are discussed. First, socio-demographic factors which have a tremendous impact on the high incidence of HIV in South African society are outlined. Second, sexual abuse of children is very common in South Africa, and not only causes physical injuries but also negatively influences health behaviour from an early age on. In the last instance a description of several studies evaluating the sexual behaviour of adolescents in South Africa is given. These results shall clarify that risky sexual behaviour even exists in these younger populations and causes a further spread of HIV in South African society. As this study is meant to examine the effects of a life skills programme on AIDS and sex education for pre-adolescent children, a theoretical model is introduced. The Social Cognitive Theory (SCT) by Bandura (1986) is presented to explain how learning processes in the interaction between individual, interpersonal, and environmental level take place, and encourage the development of health behaviour amongst the pre-adolescent participants of the programme. Finally, the research model is introduced in conjunction with its independent variable, intervention, and a range of dependent variables; the psychological indicators such as self-esteem, self-efficacy, and knowledge assess the personal level whilst social competencies on the interpersonal level are studied with regard to gender communication and social responsibility.

The foci of interest in chapter 3 are prevention strategies targeting mainly children and young people in the sub-Saharan region. Governmental and non-governmental school-based health promotion interventions, mainly life skills programmes on HIV/AIDS and sex education, are introduced as main prevention strategies to avoid HIV infection in the next generations. The last part of chapter 3 deals with the specific factors that can influence the implementation and evaluation of school-based prevention programmes, illustrated on the country South Africa.

The location of the health-promoting project was the socially-disadvantaged community "Kayamandi"; located in Stellenbosch in the Western Cape Province in South Africa (Figure 1.1). The socio-demographic conditions within the case study community are highlighted in chapter 4.

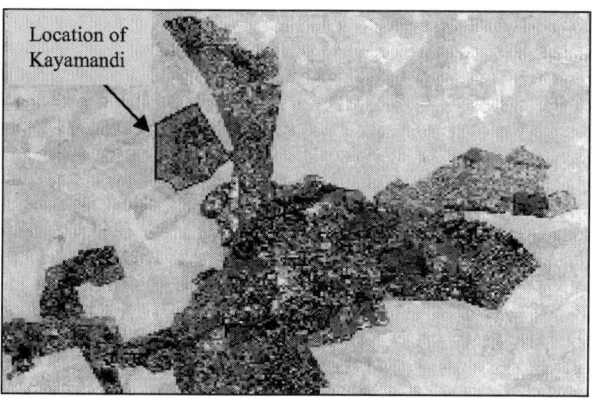

Figure 1.1. Location of Kayamandi Settlement in Stellenbosch (Dennerlein & Adami, 2004).

The description of this particular community is meant to illustrate the need for health interventions for children growing up in comparable living conditions. Thus, the chapter 4 includes a description of the geographical and political history of the case study community, as well as socio-demographic aspects, for example the health status of the population, crime rate and level of education of the population. The same chapter concludes with a description of the existing infrastructure, which can also be interpreted as a needs analysis to embed this study in its physical context.

Chapter 5 illustrates research conditions for psychology and health research in third world conditions. The aims, objectives, ethics and context of research are outlined before describing specific negotiation procedures on community, school, and personal level. Finally, challenges that arose from unanticipated events and the resulting limitations that affected the quality and design of the survey are reported.

The methodology of the study is outlined in detail in chapter 6. The study used three types of evaluation to reach an in-dept view on the personal, interpersonal and social context of the undertaken intervention. The *needs analysis*, taking into consideration the risk-resource approach (see also Hurrelmann, Klotz, & Haisch, 2004), examined risks and resources for child health in the case study community. Information for the needs analysis was drawn from regular field trips and field reports, an extensive literature review (e.g. maps, official statistics, published and unpublished articles), and accompanying photographic documentation. Main emphasis was put on the qualitative instrument of field interviews, undertaken with nine experts working in governmental and non-governmental institutions in the field of education, health, social and public welfare in the case study community. The instrument gathered data on the growing risks and resources in the socio-economic conditions and family life, as well as on the quality of educational and health care sectors. A *process evaluation* was applied with the use of the qualitative instruments of the health promotion trainers' (HPTs) reports and project documentation, and with combined quantitative-qualitative instruments of the learners' reports and participant observations of four children in the intervention group (IG). These instruments analysed the effect of the model by measuring the cognitive and emotional convictions among children (learners) and facilitators (HPTs). The *outcome evaluation* used two major instruments: a self-administered questionnaire and an opinion poll. The questionnaire, based on a quasi-experimental research design with four test phases, contains three psychological variables (self-esteem, self-efficacy, knowledge on HIV/AIDS) and two social variables (gender communication, social responsibility) which are assumed to encourage the development of cognitive and social competencies to cope with prevalent life tasks and to enhance mental and protective health behaviour, also for later life stages. The opinion poll was conducted in which learners expressed their long-term attitudes towards the programme, as well as attitudes towards their physical living environment.

Chapter 7 contains, foremost, a description of the implementation process of the evaluated intervention. A specifically designed non-governmental school-based life skills programme on AIDS and sex education for primary school children, formerly designed by the Planned Parenthood Association of South Africa (PPASA) in 1997, formed the foundation of the evaluation study. During the implementation process extensive modifications were made, so that the applied life skills programme accommodated existing cultural, contextual and developmental specifics of the participating children. A general explanation of the programme's pedagogical concept is given and linked with implementation procedures and coordination structures. Furthermore, the networking of the project with governmental and non-governmental institutions within the Kayamandi community is outlined in detail. Finally, special events such as cases of corporal punishment at school and sexual child abuse in the intervention group, which are assumed to have hindered the intervention and compromised the outcome of the life skills programme on the individual level, are discussed.

Chapter 8 describes the process assessed by health promotion trainers as part of an instrument to evaluate the quality of teaching, based on their self-confidence to teach in their position as trainers and to implement the programme in the classroom. In addition, learners' attitudes towards the programme and its methodology, and their ease with HPTs and classmates of the same and the other gender are presented. The chapter is concluded with the results from the participants' observations of the social behaviour of two girls and two boys during intervention sessions over a period of seven months. These observations illustrate the appropriateness of the intervention targeting the specific age group.

Chapter 9 contains the results of the outcome evaluation. The effects of the intervention are presented by means of the analysis of the quantitative instrument, the self-administered questionnaire. The results of the socio-demographic, psychological, cognitive and social competency research variables are presented descriptively and statistically; this is followed by a discussion of gathered quantitative data within the intervention group. An investigation into the specific segments of the model, for instance HIV/AIDS and sex education, and their learning outcomes, illustrate from a broader perspective the relevance of the intervention in terms of influencing knowledge, attitudes and skills regarding HIV/AIDS. The chapter concludes with the presentation of the results from the first part of the opinion poll that evaluated learners' long-term attitudes towards the learning programme eight months after the end of Intervention II.

Chapter 10 examines in more detail the social factors influencing child development in a disadvantaged living environment such as Kayamandi from the perspective of experts working in governmental and non-governmental organizations (NGO). The chapter revisits the literature review in chapter 4 and gives a more personal depiction of the living and growing-up conditions of children in Kayamandi. The ethnic diversity and cultural heritage of the inhabitants of the community are presented, followed by a description of the prevailing socio-demographic conditions, for example risky health conditions, prevalent childhood diseases, lack of security and socialisation pillars (families, school system). The underlying goal of the chapter is to develop an understanding of the outside factors that could have influenced the intervention unintentionally and with it uncontrolled. At the end of the chapter results from the second part of the opinion poll are presented, where children were given the chance to speak about and identify their needs and demands in their community.

Chapter 11 summarizes and discusses specific research findings regarding effects on the individual and interpersonal domain as well as the applicability of the programme and the identification of contextual conditions influencing the outcomes of such a health promoting initiative. Conclusions and recommendations are included in the argumentations and made for further research investigations on child development, as well as for the improvement of the applicability of a similar life skills programme on AIDS and sex education within the described social context.

CHAPTER TWO
Psychosocial Causes of Unsafe Health Behaviour of South African Children and Adolescents

2.1 Introduction

According to the World Health Organization (WHO), the term 'health' is defined as "a state of complete physical, mental and social well-being and not merely the absence of disease or infirmity" (WHO, 2001). To build up on the WHO's theoretical concept of health this study follows health promotion approaches (see also Hurrelmann et al., 2004), that understand health-related behaviours as being always formed by risk and protective factors which are based on three domains: physical, psychological and social. Thus, the focus of interest in chapter 2 is the presentation of an extensive literary review of different studies, especially those from South Africa. The objective of the chapter is to explain the diverse psychosocial factors pertaining to the development of mental and physical health among children and young people[1] that makes them vulnerable to HIV infection. The first part of this chapter, therefore, explains how health-related behaviour[2] develops from childhood to adolescence, and presents specific psychosocial risks and resources effecting the development of health behaviour among children and adolescents in South Africa.

The second part of the chapter describes foremost the theoretical basis and the designed model for this thesis. The Social Cognitive Theory (SCT) by Bandura (1986) forms the theoretical basis for the evaluation of the acquisition of cognitive and social competencies or rather learning processes of children participating in a specific primary preventive approach, that is, a life skills programme on AIDS and sex education. Due to an absence of research findings on pre-adolescents, the research model used and the relevance of the examined variables are explained by describing results from studies on (unsafe) sexual behaviour among South African adolescents.

---

1   In this study the terms 'youth' and 'young people' also refer to the stage of adolescence.
2   In addition, the following chapters use the term 'health behaviour' or 'risky health behaviour', and not 'sexual behaviour' as in other studies, because it is assumed that pre-adolescents have either not yet developed health behaviour or been sexually active.

2.2 HIV/AIDS Epidemic and its Impacts on the South African Society

According to the Joint United Nations AIDS Programme (UNAIDS) and the World Health Organization 40.3 million people currently live with HIV worldwide. Almost five million people were newly infected with HIV and 3.1 million died of AIDS in 2005. The sub-Saharan region has the highest number of HIV infection with 25.8 million people. This means, approximately 65% of all people infected with HIV live in this region and 77% of all infected human beings are African women (UNAIDS/WHO, 2005a). UNAIDS stated in its last report on the situation of the global AIDS epidemic that the total number of people living with HIV reached its highest level in 2005 with increasing prevalence on other continents. The conclusion reached by the same organizations in 2005 was that a reduction of the AIDS pandemic could not be foreseen (UNAIDS/WHO, 2005a).

According to UNAIDS (2002), the youth are at the centre of the global HIV/AIDS pandemic as the next generation who has to face a cumulative impact in the forthcoming years. The predictions are that a large part of the young generation, as the most infected, will be unable to raise and educate their children. The current number of 14 million AIDS orphans and terminally ill people (UNAIDS, 2002) is on the increase worldwide and without adequate treatment and care, most of them will not survive the next decade (UNAIDS/WHO, 2001). To make matters worse, most of these infected people are unaware of carrying the virus, many millions more know nothing or far too little about HIV and how to protect themselves against it (UNAIDS/WHO, 2001). Regarding taboo issues such as sex, death and illness, stigmatisation of HIV-positive people is high. Therefore, many infected people decide not to disclose their status to relatives or neighbours because they are afraid of becoming social outcasts (Campbell, 2003). The consequence of such taboos and fear is a difficulty in reducing HIV: either preventive action does not reach the most vulnerable human beings or it cannot be sufficiently and effectively implemented. Furthermore, the HIV epidemic affects mainly low- and middle-income countries, it has tremendous impacts on the stability of societies putting an additional burden on their economic, political and health systems.

South Africa has one of the highest numbers of people living with HIV worldwide. According to the National Department of Health (2004a) it is estimated that between 5.7 and 6.2 million South Africans are currently living with the virus and 1 700 more people are infected with this virus every day. The statistics on HIV prevalence in South Africa, however, consistently vary as do all statistics in this field. In the knowledge of the worldwide methodological discussion on the reliability of HIV/AIDS statistics, one resource which tends to be most valid and widely distributed is the South African National HIV prevalence, HIV incidence, behaviour and communication survey (2005). This survey was conducted in cooperation with the Human Sciences Research Council (HSRC), the Centre for AIDS Development Research and Evaluation (CADRE), and the Medical Research Council (MRC) (HSRC, 2005) and gathered its data from a cross-sectional multistage disproportionate, stratified sampling procedure. Data were obtained by collecting blood specimens.

The survey estimated the overall national HIV prevalence to be 10.8% (from 2 to 50+ years). The highest HIV prevalence can be found in the age groups 20 to 24 (15.2%), 24 to 29 (23.2%), and 30 to 34 (24.9%). Figure 2.1 shows the HIV prevalence rates clustered in age ranges and gender distribution. Statistics of the survey illustrate women in the age group 20 to 39 years are the most infected, with the most infected age group the 25- to 29-year-old group (33.3%). The survey also revealed that the highest HIV prevalence range is among African females (24.4%) and among adults, age 15 to 49 years (25.8%) living in urban informal areas (HSRC, 2005).

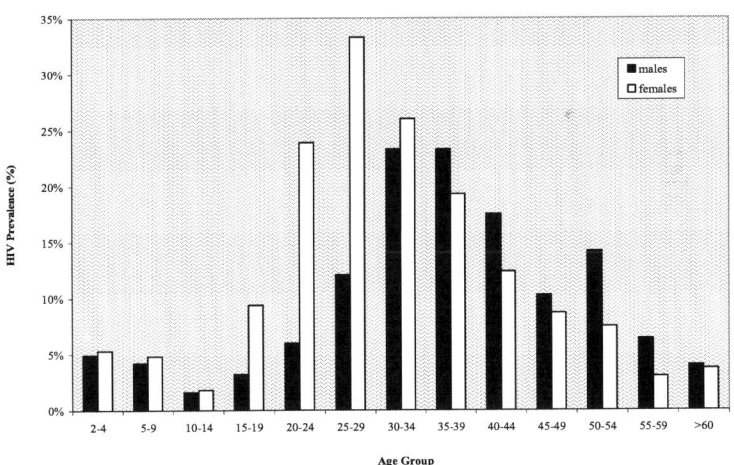

Figure 2.1. HIV Prevalence among Respondents aged two Years and older by Sex and Age Group, South Africa 2005 (HSRC, 2005).

It was difficult to assess data gathered on children aged 2 to 14. The HIV prevalence within this group was 3.3% in 2005. Compared to the survey of

2002, where 5.6% children were tested HIV positive (HSRC, 2002), the HIV prevalence decreased over the years in a confusing way (HSRC, 2005). However, the breakdown of ages makes it clear that a high number of 5- to 9-year-old boys (4.2%) and girls (4.8%) were already HIV positive. The National Household Survey of HIV Prevalence and Risk Survey of South African Children of 2004 discovered that the highest HIV prevalence was found among children living in informal urban areas (6.4%) (Brooks, Shisana, & Richter, 2004). Nonetheless, this result is alarmingly high in an age group that should show a smaller birth-related infection rate due to an absence of unsafe health behaviour (e.g. unprotected sex), which normally contributes to sexually transmitted infections such as HIV. These findings lead to a closer contemplation of the national discussion on the distribution of sexual abuse among children in South Africa (see par. 2.3.3).

In conclusion, the forecasts for the South African society as a whole are alarming. By the year 2010 South Africa will experience an overall prevalence of 25% of HIV infections. Life expectancy is predicted to drop from 65 years to 48 years due to the impact of HIV (H.J. Kaiser Foundation, 1999). A recent study on death registration has shown that deaths among people 15 years of age and older increased by 62% between 1997 and 2002, with deaths among people aged 25 to 44 more than doubling in South Africa (Statistics South Africa, 2005a). It is assumed that roughly 39% of the child population will be affected by adult morbidity and mortality (Dorrington, Bradshaw, Johnson, & Budlender, 2004).

The country South Africa experiences, besides one of the highest rates of HIV infection in the world, a non-foreseeable increase in new HIV infections among the youngest groups of society. It is also expected that the heaviest toll of this tremendous national crisis will be borne by South African children and young people because most of the people dying of AIDS will be the biologically and economically viable parts of the country. It is estimated that they will leave behind three million orphans (Gow & Desmond, 2002).

Apart from these discouraging prospects, there is still a chance to turn the tide or at least, to alleviate the heaviest burden for the human beings living in this epidemic situation. As the vast majority of children and youth under 15 years of age are not HIV-positive, they form a promising target group for prevention efforts that provide them with tools to cope with this extensive life crisis and to protect themselves against an HIV infection later in life.

2.3 Factors Contributing to the Transmission of HIV among Children and Adolescents in South Africa

The statistics mentioned above provide evidence that especially the youngest sections of South African society are exposed to specific risk factors leading to the acquisition of unhealthy (sexual) behaviour or conditions, which might make them vulnerable, for instance, to becoming infected with HIV. The following paragraphs discuss from a broader perspective what psychosocial factors influence children and youth in South Africa in their development of physical and mental health while simultaneously being influenced by the social context. These factors are considered strongly interconnected and determining in the practise of health behaviour among individuals. The complete discussion is based on scientific knowledge on common psychosocial risk and protective elements effecting the development of health behaviour from childhood to adolescence as the two main developmental phases described in this study. Specifically existing risk factors, which are scientifically proven to have a great impact on the growing up of children and young adults in South Africa, are described in the following.

2.3.1 Psychosocial Risk Factors Effecting the Development of Health Behaviour – The Starting Point

There is a conviction in the public health field that every developmental step in a human being's life from before birth until late adulthood bears specific protective or risk factors that either draw the individual towards positive outcomes or push the individual towards negative (or risky) outcomes (Richter, 2001). In other words, when trying to prevent disease and encourage the development of competences to maintain an individual's health, the best would be to encourage health even before birth or in early *childhood* (0-6 years). As Hosman and Llopis (2005) state, there is not only more development in mental, social and physical functioning during the early stages of life than in any other period, but this phase also determines a child's functioning in school later on and in the broader society, as well as relationships – with peers as well as intimate relations. However, when trying to influence health behaviour to enhance a positive quality of health, or rather to reduce negative outcomes of health effects, the developmental phase of late childhood and adolescence is regarded as a good temporary gate for health-promoting interventions, especially when preventive attempts are undertaken in cooperation with the main forms of social support, namely the family and the school.

Childhood (6-13 years) is that phase in life when body, soul and mind, together with social relationships and skills, develop within a short period of time and are subject to big changes. During this time biological disposition, learning processes and influences from the immediate environment (the family and school) interact (Bergmann & Bergmann, 2004), resulting in the creation of a personality with its individual properties, skills and behaviour (Keller, 1998; Markefka & Nauck, 1993; Bergmann & Bergmann, 2004). This process includes the completion of perception and articulation abilities, the broadening of an individual's horizon, the expansion of a role repertoire that can be used outside the family, and the development of the first signs of a social identity (Schnabel, 2004). On the basis of these developmental processes the deduction can be made that the health behaviour that is practised in childhood is very often sustained throughout life (Oerter, 1995a; Knäuper, 2002). With reference to the prevention of disease and the development of competencies that will help to maintain health, childhood is probably the most important stage in life, as most children are born healthy, meaning that the metabolism and immune system of children are sustainable and their health behaviour (or risky behaviour) has not yet been established (Bergmann & Bergmann, 2004).

The stage of *adolescence* (13-18 years), the passage from childhood to adulthood, is characterised by the exploration of new and consequently somewhat risky behaviour (Hurrelmann, 1998; Knäuper, 2002). This means that development in adolescence is an active process during which the individual takes over or establishes developmental targets and actively strives to reach these (Pinquart & Silbereisen, 2004). The developmental tasks during this stage include: reaching independence from parents, establishing relationships with peers and partners, dealing with physical development, and developing an identity (Havighurst, 1972; Pinquart & Silbereisen, 2004). During this stage the family in particular and the allocation of roles in the family function as living models (Schnabel, 2004) that are tested in relationships within the peer group and in first (intimate) partnerships. Not to be underestimated is an additional risk factor whereby adolescents generally tend to ignore potential long-term consequences of risky behaviour and consider themselves invincible – with the consequential negative impact on their health that will only present itself later in life (Knäuper, 2002). Seeing that during this phase the range of risk and protective factors changes and expands and health behaviour is established and strengthened, adolescence is regarded as another extremely important time for preventive measures (Pinquart & Silbereisen, 2004), especially in disadvantageous social conditions that encumber the realisation of developmental tasks.

In conclusion, fields of psychosocial risk and protective factors can be found in (physical) growth, (health) status, (mental) development, (social) competencies and adjustment, (school) achievement, and integration (Richter, Cameron, Norris, Del Fabro, & MacKeown, 2004). This means, for example, that child development is a matter of continual adaptation to circumstances as the balance between these factors change (Compas, Hindon, & Gerhardt, 1995 in Richter et al., 2004). In their report on children in South Africa, Berry and Guthrie (2003) identified poverty, diseases such as HIV/AIDS, and violence or child abuse as the main risk factors affecting child development, and most likely also affecting the development of health behaviour. The following three examples portray these research findings by Berry and Guthrie (2003) in more detail and, at this point, describe main risk factors which influence the development of health behaviour among South African children and young people.

2.3.2 Selected Socio-demographic Risk Factors – Poverty and Malnutrition

The socio-demographic conditions in which South African children grow up, including insecure (environmental) living conditions and malnutrition, are considered to be one of the main factors which influences the quality of child health.

In urban South Africa, the poorest strata of society are concentrated in so-called townships. Townships are relics of the apartheid past when people of African origin were concentrated in urban and semi-urban areas. In recent years, townships are growing into overcrowded areas due to extreme migration processes from rural to urban areas in the search for work. The disadvantaged areas are mainly characterised by underdeveloped infrastructures, unhygienic living conditions, lack of security, high crime rates and poverty-related physical (e.g. malnutrition) and mental (e.g. depression) diseases. Children who grow up in impoverished living conditions might be subject to health risks in four predominant areas, namely:

(1) Inadequate housing and access to water and sanitation causing overt exposure to diseases such as tuberculosis (TB) and diarrhoea (Mathee, 2004);
(2) Exposure to indoor air pollution due to the use of polluting fuels and chemicals such as lead and pesticides (Mathee, 2004);
(3) Unintentional injuries (e.g. traffic injuries, drowning, poisoning, burn injuries or road accidents) due to living in an

environment without a structured town layout or road maintenance and often inadequate care and protection (Mathee, 2004); and

(4) Intentional injuries can be caused by three categories of violence: (a) self-directed violence (e.g. suicide), (b) interpersonal violence (e.g. child maltreatment, intimate partner/group violence, sexual violence), and (c) collective violence (e.g. human rights abuse) that either result in or have a high likelihood of resulting in injury, death, psychological harm, maldevelopment or deprivation (see also Walker, Verins, Moodie, & Webster, 2005 in WHO, 2005).

Human beings living in disadvantaged, and therefore, poor living conditions are not only exposed to unhealthy and unsafe environments but also to unattained basic needs, as a result of extreme poverty. It is estimated that approximately 19.3 million South African children under the age of 18 are living in poverty and that 11 million (60%) of these are living in absolute poverty with less than R200 per month (Streak, 2002). According to Berry and Guthrie (2003), this amount corresponds with half of the amount needed to satisfy basic needs for survival and food security. Approximately 30% of the South African population experience food insecurity, which affects mainly entire families in rural and semi-urban areas (Mvulane & Proudlock, 2002; Mvulane, 2003). This food insecurity also means that a large number of children in South Africa are assumed to be undernourished, which, consequently, has long-term impeding effects on their physical and mental/cognitive development (learning ability and life task achievements).

Bray (2002, 2003) concludes that a wide range of growing risk factors on socio-economic level influence the physical, psychological and social well-being of South African children growing up in disadvantaged living conditions. Vergnani, Flisher, Lazarus, Reddy, & James (1998) agree that the living conditions or rather the socio-demographic situation of children and youth in South Africa provide major risk factors for developing unsafe health (sexual) behaviour later in life. Finally, as statistics suggest, while poverty, unemployment and inequality are on the increase in South Africa (Berry & Guthrie, 2003), the present AIDS epidemic functions like a catalytic converter that worsens the quality of life and creates a higher insecurity for the poorest strata and population groups in South Africa, especially children, who largely depend on adults and their environments.

2.3.3 The Sexual Abuse of Children in South Africa – Harmed Health

Crimes against children include kidnapping, assault, murder and attempted murder, rape and incest, amongst others (Bower, 2003b). In South Africa 72 026 crimes against children were reported in 2000, with 66 957 in 1996 (Bower, 2003a), with an increasing tendency (Office on the Right of the Child, 2001). Due to a lack of accurate statistics on children's actual exposure to the different forms of violence (Berry & Guthrie, 2003) in South Africa, only the most frequent crimes against children are known, of which the most common is common and aggravated assault, with over 36 000 reported cases (Bower, 2003a). One form of assault is where the child is the target of or witness to domestic violence; this is related to the fact that one in six relationships in South Africa is of a violent nature (Resources Aimed at the Prevention of Child Abuse and Neglect [RAPCAN], 2001). Another form of assault is the exposure to physical punishment as a method of discipline in families (Swart-Kruger, 2001) and schools. Both forms affect children's emotional and physical safety within their closer social sphere.

The second most common type of crime against children is sexual violence (Bower, 2003a) including rape, sodomy, indecent assault and sexual offence. South Africa has one of the highest rates of rape reported to the police, with 52 425 cases of women and children reported between 2002 and 2003 (Human Rights Watch, 2004a; Christofides, Jewkes, Webster, Penn-Kekana, Abrahams, & Martin, 2005) in the world. The number of reported sexual crimes against children amounted to over 25 000 in 2000 (RAPCAN, 2001; Berry & Guthrie, 2003). This means rape is among the most prevalent crimes against children, with many victims being infants or very young (Office on the Right of the Child, 2001), amounting to almost 42% of total crimes against children in 1998 (South African Police Services [SAPS], 2000). RAPCAN assumes that, in general, only one in 20 or even one in 35 rape cases are actually reported to the police (RAPCAN, 2001). This estimation might be applicable to statistics on child rape, too, because less injurious crimes than rape are far less likely to be reported (Dawes, 2002 in Berry & Guthrie, 2003). In addition, because it is unusual for children to be raped by strangers (Jewkes & Levin, 2002), the most common groups of sexual abusers of children and adolescents are male relatives, boyfriends, male acquaintances and men in a position of power, notably teachers. The conviction rate in cases of rape of children is approximately 9% (Human Rights Watch, 2004a).

According to the South African Police Service (2000) children seem to be more vulnerable to being sexually assaulted if they live in impoverished areas, in poor living conditions with parents who are often absent or do not try to protect them, or come from homes where substance abuse is a problem (National Department of Health, 2004b). Berry and Guthrie (2003) support these findings and add accompanying factors that put children at extra risk for sexually related violence, namely limited opportunities for adolescents, alienation from school (National Crime Prevention Strategy, 1996), and violence against women and children in domestic and school settings (Office on the Right of the Child, 2001). According to the Human Rights Watch (2003) the problematic nature of sexual assault has been worsened through an increasing number of AIDS orphans and child trafficking in recent years.

Apart from the statistics documented above, child rape can have an enormous impact on the child survivor. Sexually abused children suffer a variety of physical, emotional and developmental problems that can interfere with their ability to live healthy and productive lives (Bowley & Pitcher, 2002). They may have physical disorders such as sexually transmitted infections, including HIV, constipation, genital injuries, recurrent urinary tract infections, abdominal pains and behavioural problems. Psychological effects of any kind of violence shatter four basic assumptions of the self and the world: (a) the belief in personal invulnerability; (b) the view of the self as positive, and the belief that the world is a meaningful and orderly place; (c) the attitude that events happen for a reason (Janoff-Bulman, 1985); and (d) the trust that other human beings are fundamentally benign (Hamber & Lewis, 1997). Hamber and Lewis (1997, 5) conclude:

> These four assumptions allow people to function effectively in the world and to relate to others. However, after an experience of violence, the individual is left feeling vulnerable, helpless, and out of control in a world that is no longer predictable.

In regard to sexual violence, negative long-term outcomes in the psychology of the individual can be, for instance, the development of post-traumatic stress disorders or risk-taking behaviour. Research findings show that sexual abuse during childhood seems to be associated with high-risk behaviour later in life that may also increase the risk of contracting HIV (WHO, 2000). The WHO (2002) states that there are findings that teenagers and adults who were sexually abused as children are at a greater risk of substance abuse, depression, mental health problems and engaging in high-risk sexual practices. Duncan and Rock (1997) researched risk-taking behaviour among children whose health was injured by a sexual offence. They postulate that violence has come to be seen as a 'normal' condition in a society where child survivors themselves show a tendency towards violence.

In other words, many child rape victims are not only vulnerable but also already display risk-taking sexual behavioural patterns at a young age even towards other young children. In other words, they can become child rape perpetrators themselves (Jewkes & Levin, 2002).

The extent to which sexual abuse contributes to a transmission of the HIV-Virus in children is not well-known (Berry & Guthrie, 2003). Because of statistical constraints and the high incidence of underreporting of child abuse cases in South Africa it is most likely that there exists a higher proportion of undetected HIV infections among children, which are caused by a high number of acts of sexual violence committed without the use of protective barriers. Berry and Guthrie (2003) support the aforementioned assumption and resume in their report that the most likely consequence of an increase in HIV infections in the adult population, is that children will face an increasing risk of inadvertently acquiring HIV through sexual abuse.

2.3.4 Sexual Behaviour of South Africa's Young People – Complexity of Risks

As the statistics in paragraph 2.2 illustrate, the AIDS epidemic in South Africa is concentrated among the most productive section of the population, i.e. in 20- to 39-year-olds, starting at the age of 15 (Adler & Qulo, 1999; Eaton & Flisher, 2000), and mainly affects females between the age of 20 and 29, with a constant increase in numbers every year (HSRC, 2005). The following paragraphs[3] give a detailed description of the most important South African research findings of high-risk sexual behaviour among South African young people.

Sexual Debut

At least 50% of adolescents in South Africa are sexually active by the age of 16, and probably 80% by the age of 20. Boys report an earlier sexual debut than girls whilst black (African) youth are more likely to start sexual activity in early adolescence than other ethnic groups (Eaton, Flisher, & Aaro, 2003).

---

3 Studies with young adolescents in primary schools are generally underrepresented (Kaaya et al., 2002). This literature review on unsafe sexual behaviour will therefore only focus on studies with adolescents older than 12 years.

Condom Use

In their study, Eaton et al. (2003) report that a maximum of 86% of sexually active respondents have used a condom. A maximum of 55% of youth use condoms at every sexual encounter. An overall estimate of 50% to 60% (the number varies between 23% and 85% in other studies) of the youth do not use condoms at all (Eaton et al., 2003). In Peltzer and Promtussananon's study (2005) one third of the learners stated that they had not used a condom at their first sexual encounter. Despite the fact that unprotected sex among youth places them at risk of unwanted pregnancies and STIs, including HIV/AIDS, the majority of sexually active adolescents in South Africa use condoms irregularly. Certain factors contribute to the non- or irregular use of preventive barriers. Campbell (2003), for example, found that women are being prevented from taking the sexual initiative, the focus being mainly on male desire and the satisfaction of male needs, also regarding the use of condoms. Women thus find themselves in a relatively powerless position. She explains this by defining the role of the female, especially the women with African ancestry in South African society, whose respectability is strongly associated with the role of wife, mother and homemaker, as well as with behaviour that reflects sexual fidelity (Campbell, 2003). In the same study, on the other hand, some of the men reported to be exposed to peer pressure and explained that male peers would sneer at them and belittle them if they decided to use condoms (Campbell, 2003). Further behavioural factors that contribute to risky sexual practices are drug and alcohol abuse, stress and various forms of violence, including peer pressure and sexual harassment (Everatt & Orkin, 1993; Duncan & Rock, 1997; Vergnani et al., 1998; Angless & Shefer, 1997; Magwaza, 1997).

Sexual Partnerships and Age Mixing

Eaton et al. (2003) report in their study that between 10% and 30% of sexually active youth have more than one sexual partner at a given time, with more men than women engaging in a concurrent multiple-sex relationship. While boys seem to engage with more sexual partners, girls report sexual relationships with much older partners than boys. Peltzer and Promtussananon (2005) found that 25.6% of the learners had had sex with someone much older than themselves (above 30 years). Significantly more females (31.2%) than males (22.9%) made this statement (Peltzer & Promtussananon, 2005). One possible assumption is that such relationships are linked to impoverished living conditions that put young people in a position where they have to grant sexual favours in exchange for gifts in order to be able to pay their school fees, for example. In this regard Peltzer and Promtussananon (2005) reported that 27% of the learners had had sex in exchange for gifts. Nair (2005) undertook a study in a South African semi-urban community on how social exclusion of children and youth can encourage HIV transmission. Again, he reports that in conditions of poverty, girls in particular often depend on sexual partners for gifts such as money or clothing, and consequently have limited power to insist on condoms in such situations (Nair, 2005). For older men, preference for adolescent girls is partly driven by the belief that the girls are free of AIDS (UNAIDS/WHO, 2005b). However, these men have usually had a number of sexual encounters and are more likely to be infected with HIV and consequently transmit the virus to the younger female sexual partner.

Access to Information

Another factor that contributes to risky sexual behaviour among youth is the difficult access to clear and unbiased information and services. Possible sources of information for the youth are parents, media, clinics, and schools; however, these sources of information are problematic. Firstly, South African adolescents report poor communication with parents about sexual matters (Boult & Cunningham, 1991; Kau, 1991; Kelly, 2000; Kelly & Parker, 2000; Visser, Roos, & Korf, 1995; Wood, Maepa, & Jewkes, 1997). The strategy intended to encourage abstinence and underline the message "sex is taboo", not only caused teenage sexual activity to be greatly denied (Campbell, 2003; Yoro Badat, 2004), but also to be practised with the added danger of secrecy. Secondly, youth in rural and poor areas where media distribution is low, clearly require alternative sources of information (Flisher et al., 1993). The third problematic source is the community clinic. Clinics are not regularly used by the youth as a resource centre for health and prevention because young people report that clinic staff sometimes scold or mock them when they go there to obtain condoms (McPhail & Campbell, 2000; Richter, 1996; Wood et al., 1997; Eaton et al., 2003). A visit to the clinic often is the beginning of being exposed to gossip and a bad reputation within the community (Campbell, 2003).

Specific Historically-based Factors

Socially related risk factors that encourage highly unsafe sexual behaviour among South African youth are found in historical marginalisation and disadvantages (Dryfoos, 1991; Vergnani et al, 1998) in colonial times, during apartheid, as well as in current transformation processes in the social, political and economic system of a young democratic state. Gow and Desmond (2002) identified special socio-demographic conditions that determine young people's lives by increasing their risk of being exposed to diseases: the high level of poverty and unemployment, social and familial disruption through urbanisation/migration processes and the related migrant labour system, regular commercial sex practises, the low level of education in large sectors of society, and the low position of women in relationships and in society.

In their respective studies, Peltzer (2002a) and Campbell (2003) confirm that some of these risk-taking sexual behaviours, described on the case of condoms use, are affected by a wide range of situational, interpersonal and structural factors (peer norms and gender relations), such as knowledge about AIDS (access to information), behavioural intention, perceived vulnerability, perceived barriers (adults' disapproval of young people's sexuality or access to condoms), self-efficacy, demographic factors, and economic constraints. This means that all the psychosocial factors listed above strongly influence the health behaviour of South African children and youth.

2.4 Learning Processes to Enhance Health – The Application of the Social Cognitive Theory by Bandura (1986)

Social and behavioural scientists have developed a number of cognitive and decision-making theories and models to explain and predict (health) behaviour of individuals and groups. A number of theories have specifically been used in the field of health promotion, namely the Health Belief Model (HBM) (Becker, 1974; Janz & Becker, 1984; Rosenberg & Rosenstock, 1966), the Theory of Reasoned Action (Ajzen & Fishbein, 1970), the Theory of Planned Behaviour (Azjen, 1985) and the Social Cognitive Theory (Bandura, 1986, 1991). One of the most important, widely used and proved practical theories (see also Elkins, Maticka, Kuyyakonond, & Miller, 1997; Schinke, Botvin, Orlandi, & Schilling, 1990; Klepp, Ndeki, & Seha, 1994; Shuey, Babishangire, Omiat, & Bagarukayo, 1999) to promote condoms in particular (Aaro, Flisher, Kaaya, Onya, Fuglesang, Klepp, & Schaalma, 2005), is the construct of the Social Cognitive Theory (Bandura, 1986).

The SCT, as part of a static motivational theory, explains how cognitive and social factors determine human health or rather human disease. This theory attempts to explain human behaviour by using a broad social perspective which is based on a triadic reciprocal determinism in which behaviour, personal factors (such as cognitive factors) and environmental events (environmental and internal forces) operate as interacting determinants. Here, the term 'reciprocal' refers to the mutual action between the factors, while 'determinism' refers to the production of effects by certain factors. The strength of the reciprocity between factors can vary according to the person and the situation and is subject to change over time as a function of maturation and experience. In other words, changes in any of these three factors are hypothesised to produce changes in the others.

In more specific terms, the *person-behaviour* interaction involves the bidirectional influences of one's thoughts, emotions, and biological properties and one's actions (Bandura, 1986). A bidirectional interaction also occurs between the *environment and personal* characteristics (Bandura, 1986). In this process, human expectations, beliefs, and cognitive competencies are developed and modified by social influences and physical structures within the environment. These social influences can convey information and activate emotional reactions through such factors as modelling, instruction, and social persuasion (Bandura, 1986). The final interaction occurs between *behaviour and the environment*. Bandura (1986) argues that people are both products and producers of their environment meaning a person's behaviour will determine those aspects of their environment to which they are exposed, and behaviour is, in turn, modified by that environment. Humans evoke different reactions from their social environment as a result of their physical characteristics, such as age, size, race, sex, and physical attractiveness.

One of the key concepts in the SCT is the environmental variable *observational learning*. In contrast to earlier behavioural theories, the SCT considers the environment as not just a variable that reinforces or punishes behaviours, but one that also provides a milieu where an individual can observe the actions of others and/or learn the consequences of their behaviour (Bandura, 1986). This means the SCT adds a cognitive component by identifying that people can also learn from the experiences (observation) of others (e.g. living models) and takes into account how the people's perceptions of their environment affect their decisions (Rotter, 1954; Bandura, 1977).

In other words, the SCT specifies factors which determine and drive competencies (e.g. self-efficacy), which in turn also influence physical and emotional well-being as well as self-regulation of health behaviour (e.g. health habits.) (Dohnke, 2003). Thus, the theory distinguishes between four psychosocial determinants: (a) self-efficacy, (b) outcome expectations, (c) goals, and (d) impediments (see also Figure 2.2). The two central cognitive determinants of intentions and health behaviour are self-efficacy and outcome expectation (Abraham, Sheeran, & Johnston, 1998; Armitage & Conner,

2000 in Dohnke, 2003). Bandura assumes that subjective expectations such as outcome expectations and self-efficacy strongly influence cognitive, motivational, emotional and active processes taking place within an individual (Knoll, Scholz, & Rieckmann, 2005).

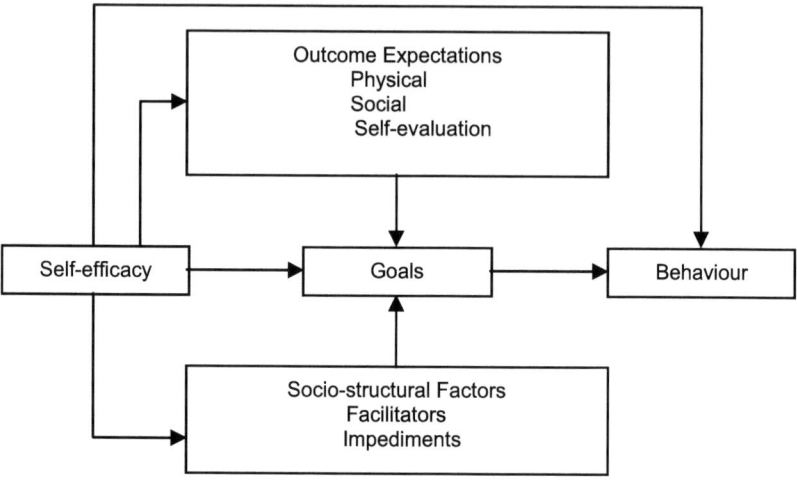

Figure 2.2. Bandura's Model of the Social Cognitive Theory (1998).

Self-efficacy, hereby, holds a key position in the SCT (Dohnke, 2003). This determinant refers to the perception that a person has the capacity to perform a behaviour (Skinner, 2000) and is presumed to have a direct or indirect (over other determinants) effect on behaviour (Dohnke, 2003). This means in the process of the behavioural change self-efficacy influences the range of specific situations, goals and actions (behaviour), the investment of efforts, persistence regarding experienced difficulties and barriers, recovery of setbacks, as well as degree of success (Bandura, 1997, 1998; Schwarzer, 1996 in Dohnke, 2003). Bandura (1986) names four sources for the development of self-efficacy within an individual, listed from the strongest to the weakest source: (a) mastery experience, (b) vicarious experience, (c) symbolic experience, and (d) emotional arousal (Dohnke, 2003) encouraged through observing a model.

The second most important cognitive determinant, outcome expectations, predicts health behaviour by directly influencing goals (intention) or indirectly influencing goals (Dohnke, 2003). The development of positive (incentives) and negative (disadvantage) outcomes, which can be physical, social and self-regulatory, is always influenced by self-efficacy. The last two cognitive determinants of the SCT are goals (here also intentions) and impediments. Both determinants are influenced by self-efficacy. The determinant goals contain additional self-incentives to influence certain behaviour whilst the impediments are not only grounded in an individual but can also be determined by specific socio-structural factors.

In summary, the Social Cognitive Theory is a multidisciplinary approach that incorporates a wide range of psychosocial phenomena that can be fashioned by direct and observational experience into a variety of forms within biological limits. As it encompasses attention, memory and motivation it spans both cognitive and behavioural frameworks. In his theory of social learning, Bandura (1986) formulated conditions in which (positive and critical) behaviour is learned by social interaction, or in other words, the desired social behaviour is specifically practised and positively encouraged (Bühringer & Bühler, 2004) with the help of a model (intervention).

With regard to the prevention of HIV infection within individuals, the SCT has been applied extensively to understand the theoretical foundation of the technique of behavioural modelling. The theory is widely used in training programmes because it allows trainers (facilitators) to identify the environmental conditions that lead to the acquisition and preservation of behaviour and encourage behavioural change (Skinner, 2000). As the aim of this study is to enhance health promoting behaviour to reduce the risk of HIV infection among pre-adolescents (also later in life), the SCT (Bandura, 1986) forms the theoretical basis in the evaluation of cognitive and social variables among participants through a specific school-based life skills programme on AIDS and sex education (model).

2.4.1 *The Research Model and Underlying Assumptions*

According to Gibney (1999), the following main components of the SCT should be reflected in any HIV prevention approach: (a) the promotion of knowledge about risks and prevention, (b) the acquisition of skills and competencies regarding the reduction of an HIV infection, (c) the increase of self-efficacy, and (d) the promotion of peer norms reflecting protective behaviours (Gibney in Peltzer, 2002b). Furthermore, any intervention undertaken to increase competencies and to enhance the development of protective health behaviour should incorporate the following processes: (a) cognitive processes (knowledge, self-efficacy, self-esteem, reasoning and problem-solving skills, learning ability and achievement), (b) emotional processes (trust, empathy, positive social relationships, supportive social network), (c) affective processes (reduction of discrimination and fear), and (d) motivational processes (impulse control, constructive coping and goal-directed behaviour, development of social responsibility and interpersonal communication).

Therefore, a specific research model for this study is applied to examine the participating pre-adolescent age group, who are in their early phases of developing an attitude and value system. This model is set to encourage skills and competencies to cope with current prevailing life tasks and to prevent risk factors or increase protective factors to enable pre-adolescents to apply health behaviour later in life. Figure 2.3 illustrates the presented model in combination with underlying assumptions.

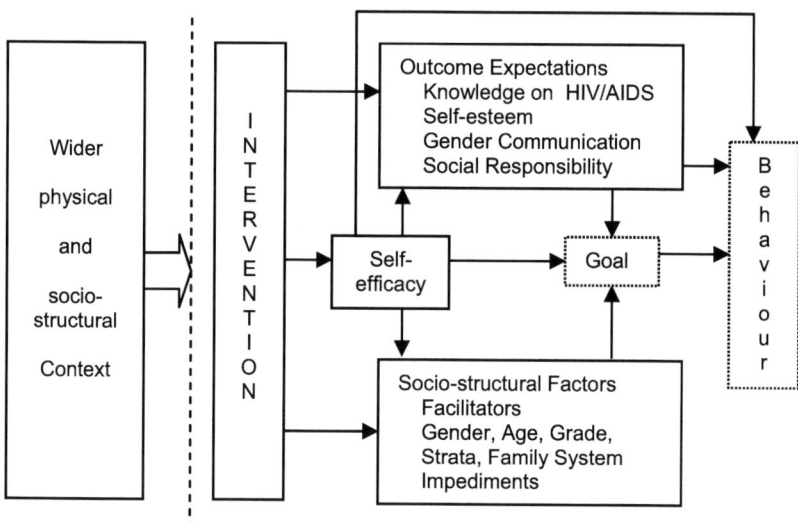

Figure 2.3. Research Model for Organizing the Relationship between psychological Competencies, interpersonal Conditions, and environmental Factors.

The research model depicts a reciprocal one-way process, in which individuals (participants, facilitators) in interpersonal relations act in an intervention (life skills programme on HIV/AIDS and sex education), or model (Bandura, 1998), in their closer environment (classroom). The intervention itself, as an independent variable, is an opportunity to encourage the individual to learn by experience (activity) and by the observation of others, and strengthens and reinforces individual behavioural capabilities such as symbolising, forethought, and vicarious, self-regulatory and self-reflective behaviour. The underlying assumption is that learners, first of all, acquire and experience their own cognitive and social competencies in a specific learning model. The used dependent variables are regarded to reinforce cognitive and social competencies on the individual and interpersonal level by encouraging certain health-related outcome expectations among participants.

First, the development of general biological-medical *knowledge on HIV/AIDS* and ways of transmission is assumed to raise awareness towards this particular health risk among participants. Second, *self-efficacy* is assumed to represent the individual's conviction in his/her own competencies to be able to keep goals while confronted with impediments that influence outcome expectations, goals, and socio-structural factors. The variable *self-esteem* is assumed to be a psychological motivating stimulus to enhance the individual's confidence in his/her own competencies. The psychological factors in particular, such as self-esteem and self-efficacy, are assumed to critically affect interpersonal factors that represent social competencies such as gender communication and social responsibility.

The encouragement of social responsibility and gender communication is assumed to form the basis for personal outcome expectations in relation to the establishment of positive relations to and with other peers of the same and other gender; with gender being viewed as both a physical and psychological term. The variable *gender communication* refers mainly to the quality of interaction between boys and girls in the class. Communication in the group or with other individuals about different topics will teach communication skills such as listening and discussion; the skills will in turn encourage the ability to trust and empathise with other individuals and promote an understanding of non-violent and communicative social relationships (e.g. family, friends). *Social responsibility* encompasses the development of the child's social skills, while enabling him or her to be an active and responsible member of his/her closer (class) and wider social community (Berman, 1997). Social responsibility as a variant is also examined, because it is assumed to have an effect on the children's cognitive development outside the intervention setting. Socio-structural factors, such as the quality of relations to health promotion trainers (facilitators) or other classmates (living models) are examined to broaden the understanding of underlying processes that influence the cognitive development of the participants.

Other socio-structural determinants such as gender, age, grade, strata, and family systems function as a filter to identify possible subgroups within the group structure. The physical and socio-structural environments encompass the wider learning environment (school), as well as the living environment of the participants (case study community). According to the SCT, all these factors are potentially equally determining (Bandura, 1991; Eaton et al., 2003).

Furthermore, there are several weaknesses of the research model. First, the SCT puts great emphasis on the assessment of attitudes related to, for instance, HIV/AIDS and sex. Attitudinal items that enquire about intimate convictions could not be formulated due to the young age of the samples and several contextual reasons as well as cultural convictions which are outlined in more detail in chapter 5. Goals (intention) were not examined. The absence of intention is assessed as a factor that reduces the effectiveness of the research model used, because intention is seen as an important predictor of attitudes and behaviour in the field of health behaviour, and because intention, planning and other self-regulative capabilities seem to increase the effectiveness of self-efficacy (Schwarzer, 2002). Finally, behaviour could not be assessed because the examined participants were in the stage of pre-adolescence; the samples therefore were only in the formation process of developing health behaviour.

2.4.2 Depiction of Research Variables

In the following section the research variables in conjunction with findings from other surveys are explained. Those findings shall well support the importance of research variables in the analysis of the effectiveness of the model. In the absence of studies with pre-adolescents, most of the presented results are gathered from studies examining adolescents.

Knowledge of HIV/AIDS

Sufficient public knowledge about HIV/AIDS and prevention measures is an essential requirement for any society trying to limit the spread of HIV. According to Peltzer and Promtussananon (2005), knowledge is only part of what is needed to develop an adequate response to HIV/AIDS but it is certainly a commodity that has to be taken into consideration. Eaton and Flisher's (2000) literature review on knowledge about HIV/AIDS among South African youth shows two key findings.

The first finding is that most young people in South Africa have heard of AIDS. The percentage ranges from 85% (Richter, 1996) to 100% (Strebel & Perkel, 1991; Van Wijk, 1994; Varga & Makubalo, 1996). In a study of urban black youth (Richter, 1996), 73% of young men and 75% of young women had heard of HIV, compared to 92% and 85% respectively having heard of AIDS. In a sample of 141 street youth (Van Wijk, 1994), nearly all had heard of AIDS, but none had heard of HIV. The second key finding is that, despite an overall high awareness of AIDS, the youth show highly variable actual knowledge about the illness itself. Some researchers concluded that their subjects had a good overall knowledge about AIDS; however, they also reported that knowledge was mediocre, that is, 40% to 60% as measured by knowledge tests (Everatt & Orkin, 1993; Kruger & Richter, 1996; Friedland, Jankelowitz, De Beer, De Klerk, Khoury, Csizmadia, Padayachee, & Levy, 1991; Heunis, 1994). Other studies reported that the majority of the subjects were very ill-informed about HIV and AIDS (Friedland et al., 1991; Ratsaka & Hirschowitz, 1995). Peltzer and Promtussananon (2005) revealed in their study that respondents showed less knowledge when assessed with open, rather than set-choice questions, suggesting low levels of spontaneous memory of AIDS information without a significant gender difference ($t=1.49$).

In South Africa, as elsewhere, results differ in studies on the relation between HIV/AIDS knowledge and gender (Peruga & Celentano, 1993; Eaton & Flisher, 2000). Two studies reported gender differences. A study among university learners found that female learners were significantly more knowledgeable about HIV/AIDS than their male peers (Strebel & Perkel, 1991). In a small study among adolescents the opposite was found, with the young men being significantly more knowledgeable than their female peers (Kaplan & Van den Worm, 1993). Three studies reported no significant differences regarding gender (Coughlan, Coughlan, & Jameson, 1996; Elkonin, 1993; Perkel, 1991).

On the other hand, Peltzer and Promtussananon (2005) report significant differences between genders in various HIV knowledge items. For example, more male than female learners believed that "People who have been infected with HIV quickly show serious signs of being infected". In addition, the same study reports that English-speaking learners and learners from urban schools are much better informed than African learners from non-urban schools (Peltzer & Promtussananon, 2005). Peltzer and Promtussananon (2005) conclude that knowledge of HIV/AIDS was not satisfactory enough to sustain adequate HIV/AIDS response in a context of high and widespread HIV/AIDS prevalence, and suggest that lower levels of knowledge in younger persons, gender, as well as racial and urban-non-urban differences should be clearly addressed by AIDS education efforts.

Finally, knowledge of HIV/AIDS seems to increase from childhood to adolescence and then appears to reach a plateau during adolescence, with no appreciable gains during adulthood. This may be because school guidance programmes and adolescents' increasing interest and participation in sexual activity enable teenagers to acquire knowledge on HIV/AIDS (Eaton &

Flischer, 2000). Once young people possess a basic knowledge, there may be little incentive for them to seek additional information, especially since most young people do not perceive themselves as being at a high risk of contracting HIV/AIDS (Blecher, Steinberg, Pick, Hennick, & Durcan, 1995; Everatt & Orkin, 1993; Friedland et al., 1991; National Progressive Primary Health Care Network [NPPHCN], 1996; Perkel, 1991; Ratsaka & Hirschowitz, 1995; Strebel & Perkel, 1991).

In South Africa, interventions that attempt to curb the spread of HIV are generally aimed at imparting knowledge about AIDS and promoting condom use (Eaton & Flisher, 2000). However, most studies clearly illustrate that gender tendency to use condoms and being sexually active have no significant relation to levels of knowledge (Peltzer & Promtussananon, 2005). An explanation is given by Campbell (2003) who states in her study that knowledge about HIV/AIDS seems to be far more complex and reflect local ideas of health, sexuality, traditional values and healing systems. Furthermore, she explains that such facts are embedded within a range of doubts, qualifications, contradictions and uncertainties, and are constructed in social conditions that shape and constrain individual sexual choices. These conditions serve to blunt the factual messages imparted by the programmes (Campbell, 2003). This also means that health education messages compete with alternative beliefs, experiences and logics that may be more compelling than the information health educators seek to impart (Campbell, 2003).

Global Self-Esteem

Self-esteem theorists Rosenberg (1979) and James (1983 in Hamber & Lewis, 1997) have suggested that self-esteem is a dynamic, changing construct. James (1983 in Hamber & Lewis, 1997) views self-esteem as the ratio of one's successes and pretensions, whereas Rosenberg (1979, p. 31) refers to self-esteem as a "positive or negative evaluation of the self". A combination of these two perspectives leads to the following proposition: "A positive evaluation of the self stems from having more success than expected, whereas a negative evaluation stems from having fewer successes than expected" (Rosenberg, 1979, p. 31). Clearly, this interpretation suggests that a person's self-esteem is not constant over time, but dynamic instead, depending on the individual's successes and expectations (Baldwin & Hoffman, 2002).

As noted by developmental theorists, these ebbs and flows of self-esteem are probably felt most strongly during the adolescent years. Long-term studies of adolescent self-esteem have revealed a decline in self-esteem at the age of 11, a low between the ages 12 and 13, and a gradual, systematic improvement in self-esteem between ages 18 and 19 (Demo & Savin-Williams, 1983; Eccles, Midgley, Wigfield, Buchanan, Reuman, Flanagan, & Maclver, 1993; McCarthy & Hoge, 1982; Rosenberg, 1986). Cairns, McWhirter, Duffy, and Barry (1990), Chiam (1987) and O'Malley and Bachman (1983) support these findings and report that self-esteem is inconsistent during adolescence. However, some cross-sectional studies contradict these findings and have found that self-esteem either declines during the adolescent years (Brack, Orr, & Ingersoll, 1988; Brown, McMahon, Biro, Crawford, Schreiber, Similo, Waclawiw, & Striegel-Moore, 1998; Simmons & Rosenberg, 1975) or remains static (Bolognini, Plancherel, Bettschart, & Halfon, 1996; Chubb, Fertman, & Ross, 1997; Nottelmann, 1987; Savin-Williams & Demo, 1984; Simmons & Blyth, 1987; Wylie, 1979).

Despite all contradictory results about whether or not self-esteem changes significantly during adolescence (Baldwin & Hoffmann, 2002), it is safe to say that self-esteem during the adolescent years appears to undergo a process of metamorphosis (Quatman & Watson, 2001). Adolescence brings with it an increased differentiation in self-concept as well as an increased cognitive capacity for abstraction and self-reflection (Harter, 1990a, b). These changes, says Simmons and Blyth (1987) comprise the increase in self-determination, peer orientation, self-focus, self-consciousness, concern over opposite-sex relationships, and the capacity for abstract cognitive activity. All of these issues, which are salient in adolescence, occur simultaneously with bodily changes at the onset of puberty and gender intensification pressures (Hill & Lynch, 1983). Quatman and Watson (2001) argue that these issues mutually create significant challenges to a young person's self-esteem. Adolescence is clearly a pivotal and change-related time in the context of self-esteem, and has a unique transitional nature (Eccles et al., 1993) that necessitates adjustments to and changes in self-definition that appear to disturb global self-esteem (Wigfield & Eccles, 1994).

According to Polce-Lynch et al. (1994) global self-esteem, which refers to a person's general sense of worth or acceptance (Wylie, 1979), is recognised for its critical role in mental health and psychopathology (Bednar, Wells, & Peterson, 1989; National Advisory Mental Health Council [NAMHC], 1996; Rosenberg, 1979). Their study revealed that socio-cultural influences (peer and family relationships, gender harassment, and the media) might be associated with body image, and that these in turn are related to self-esteem (Polce-Lynch et al., 1994). Other studies (Goliath, 1995; Perkel, Strebel, & Joubert, 1991) on self-esteem in the context of sexual behaviour have found that a low self-esteem is associated with an earlier onset of sexual activity and having multiple sex partners. It has been hypothesised that a person with a poor sexual self-concept may rely on others for affirmation. This may lead him or her to search for external affirmation in multiple sexual encounters. South African studies also indicate that young people with a low self-esteem may be more concerned with what their partners think of them; they also tend to avoid displeasure of or rejection by partners and people with more positive, self-affirming self-concepts (Perkel et al., 1991). A person with a low self-esteem is therefore more likely to think that condoms are offensive to their partner, that using condoms may make their partner think they are dirty, or to feel embarrassed about using condoms, and therefore are likely to have a negative attitude towards condoms (Perkel et al., 1991; Eaton et al., 2003). Low self-esteem also seems to undermine abstinence or monogamy (Eaton et al., 2003), which puts the individual at extra risk of becoming infected with HIV or any other STIs.

Perceived Self-Efficacy

Perceived self-efficacy refers to the perception that a person has the capacity to perform health-related behaviour and; consequently, a person's sense of his/her self-efficacy can influence his/her sense of capacity to be able to maintain safe behaviour. This capacity explicitly refers to one's competence to deal with challenging encounters (Schwarzer, 2001).

It is assumed that a higher self-efficacy promotes the chance of positive behaviour being performed, both of the person and that of others (Skinner, 2000). This perception of self-efficacy is adjusted over time by the person's experience in attempting different tasks, and observing other (similar) people doing tasks, through persuasion and personal changes. Success or failure is attributed to four factors, namely ability, effort, difficulty of the task or situation and luck (Leviton, 1989). Greater self-efficacy facilitates disclosure of an HIV-positive status to partners (Kalichman & Nachimson, 1999) and was also found to be relevant if women develop a capacity to insist on safer sexual practices (Soet, Dudley, & Dilario, 1999) in an intimate relationship.

Skinner (2000) criticises the concept of self-efficacy in relation to HIV in two ways. While self-efficacy does assist a person's capacity to perform the behaviour, on the one hand, it does not necessarily improve his/her desire to use safer sexual practices. On the other hand, self-efficacy may also be easily reduced when faced with a situation over which the person has reduced control. Campbell (2003) supports these findings in her study and argues that because of gender-specific socialisation in patriarchal societies such as South Africa, men are often encouraged to be macho risk-takers and have multiple sex partners whereas women are often hindered to take assertive control of their sexual health. Such critical points are assumed to be reduced if HIV interventions focus on self-efficacy and increase the latter by providing education on how to perform safer behaviour and by providing support in the performance of such behaviour (Leviton, 1989; Soet et al., 1999; Sanderson, 1999). In contrast, two South African studies among young adults established that increased self-efficacy is indeed linked to higher self-reported condom use (Peltzer, 1999; Reddy, Meyer-Weitz, Van den Borne, & Kok, 2000), therefore, it can be posited that people consider positive and negative features when changing preventive behaviours. Weighing one feature against the other will influence their behaviour and perhaps determine the outcome.

In a study on motivation, attributions and self-efficacy among children, Smith (2002) found that children with a higher sense of self-efficacy showed higher levels of persistence and effort. He noticed that it takes time and practise for most individuals to gain proficiency in a new skill and to progress through the learning stages (cognitive, associative, and autonomous); if individuals give up quickly and easily, their learning stage will never move on to the associative or autonomous stage. Results from this study (Smith, 2002) support the assumption that individuals with higher self-efficacy believe their failures are due to a lack of *effort* and that those with lower self-efficacy believe their failure is due to a lack of *ability*. Smith (2002) states the reasons children give for failing are important to their future self-efficacy and motivation. If they believe they cannot change their ability, they probably will not want to continue to try to improve. Children should understand the role of effort, preparation and ability to learn and recognise that they are in control of their ability and that failure in a task may merely be due to a lack of effort or preparation (Smith, 2002).

Inter-Gender Communication

Communication with a partner about the risk of STIs or condom use has been found to be strongly correlated with the willingness to use condoms and self-reported use (Reddy et al., 2000). Open discussion and mutual agreement to behavioural change can strengthen the relationship, increase partners' respect for each other, confirm that they care about each other's well-being, and enhance their sexual intercourse by removing any anxiety about the risk of infection (Wood & Foster, 1995; Eaton et al., 2003). However, sexual negotiation of any kind, be it about condom use, faithfulness, or about the nature and frequency of sexual intercourse, is missing from many sexual relationships between young South Africans (Eaton et al., 2003).

Studies have noted that pervasive, culturally entrenched gender discrimination especially increases the risk of HIV infection for South African women (Eaton et al., 2003). In certain communities, young South

Africans' heterosexual relationships frequently involve sexual pressure on, and violence towards, the female partner. In such relationships, the male partner largely controls sexual activity. The threat of violence or rejection prevents girls and women from insisting on condom use as a result (Meyer-Weitz, Reddy, Weijtz, Van den Borne, & Kok, 1998; Varga & Makulabo, 1996). While young women in such relationships may be violently punished for perceived unfaithfulness (McPhail & Campbell, 2000; Meyer-Weitz et al., 1998; Reddy & Meyer-Weitz, 1997; Whitefield, 1999), their boyfriends claim the right to have multiple sex partners (Meyer-Weitz et al., 1998; Reddy & Meyer-Weitz, 1997; Richter, 1996).

Other factors that were found to be closely linked with the ability and quality of protective communication, are peer pressure and harassment, as well as the quality of relationships with peers, family or intimate partners. For example, South African research has addressed the issue of peer pressure mainly in studies of black youth (Buga, Amoko, & Ncayiyana, 1996; Cassimjee, 1998; NPPHCN, 1996). This research indicates that both girls and boys experience considerable same-sex peer pressure to be sexually active. For boys, the pressure has to do with proving masculinity; having many sexual partners wins a young man status and admiration (Blecher, Steinberg, Pick, Hennick, & Durcan, 1995; McPhail & Campbell, 2000). For girls, pressure sometimes comes from sexually experienced peers who exclude inexperienced girls from group discussions because they are still 'children' (Wood et al., 1997). However, peer pressure does not have the same negative influence on all youth. Individuals differ in their susceptibility (Perkel, 1991), and young men appear to be influenced to a greater extent than young women (MacPhail & Campbell, 2000). Peer pressure does not necessarily have to be a negative influence; positive examples set by friends and role models can promote safer sexual behaviour (Perkel, 1991) and are deeply linked to the quality of communication and the information conveyed.

Social Responsibility

The concept of responsibility encompasses the developing of adolescents' social skills that enable them to be active and responsive members of their society and family (Berman & La Farge, 1993; Berman, 1997). Responsibility involves being accountable for things that need to be done and to fulfil one's duties and obligations to oneself and others (Flexner, 1980). In regard to health-related behaviour, therefore, social responsibility functions as a social competency that, on the one hand, strives to ensure personal health and, on the other hand, strives to ensure that the partner or other people will be protected by one's own actions.

Polk (2002) assumes that responsibility includes, among others, the recognition and acceptance of the consequences of one's actions, caring attitudes towards self and others, recognition and acceptance of basic human rights of self and others, resolving conflicts peacefully, or the development of leadership, communication and social skills. The ability of adolescents to identify and define social responsibility is important in defining who they are, where they fit in the social world, and for building confidence (Berman, 1997). Children and adolescents learn responsibility and social skills through interaction with their families, peers, mentors and communities. When adolescents are offered participatory experiences that are meaningful, and when they are allowed to discover their potency and to assess their responsibility, they acquire a sense of commitment to a moral-ethical ideology (Youniss, McLellan, & Yates, 1997; Youniss & Yates, 1997). According to Davis and Palladino (2000) responsible youth are those who feel accountable for their actions and activities in their classes, at school and at home; they strive hard to achieve the goals they set and regulate their behaviour in directions that help them attain their goals.

2.5 Conclusion

According to the WHO (2005) mental health and mental illnesses are determined by multiple and interacting social, psychological and biological factors. In accordance with the WHO's definition of health, chapter 2 explained the interconnection of factors that influence the child's physical and mental development and also contribute to the wide distribution of HIV, especially among the youngest segments. Here, statistics show that more than 15% of infected people in South Africa are between the age of 20 and 24 (HSRC, 2005).

Identified risk factors for child health are the high level of poverty, the high number of sexual child abuse cases, and risk-taking health behaviour among youth. Poverty-related migration, for instance, forces large sections of the population to move from rural to often overcrowded, chaotic, and disadvantaged urban areas and lifestyles. Urbanisation and modernisation have not only prompted welcome shifts in gender roles and obligations of adults towards children (Barbarin & Richter, 2001), but have also caused confusing transmission processes of value systems for human beings and exerted pervasive influence regarding sexual and general health behaviour especially on children and youth who already experience confusing developmental processes in unstable social settings where the risk of HIV infection is high (Eaton et al., 2003). Furthermore, the widespread occurrence of rape and the low status of women in society and in relationships make it even more difficult for children and women to protect themselves in (sexual) relationships, leading to an increased risk of being exposed to diseases such as HIV.

From the list of different risk factors presented at the beginning of this chapter it becomes clear that South African children and adolescents, especially those from the lower strata of society, are faced with a multitude of difficult life tasks and are, therefore, at higher risk in unhealthy conditions. The WHO (2005) confirms this finding and states that child development is more exposed to psychosocial risks in a surrounding with a multitude of socio-structural and socio-economic constraints (WHO, 2005). It can be argued, based on findings, that the health risk for children will become even higher during adolescence if no positive action is taken. This study thus assumes that it is extremely important to influence health behaviour among adolescents in an early stage of their lives. As is assumed that HIV infection is rare among children in South Africa below the age of 15, this age group should be the target of primary prevention.

Thus, to evaluate the effect of such a preventive approach, a life skills programme on AIDS and sex education for pre-adolescent children and a specific research model were applied theoretically based on the Social Cognitive Theory (Bandura, 1986). The examination of the individual (psychological) learning processes and interpersonal interactions, with its underlying assumptions, are at the centre of this study. Some psychological variables (self-esteem, self-efficacy, knowledge on HIV/AIDS) and social variables (gender communication and social responsibility) are used to equip individuals with learning processes with the purpose of encouraging skills and competencies so that they can cope with prevalent life tasks and so strengthen protective factors that will ultimately enable pre-adolescents to apply appropriate life-enhancing health behaviour later in life.

CHAPTER THREE

Life Skills Interventions on HIV/AIDS in South Africa

3.1 Introduction

As explained in chapter 1, the International Convention on the Rights of Children and Youth declares that access to and fulfilment of education and information form a fundamental basis for the development of the social, psychological and moral welfare and the physical and psychological well-being of the next generation (UN, 1989, par. 28, 17). According to the UN's (1989) declaration, it can be proposed that children and young people are especially in need of access to information because they know less of human nature and have fewer life experiences; they should therefore receive information before they are exposed to risky health situations. The WHO (1999a) agrees with the above conviction and refers to primary preventive approaches as an effective method to protect children's rights to enable them to live a healthy life. Life skills programmes, as health promoting instruments, are expressly recommended by the WHO (1999a) in the context of specific risk situations and situations where, for example, children and adolescents need to be empowered to promote and protect their rights.

The following reviews present exclusively selected evaluations of school-based life skills interventions regarding AIDS and sex education in the sub-Saharan region that targeted upper primary school children. This discussion is followed by a description of one specific South African case. The chapter is concluded by a discussion on growing problems on personal, interpersonal, socio-cultural and socio-economic level problematic to the implementation of highly standardised life skills programmes and their proposed outcomes.

3.2 Sub-Saharan School-based Life Skills Initiatives on HIV/AIDS with Pre-Adolescents

In recent years, behavioural training to enhance competences (life skills) for the prevention of HIV/AIDS in schools has turned out to provide a particularly efficient and varied form of intervention (see also WHO, 1999a; Jerusalem, 2002a; Bühringer & Bühler, 2004; Pinquart & Silbereisen, 2004). Life skills programmes claim to develop and to positively support the mental and physical health of individuals in their preparation for the developmental tasks and demands in life they are exposed to. Because learning about health and experiencing individual behaviour is promoted in social learning situations, these programmes have to equally combine teaching on health and the promotion of positive attitudes and values in a supportive learning environment (WHO, 1999a). Furthermore, this form of intervention has to cover a wide range of topics (e.g. teenage pregnancy, violence, and HIV/AIDS) and combine the conveying of information with the teaching of life skills in order to help the target group to adequately deal with specific developmental and life tasks designed for them. The range of topics are considered to function best if learning methods are participatory and convert real life situations into a social learning process that includes: (1) explanation of the skill in question, (2) observing the skill (modelling), (3) practising the skill in selected situations in a supportive learning environment, and (d) receiving feedback about the individual performance of skills (WHO, 1999a).

Schools are considered a most suitable setting for health promoting initiatives. Because the majority of young people are of school-going age they can be better reached at this location. Schools constitute a main pillar of the socialisation of children and are therefore a better accessible setting for health-promoting interventions like life skills programmes. Furthermore, they provide frameworks in which additional learning programmes can be better implemented, for example, school hours, mode of operations, mechanisms for introduction of new programmes, number of learners, and measures for the assessment of participants (Gallant & Maticka-Tyndale, 2004). Primary schools in particular are considered to be good locations, especially in the developing world, because they accommodate the majority of children and youth (approximately 50%) (Gallant & Maticka-Tyndale, 2004), with reduced numbers in higher grades; 70% enter primary school and only 67% do still attend grade 5 (UNICEF, 2001). In their assessment of the effectiveness of AIDS reduction strategies, Stover, Walker, Garnett, Salomon, Stanecki, and Ghys (2002) identified school-based programmes as a necessary basis for other programmes to enhance and encourage mental and physical health amongst attending individuals.

Considering the scope of the AIDS pandemic and its related dangers for physical health and mental well-being, the implementation of such health promotion initiatives is considered to be of special importance. In an extensive literature review by Gallant and Maticka-Tyndale in 2004, 32 reports on evaluated school-based intervention programmes were identified based on specific research criteria, namely that the programme (1) be designed to affect a change in AIDS-related knowledge, attitudes, behavioural intentions, and/or behaviours; (2) be evaluated using quantitative data; (3) be reported in a peer reviewed journal between 1990 and 2002; (4) targets youth under the age of 25; and (5) reports on school-based programmes implemented in sub-Saharan Africa. Only 11 of the reviewed studies[4] fulfilled these research criteria; only four learning or pedagogical theory-based programmes were found (Dalrymple & DuToit, 1993; Harvey, Stuart, & Swan, 2000; Klepp, Ndeki, & Seha 1994/ Klepp, Ndeki, Leshabari, Hannan, & Lyimo 1997; Shuey, Babishangire, Omiat, & Bagarukayo 1999) and only two studies out of eleven (Klepp et al., 1994, 1997; Shuey et al., 1999) that met the parameter of school-based sexual health interventions in sub-Saharan Africa in a primary school (see also Table 3.1 to 3.4).[5] With reference to these research findings (Gallant & Maticka-Tyndale, 2004), only a relatively small number of utilisable evaluated studies have so far been carried out on school-based HIV/AIDS educational programmes in sub-Saharan Africa.

According to the literature review in Gallant and Maticka-Tyndale (2004), an important determinant that influences programme outcomes appears to be the stage of sexual development amongst the participating individuals. In Africa it was measured that sexual debut amongst boys ranges from 12 to 15.5 years, while the corresponding range amongst girls is 13.6 to 15.9 years (Kaaya et al., 2002a, 2002b; WHO, 1992a). This means that the commencement of sexual activity starts with the entrance into adolescence.

Consequently, the age of 13 to 14 years seems to be an important transition point for interventions that aim to delay the debut of sexual activity amongst the younger population, and to increase the adoption of risk reduction strategies in older populations (Kaaya et al., 2002a). Programmes targeting younger school children, for example lower secondary level, confirm these assumptions and were found to have had greater success in influencing sexual behaviours than those targeting older children, namely upper secondary level.

---

4   Another review by Kaaya et al. (2002a) found in their literature study 47 articles reporting sexual behaviour of learners aged between 14 and 24 years and conducted between 1987 and 1999. Not one of those presented a health initiative targeting children in primary school-going age.

5   Another school-based intervention undertaken in Kenya (Maticka-Tyndale, Wildish, & Gichuru, 2004) fulfilled most of the research criteria set by Gallant and Maticka Tyndale (2004). This study is not included in the list of studies as it had not yet been published at the time this literary review was compiled. However, most of its published interim-outcomes are summarized in paragraph 3.2.3.

Table 3.1.
Characteristics of Sub-Saharan School-based Life Skills Initiatives on HIV/AIDS and Sex Education – Four Examples.

Evaluated by	Theory	School level	Implemented in x school	Community involved in design	Content		Form		Implementation		
					Targeted behaviour	Main activities	In/after school	Total exposure	Instructor	Instruct. training	Monitored
Knowledge only											
Dalrymple & duToit (1993) Tanzania	Theories of play	Secondary	Not specified	KABP and participatory research		Participatory educational drama	In	DK	Teachers and University Drama Team	Not specified	No
Knowledge, attitudes and intentions											
Klepp et al. (1994, 1997) Tanzania	TRA, SLT	Primary (M=14yrs)	18	Local health educator and community participation	A	Activities infused, includes peers, educators	In	20 h	Teachers	1 week	DK
Knowledge, attitudes and behaviour											
Harvey et al. (2000) South Africa	Drama-in-education and an applied behaviour change framework	Secondary (STD 8) (M=17.6yrs)	770 (tested in 14)	No	A and C	Drama in education (3 phases)	In	DK	Teachers	Not specified	No
Shuey et al. (1999) Uganda	SLT implied	Primary (age range 13-14 yrs)	95 (tested in 37)	Community sensitization and input	A[a]	Activities infused, School Health Club, peer led, question box	In	>100h	Teachers	Teachers 1 week, head teacher 1 day	Yes

Note. DK = Do not know. Theories: TRA = Theory of Reasoned Action; SLT = Social Learning Theory; Targeted outcomes: A = Abstinence; C = Condoms. Main Activities: Activities infused: Multiple activities are infused throughout the curriculum. [a]Goal was a shift to rational decision-making about sexual activity. (Gallant & Maticka-Tyndale, 2004, extract).

Table 3.2.
Summary of Evaluation Methods on Sub-Saharan School-based Life Skills Initiatives on HIV/AIDS and Sex Education – Four Examples.

Evaluated by	Design	Sampling strategy	N base/post	Control group	Experimental/Control contamination	Time to evaluation	Local input in design	Pre-test	Base effects controlled	Statistical procedures	Statistics or interpretation appropriate	Corrected alpha level
Knowledge only												
Dalrymple & duToit (1993)	Longitudinal Panel	Purposive [a]	72/72	No	n/a	Immed	n/s	Yes	n/a	T-test	Yes	n/a
Knowledge, attitudes and intentions												
Klepp et al. (1994, 1997)	Repeated cross section	Multi-stage random	2025/1772, 814	Yes	No	6 mos, 12 mos	Yes	Yes	Yes	ANOVA	Yes	n/a
Knowledge, attitudes and behaviour												
Harvey et al. (2000)	Longitudinal panel	Multi-stage random	1080/699	Yes	No	6 mos	Yes	Yes	Yes	Bivariate linear regression	Yes	n/a
Shuey et al. (1999)	Repeated cross section	Multi-stage random	400/400	Yes	No	24 mos	Yes	Yes	Yes	Chi-square	Yes	n/a

Note. [a] = Selected schools from the community where the university was located. (Gallant & Maticka-Tyndale, 2004, extract).

Table 3.3.
Summary of Results on Knowledge, Attitudes, and Intentions on Sub-Saharan School-based Life Skills Initiatives on HIV/AIDS and Sex Education – Four Examples.

Evaluation	Knowledge			Attitudes towards			Intentions		Other		
	General	Abstinence	Condom use	PHAs	Abstinence	Condom use	Abstinence	Condom use	Perceived Susceptibility	Self-efficacy	Close friends sexually active
Knowledge only											
Dalrymple & duToit (1993)	+										
Knowledge, attitudes and intentions											
Klepp et al. (1994, 1997)	+/+			+/+	0/+0		+/+				
Knowledge, attitudes and behaviour											
Harvey et al. (2000)	+			+	+				0	+	
Shuey et al. (1999)	+										+

Note. + = A statistically significance programme effect ($p<0.05$) in the desired direction; 0 = no statistically significant programme effect; / to left = is result at 6 month post-programme; / to right = is result at 12 month post programme (Gallant & Maticka-Tyndale, 2004, extract).

Table 3.4.
Summary of Results on Communication and Behaviour on Sub-Saharan School-based Life Skills Initiatives on HIV/AIDS and Sex Education – Four Examples.

Evaluation	Commu-nication	Sexual intercourse behaviour			Condom use behaviour		
		Ever sex	Recent sex	No. of partners	Ever use	Use at last sex	Always use
Knowledge only							
Dalrymple & duToit (1993)							
Knowledge, attitudes and intentions							
Klepp et al. (1994, 1997)	+	0					
Knowledge, attitudes, intentions and behaviour							
Harvey et al. (2000)		0		0	+		0
Shuey et al. (1999)	+	+		–	+		

Note. + = statistically significance programme effect ($p<0.05$) in the desired direction; 0 = no statistically significant programme effect; – = a statistically significant programme effect opposite to the desired direction. (Gallant & Maticka-Tyndale, 2004, extract).

Likewise there appears to be a differential success amongst youth who were virgins at programme initiation compared to those that were already sexually active (Shuey et al., 1999; Stanton, Li, Kahihuata, Fitzgerald, Neumbo, & Kanduuombe, 1998). With this in mind, school-based HIV prevention programming that start as early as primary school has been viewed as a necessary step to protect the general population from further infection (Barnett, de Koning, & Francis, 1995; Finger, Lapetina, & Pribila, 2002; Grunsheit, 1997; Kaaya et al., 2002b; World Bank, 1993).

To give a more detailed view on research findings regarding the outcomes of life skills programmes targeting pre-adolescents, three studies working with upper primary school or lower secondary school learners are presented together with their outcomes in the following paragraphs.[6] The first

---

[6] The presented literature review does not include the 'South Africa and Tanzania Project' (SATZ) school-based HIV/AIDS intervention undertaken in South Africa and Tanzania (Aaro et al., 2005) because the study was still in progress at the time of the implementation and analysis phase of this survey.

two programmes, also listed in Gallant and Maticka-Tyndale's literature review (2004), were undertaken in Tanzania (Klepp et al., 1994, 1997) and Uganda (Shuey et al., 1999). The third programme was a school-based evaluation programme undertaken in Kenya (Maticka-Tyndale et al., 2004). The Kenyan (Maticka-Tyndale et al., 2004) and Ugandan (Shuey et al., 1999) programme controls were aimed at the standard national school health and educational curriculum. The Ugandan and Tanzanian programmes (Shuey et al., 1999; Klepp et al., 1994, 1997) were implemented with the support of health educators in cooperation with teachers and schools while the programme in Kenya (Maticka-Tyndale et al., 2004) trained specific teachers and community representatives in an excessive two-cycle workshop on the content of the programme. All three programmes employed the greatest diversity of activities, namely health club, secret box, and multiple learning activities (Gallant & Maticka-Tyndale, 2004; Maticka-Tyndale et al., 2004), and had sound programme and evaluation designs (providing confidence in their findings). The studies were carried out for one or two years respectively, before their outcomes were evaluated.

3.2.1 The Tanzanian Evaluation

Klepp et al. (1994, 1997) evaluated an intervention programme which was carried out in Tanzania amongst learners with a mean age of 14 years. Their study was based on the Theory of Reasoned Action and Social Cognitive Theory. The study was designed to evaluate the knowledge, attitudes and communication regarding AIDS, susceptibility and condom use; however, sexual behaviour was not examined (Klepp et al., 1994, 1997). Changes in the desired directions were recorded in all of these areas. The study noted a significant effect on subjects exposed to AIDS information, who displayed positive changes in their attitudes towards persons with AIDS; communication on HIV/AIDS between the participants was found to have increased (Klepp et al., 1994).

3.2.2 The Ugandan Evaluation

The second study was conducted by Shuey et al. (1999) in Uganda amongst learners aged 13 to 14. They employed a Social Cognitive Learning Theory approach. The study revealed that learners subjected to experimental conditions were more than three times less likely to be sexually active at posttest, regardless of location, with no significant changes in self-reported sexual activity amongst learners subjected to standard conditions. The same study found a significant desirable improvement in reports of sexual initiation and number of sexual partners (Gallant & Maticka-Tyndale, 2004). Learners that have been subjected to experimental conditions reported significantly more communication on issues of sexual health than those subjected to standard conditions. More favourable attitudes towards premarital abstinence were reported amongst experimental participants during post-intervention phases compared to control learners, the reasons for their abstinence being based on rational decision-making (Shuey et al., 1999; Mukoma & Flisher, in press).

3.2.3 The Kenyan Evaluation

The third study was undertaken in primary schools in Kenya, called the Primary School Action for Better Health (PSABH) (Maticka-Tyndale et al., 2004). The intervention was undertaken with primary school learners with an approximate age range of 11 to (even) 16, teachers who attended a workshop on the programme content and messages, and people from the community (e.g. parents and head teachers). The Kenyan project evaluated knowledge, attitudes, intentions and behaviour. The study revealed that a significant increase in communication could only be reached in communication with others; no other significant changes were found. Although modes of abstinence were based on the A(bstinence), B(e faithful), C(ondom), and D(elay) approach, for example, no significant changes have been found in either the abstinence level or in condom use. However, Maticka-Tyndale et al. (2004) report that there was evidence that significantly fewer pupils, who completed the survey at the six-month evaluation stage, had initiated sexual activity compared to pupils who completed surveys prior to PSABH programming. The absence of a significant difference between control and target schools in sexual initiation makes it impossible to credit this change specifically to PSABH (Maticka-Tyndale et al., 2004).

The studies by Klepp et al. (1994, 1997) and Shuey et al. (1999) met almost all of their objectives regarding changes in sexual behaviour and particularly the number of learners initiating sexual activity (Gallant & Maticka-Tyndale, 2004) as compared to other studies with older target groups. Gallant and Maticka-Tyndale (2004) attribute the less positive results to the fact that the participants were older and that a larger number of them had already been sexually active. Kaaya et al. (2002a) support this finding and conclude that studies amongst pre-adolescents are essential to explore determinants of delayed sexual debut and to cast light on the appropriateness of primary school settings for sexual health interventions. The importance of initiating long-term prevention programmes in primary schools is evident from the conclusions of reviews of interventions, which demonstrate that programmes conducted prior to sexual debut are the most effective in reducing rates of sexually transmitted infections (see also Grunsheit, 1997).

3.3 A Case of a School-based Life Skills Programme on HIV/AIDS in South Africa

As outlined in the HIV/AIDS/STD Strategic Plan for South Africa (HIVSP) (2000-2005), the primary focus of every preventive strategy to avoid a further spread of HIV in the South African society should be (1) to reduce the number of new infections (especially amongst youth) and (2) to decrease the impact of HIV/AIDS on individuals, families and communities (Smart, 2002). Within the HIVSP for 2000 to 2005, life skills programmes should meet suggestions from the WHO (1999a), and are seen as a main preventive strategy to target young population groups in South Africa in particular.

Until 1997, school-based HIV/AIDS prevention and sex education programmes in South Africa were organised and managed by many non-governmental organizations such as the PPASA or Love Life. Other well-published school-based interventions were designed and implemented by the Department of National Health and Population Development (Meyer, 1989; Visser, 1996) and by independent professionals (Mitchell, 1994; Page, 1990; Flisher et al., 2000) like the famous Drama Approach to AIDS Education (DramAide) (Harvey et al., 2000). These listed health promoting initiatives foremost targeted adolescents in impoverished communities, raised awareness of HIV/AIDS and offered peer education outside of or in cooperation with schools. Discrete projects, targeting in-school youth as well as out-of-school youth, offered hopes of success, but these had not been applied on a large scale to reach more children and young people.

Given this background, it became clear that the impact of such programmes in concurrence with the increasing number of young people infected by HIV could only be increased by implementing a national life skills and AIDS prevention programme as part of the curriculum in South African schools. The intention behind this plan was to expand the application of the programme to reach as many children and young people as possible to inform them about and protect them against HIV infection, and to prevent the further transmission of HIV in the South African society. Against this setting, the South African National Department of Education (NDOE) in cooperation with the South African National Department of Health launched a national life skills programme on HIV/AIDS and sex education in secondary schools that was managed by the provincial departments in 1997/1998 and funded by the European Union (EU) (73%), the National Department of Health (16%) and the National Department of Education (5%) (Magome, Louw, Motlhoioa, & Jack, 1997/1998). The pedagogical basis of the government programme and papers from the Love Life campaign formed the teaching manual of the life skills programme on AIDS and sex education from the Planned Parenthood Association of South Africa (1997). An extensive plan was developed to implement the programme in 27 864 primary and secondary schools, and to design learning materials and media for teacher and learner training (Magome et al., 1997/1998).

In actual fact, there is little data available on the national impact of the life skills programme, especially on primary school level. In an evaluation of the impact of the life orientation (life skills) programme on HIV/AIDS in Gauteng schools 16 secondary schools and four primary schools were interviewed. The survey revealed that only 70% of the schools had implemented life orientation in every grade; 30% have not implemented it at all or only taught it in higher grades (8-9) (Bhana, Brooks, Makiwane, & Naidoo, 2005). Given that in Gauteng, one of the most developed regions in South Africa, the implementation of the programme is still being carried out, it is assumed that the full implementation of the programme should be even more difficult in very poor provinces such as the Eastern Cape Province. Other studies conducted in 12 schools and six communities across South Africa in 1999 and 2001 showed that education on HIV/AIDS was conducted erratically and that in these contexts, life skills education is skeletal at best (Kelly & Parker, 2001; Kelly, 2001). With regard to the above mentioned findings, the existence of underlying obstacles, as well as little practical and adequate delivery of life skills education in the classroom, delays the full implementation of the programme at primary and secondary school level. The underlying obstacles are explained further in the following paragraph.

3.4 Factors Influencing the Implementation at School Level

According to a report by the University of Sussex on the impact of school-based HIV/AIDS education at elementary and secondary schools in Botswana, Uganda and Malawi, there is "little hard evidence" to show that these primary preventive initiatives have a major impact on sexual behaviour (change) (Berger, 2002). The same report states that inappropriate implementation is due to a lack of time, resources and training of educators.

In this report, researchers reported that curriculum-based education as well as counselling and peer education was inadequate because of inappropriate training of teachers in the programme topics, insufficient resources at schools, and an overloaded and examination-driven curriculum (Berger, 2002). Farquhar and Kanabus (1998) confirm that these findings are pertinent for the implementation of programmes in South Africa, and mention difficulties in the provision of life skills education that either lead to inadequate or inappropriate conditions of or significant institutional, political, religious and cultural barriers to school-based life skills education in particular and preventative education in general.

3.4.1 Minimal Resources in Public Schools

In 2000, nearly 12 million learners were enrolled in South African schools (Education Atlas, 2000). A national audit of these public schools found them in poor condition and without the necessary amenities available on site (Education Atlas, 2000). A key problem in South African public schools is the high teacher-learners ratio; classes with 70 learners and more is not a rare occurrence, especially in poor provinces. The schools lack teaching materials and facilities. In addition, government schools in disadvantaged settings face a multitude of problems related to high drop-out rates, poverty and malnutrition, and crime and violence. Visser (1996) states that as long as schools are poorly equipped, teachers will find difficulty in fulfilling their task of bringing basic education to children, apart from implementing further programmes such as life skills programmes on AIDS and sex education. Other barriers to the implementation of health promoting programmes are the decline in teachers that results from teacher transfer, illness, absence, or death (including death by HIV/AIDS) (World Bank, 2002).

3.4.2 Work-overstrain and Attrition of Teachers

There are excessive demands relating to low-level educational standards for teachers and the complete remodelling of the South African educational system in regard to Curriculum 2005. The national reform creates a working and learning system that easily overburdens or even burns out teachers with psychosocial, structural and organizational demands in school work and contributes to a high attrition rate among those professionals. A comprehensive survey of factors determining educator supply and demand in South African public schools supports these assumptions (Phurutse, 2005) and has found that educators are leaving the profession in large numbers for the following reasons: low morale; low job satisfaction and stress and a correspondingly high absenteeism rate; AIDS and other diseases; and premature death (Education Labour Relations Council, 2005).

In relation to the HIV status of teachers it was found that especially African educators were very likely to be HIV positive compared with other groups working in rural and disadvantaged school environments. From this, it follows that they seem to be exposed to risk factors regarding their personal health (Education Labour Relations Council, 2005). A World Bank report suggests that at least 12% of the country's teachers are HIV positive (Education Foundation Trust, 2002). This, together with the psychological impact of the illness, reduces contact time, performance and the quality of teaching and worsens the learner-teacher ratio (Badcock-Walters, 2002). These conditions decrease the chance of high quality education amongst children from disadvantaged communities and their access to life-prolonging and protecting information that result in a lowering of their future expectations.

3.4.3 Resistance to Teach about Condom Use

Information barriers from teacher to learner level are considered another hurdle for the implementation of school-based life skills programme on AIDS. Visser (1996) mentions that teachers did not address some of the major HIV/AIDS prevention issues due to their fear of community disapproval, their reluctance to discuss sex and HIV, curriculum overload, and their general preference for doctrinaire instruction. The same was found in many other sub-Saharan studies (Kinsman, Nakiyingi, Kamali, Carpenter, Quigley, Pool, & Whitworth, 2001; Klepp et al., 1994, 1997; Shuey et al., 1999). Furthermore, this resistance can be linked to existing community norms and the strong beliefs that education on condoms implicitly condones or encourages sexual activity (see also Visser, 1996) or addresses high levels of learners' sexual activity (Fawole, Asuzu, Oduntan, & Bieger, 1999). Maticka-Tyndale et al. (2004) support these findings and report that teachers in their programme held true to the community focus on abstinence as the only acceptable method of prevention reinforced by fear (i.e. if you don't abstain you will die of AIDS). According to Gallant and Maticka-Tyndale (2004), there were, however, two exceptions. These are the only two reported programmes which successfully included condom presentation as an element in prevention programmes outlined in cooperation with 'non-teachers': one programme evaluated by Harvey et al. (2000) in South Africa and the second, a post-school programme, evaluated by Fawole et al. (1999) in Nigeria.

3.4.4 School Atmosphere and Violence Levels

Another very important obstacle for a highly holistic physical and mental health promoting approach, such as life skills programmes, is the widespread presence of emotional, physical and sexual violence in South African schools. Morrell (2004) calls this condition a "Culture of Silence" to conflict sharply with the official frequently used slogan "Breaking the Silence" about AIDS. Morrell (2004) applies the term silence to the suppressed discourse about taboo-related issues surrounding gender-related issues and violence, sexuality or sex, and the stigma of AIDS at school. A violent school atmosphere does not only tremendously influence any kind of AIDS prevention initiative by blocking its message but puts teachers and especially learners in a situation where power is unequally distributed (Morrell, 2004).

Two examples shall be given at this point to clarify what is meant by an 'atmosphere of silence' and 'unequal power' in school settings. First, as Morrell (2004) states in his article, Calvinist traditions combined with the authoritarianism of apartheid produced a silent society that existed until the end of Apartheid in 1994. Schools were the main pillar of socialisation of future 'valuable' citizens in the system; however, instruments such as corporal punishment were used to oppress any signs of curiosity or independence which were understood as impertinence (Morrell, 2004). At present, the South African Schools Act 84 of 1996, Section 10, prohibits corporal punishment in schools and imposes criminal sanctions. However, positive attitudes to and beliefs in those methods of education are still prevalent and practised, as several studies uncovered (see also Dawes, Kropiwnicki, Kafaar, & Richter, 2005; Morrell, 2001; Human Rights Watch, 2001). Corporal punishment[7] has harmful effects on the physiognomy and psychology of individuals. As Bower (2005) states, physical insurance can be accompanied by bruises and cuts, broken bones, knocked-out teeth, permanently disfigurement or disabling or even death. Mental outcomes, on the other hand, can include antisocial behaviour which results in the escalation and encouragement of violence in school settings; this stand in sharp contrast to interventions that aim to enhance the mental and physical health of individuals.

Second, in regard to sexual violence and harassment at South African schools, a Human Rights Watch study (2001) undertaken in three South African provinces revealed multiple forms of sexual violence at schools, committed most often by fellow learners or teachers. Another study by the

---

7 Emotional abuse will not be described in this study. It is recognised as most prevalent and inherent in physical and sexual abuse.

National Department of Health (1998) underlined those findings and revealed that 38% of rape victims said that they had been raped by a schoolteacher or principal (Kenyon et al., 2000). Brooks, Shisana, and Richter (2004) agree that sexual harassment in South African schools is a serious problem. They report in their survey that 40% of the children surveyed said that boys sexually harassed girls and 15% of the children reported that male educators proposed relationships with girl learners. This survey was based on results amongst 12- to 14-year-old primary school learners (Brooks et al., 2004). Other studies have reported girl learners having their school fees paid by a teacher in exchange for sex (Jewkes & Abrahams, 2002; World Bank, 2002). A disturbing finding by Kinsman et al. (2001) indicated that such problematic structures influence life skills programmes too. According to this study a teacher attending a life skills programme on AIDS was found to have impregnated a female learner and was imprisoned.

From the previous description it is clear that barriers and hurdles to adequately implement and produce outcomes amongst individuals participating in school-based life skills programmes on AIDS and sex education are manifold and varied in nature. Badcock-Walters (2002) concludes that irrespective of the quality of curricula and education-driven interventions, the success of these programmes will be limited by the structural stability and comparative functionality of the system in which they take place. In addition, Kenyon et al. (2000) deduce that the quality of a life skills programme depends on adequate initial teacher training and/or continued teacher support, cooperation with other teachers at the school and open-minded ideologies and practices, amongst others. Under-resourced public school settings, the daily management of social and psychological problems, and the existence of emotional, physical, and sexual violence make it necessary to consider the actual implementation of life skills programmes on AIDS and sex education by school personnel. Personnel are often expected to act in conflicting and overburdened learning and operational settings without external conducive support. Many of the factors listed above have been cited as barriers to the effectiveness of HIV/AIDS intervention, not only in South Africa and the rest of the sub-Saharan region, but worldwide (Applegate, 1998).

3.5 Conclusion

Twenty years after the existence and effects of HIV/AIDS on individuals and societies became known all interventions tackling HIV/AIDS in sub-Saharan

Africa seemed to experience wide-ranging problems to fully and effectively implement programmes at school level. Currently, the only instruments to deal with this pandemic are those offered by health promotion methods such as life skills programmes. However, the quality of implementation and the outcomes of every intervention strongly depend on the interrelation of the distal, proximal and individual domain, which can be immense when such programmes are implemented in a setting with a magnitude of socio-economic and socio-structural problems.

Eleven studies fitting the research criteria set by Gallant and Maticka-Tyndale in a literature review in 2004 have been conducted on school-based life skills programmes on HIV/AIDS and sex education in the sub-Saharan region. Only three of the evaluated programmes also targeted children under the age of 12 despite the research finding that preventive approaches are more effective if implemented at an early life stage and before sexual debut (viz. Polce-Lynch, Myers, Kliewer, & Kilmartin, 2001). In other words it is proposed that the most appropriate time for the implementation of intervention programmes targeting primary school children is early adolescence and before the onset of unsafe behaviour.

Other factors that were found to hinder the implementation of school-based life skills programmes or affect the outcomes of such health promoting initiatives are highlighted by Kelly, Ntlablati, Oyosi, Van der Riet, and Parker (2002): (1) problems of prioritising life skills programmes; (2) intensive activity in an environment where there is much pressure to improve school performance; (3) lack of follow-through on the mandate to provide life skills education; (4) lack of follow-up training of teachers; (5) little promotion of the value of the concept of teaching life skills amongst teachers; and (6) perceptions that it is a soft teaching option which is not highly appreciated amongst teachers.

These findings may suggest that the focus of studies should not only be on methodological aspects and outcomes of interventions, but also on socio-demographic and proximal psychosocial determinants of various sexual and risk reduction practices in order to provide a broader framework within which adolescent sexuality in the region can be understood and more realistically addressed (Kaaya et al., 2002a). Furthermore, Kaaya et al. (2002a), amongst others, suggest that method triangulation of both quantitative and qualitative data sources be used to explore local contextual factors in order to enhance the adaptation of instruments to suit local circumstances.

CHAPTER FOUR
A Needs Analysis for Health Interventions – Case Study of Kayamandi

4.1 Introduction

In the 1980s, the WHO emphasised that health and well-being of individuals are closely connected with social, cultural, physical, economic and other factors inside living areas or towns (Burlington, 2005). Against this background, it can be assumed that individuals living and growing up in extremely impoverished settings should therefore have the greatest need for health interventions that will enhance and strengthen their health and well-being. In regard to the intervention presented in this thesis, and undertaken in a very impoverished community, a needs analysis was outlined beforehand to (1) identify prevalent risks and resources in the specific setting, (2) immure the intervention in its surrounding and (3) adequately adjust the life-orientated modules for its participants.[8]

The following section describes the particular case of Kayamandi (translated as 'pleasant home') in order to highlight the social, health, security and educational infrastructures in a disadvantaged community[9] in South Africa that have resulted from historic, socio-economic, as well as political processes in the country.

---

[8] The information for the needs analysis was drawn from regular field trips and field reports, an extensive literature review (e.g. maps, official statistics, published and unpublished articles), and photographic documentation. The methodology for the needs analysis is described in chapter 6.

[9] Community is hereby defined as everyone living or working in a specific geographical area (Campbell, 2003).

4.2 The History and Geographical Development of Kayamandi

The town Stellenbosch is located 30 kilometres east of Cape Town in the Western Cape Province. It is the second oldest town (founded in 1679) in South Africa (Dennerlein & Adami, 2004), and historically a centre of Afrikanerdom during Apartheid in which the university played a central role in educating the Apartheid elite. The economic pillars of the town are wine and citrus farming. Light industry and tourism have assumed growing economic functions (Donaldson, 1990) in recent years.

Stellenbosch's 79 000 inhabitants predominantly live in three sections, according to the standardised town structure during Apartheid. The centre of Stellenbosch comprises of various neighbourhoods as well as the university campus, and accommodates mainly students of the university and people of European (white) origin. The so-called coloured population predominantly lives in the areas of Idasvalley and Cloetesville. During the Apartheid era these areas formed the buffer zone between 'white' and 'black' areas. The third area comprises mostly of people with African origins. This part of town is called Kayamandi and is situated on the north-western side of Stellenbosch along an arterial road.

This type of town structure, which represented a visual and local separation of people on the basis of race, came about during the Apartheid era and ultimately led to different standards of living. The present town structure of Stellenbosch has not changed significantly since the democratisation of South Africa in 1994, and currently encourages the separation of social strata within the population by means of social affiliation.

4.2.1 The Establishment of a Township Structure (1930s until mid-1980s)

In the 1930s, before the Group Areas Act (1950) that distributed living areas in order to separate racial groups, the Municipality of Stellenbosch introduced separation and control measures. They relocated the group of African people living in Stellenbosch at the time, to another area at the edge of town. Therefore, Kayamandi can be regarded as the second oldest township in South Africa. At this time, approximately 80 black people lived as housekeepers or farm workers in Stellenbosch. From 1930 until 1940, the farm Platte Clip accommodated the African community of Stellenbosch. In 1940 people were moved from Platte Clip to the current site of Kayamandi on the north-western outskirts of Stellenbosch (Figure 4.1). Then, the area had fixed borders and a surface of 7.5 ha.

The residential area was planned to accommodate mainly single men who were farm workers on the nearby wine farms. At that time, blacks were admitted to urban areas only if they had work contracts; their wives and children had to stay in designated territories, which later led to the degeneration of family structures and severe and widespread poverty (Peires, 2005). Fifty-five hostels, i.e. houses exclusively for single men, were built, where ten men stayed in rooms with double-bedding and shared one toilet and one kitchen. However, ninety-six detached houses were built for families (318 people) that already lived in the community. The detached houses had one room, an indoor shower, a kitchen, and were surrounded by a small garden (Dennerlein & Adami, 2004). In the early 1940s, private companies built more hostels. These new buildings accommodated sixteen men who lived in basic units with one shower, one toilet, one small kitchen, and tiny bedrooms for up to three men.

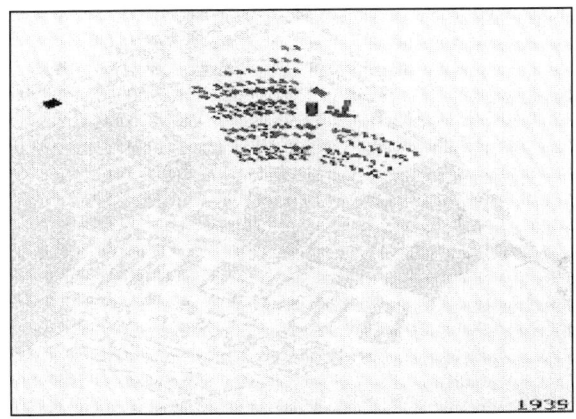

Figure 4.1. Kayamandi Structure in 1939 (Dennerlein & Adami, 2004).

In 1948 Apartheid was officially established as the new South African form of government. The Segregation Law, one of the main segments of Apartheid regulations, separated public and private life for all South African inhabitants on racial grounds. Legalised township structures, such as Kayamandi, were established as living areas. In the 1960s, the Municipality of Stellenbosch considered moving the residents of Kayamandi to another industrial area further away from town. The relocation to a distant area was intended to visually and geographically separate the black township from Stellenbosch.

In the end, the municipality's intention was abandoned because it was feared that the relocation would traumatise the people and restrict their ability to work. In the 1970s until the 1980s Kayamandi's structure was formally divided into areas for hostels and areas for detached houses with gardens. During that decade, a conflict between long-term residents and hostel dwellers turned into violence within the township.

4.2.2 Migration and Population Growth (1989 until 2004)

Since the abolishment of Influx Control in 1986, together with the Segregation Law and the Group Areas Act in 1991 there has been a considerable growth in African communities especially in the period between 1989 and 1991. Because migration streams are primarily shaped by human flows from distribution areas of relative poverty like the Eastern Cape Province, immigration mainly happens to areas of relative affluence like the Western Cape Province and the Cape Metropolitan Area. People who migrate to these areas mostly belong to rural and unskilled Xhosa speaking households pushed by rapidly deteriorating conditions in the former homelands of Transkei and Ciskei (PGWC, 2001). In 2001, a socio-economic survey conducted in Kayamandi asked residents to state their date of migration into the Stellenbosch area, and the source area. Most of the in-migration took place in 1998 (6.3%). The majority of people (74.4%) came from the Eastern Cape Province (Transkei/Ciskei). The majority of the rest (23%) came from other areas of the Western Cape Province, e.g. 10% from the Cape Metropolitan Area (Guguletu, Khayelitsha, Langa) (University of Stellenbosch, 2001).[10]

Migration from the rural areas to the semi-urban area of Kayamandi changed the township structure from formal to informal and caused dense living and housing conditions. The shortage of formal housing forced immigrants to stay either in the hostels, where they lived with sixteen other families, or to build informal houses. The first squatters (builders of informal housing) settled on the rugby field in the community and then in the early 1990s began to fill all other vacant areas, thereby forcing the community boundaries (Skinner, 2000). Since 1991 the most rapid increase in population has occurred in the squatter area; a continuing trend at present (Dennerlein & Adami, 2004). Another fact, confirmed by the PGWC (2001), is that the metro-born section of the African model is closely connected to the long-

---

10 The results are assumed to be not representative for the Kayamandi population because most of the people asked refused to answer this question.

established African townships, whilst the population of the informal settlements consists almost entirely of in-migrants. In most recent years, the uncoordinated influx and overcrowding deepened the long-term conflict between old residents and new arrivals; a conflict that characterises the atmosphere within Kayamandi at present.

However, apart from the migration flow into the township, there seems to be an even stronger migration process within Kayamandi itself, another fact that contributes to a tense atmosphere. Zone F, an informal settlement area, for example, consists mainly of people (74%) that have moved into Kayamandi in 2001 and have recently moved to this informal area from other areas in Kayamandi because they were unable to afford high rents for backyard shacks or rooms (Development Action Group, 2002). This means, the lack of space seems to force people to move between already densely populated areas in Kayamandi in order to identify free plots.

The demographic data for Kayamandi varies considerably due to these migration processes. In 1989 a macro plan of Stellenbosch was drawn up by the Provincial Administration of the Western Cape (PAWC) and the Kayamandi Town Council (KTC) (PAWC & KTC, 1989), that estimated the population at 6 524. In 2002, whereas the Stellenbosch Town Engineer was convinced that a total of 14 000 people lived in the township, the latest independent census in Kayamandi undertaken in 2004 estimated the number of inhabitants at 28 000 (Dennerlein & Adami, 2004) (Figure 4.2).

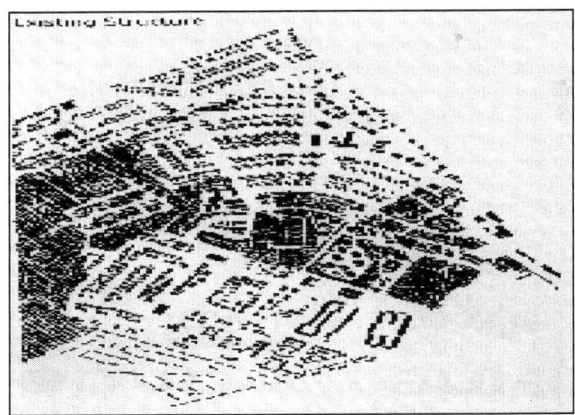

Figure 4.2. Kayamandi Structure in 2004 (Dennerlein & Adami, 2004).

This census also indicated that 35% of the inhabitants of Stellenbosch lived on one eighteenth (1/18) of the total area of the town. This also means that

2 980 people on 1 km², with an influx rate of about 150 people per month (Dennerlein & Adami, 2004), which makes a decline in in-migration in the near future unlikely. The reasons for the increase in population in Kayamandi are rooted in political and demographical dimensions. The abolition of Influx Control (1986) and the Segregation Law (1991) in particular, allowed people to choose freely their living locality and work place even though the township structure was not prepared for the high and uncontrolled influx. The demographical dimension included two factors: First, the high growth in the internal birth rate and second, the growing number of immigrants who had been rooted in increasing poverty in deprived provinces or rural areas. The extreme increase in population without a parallel increase in territory caused a high population density within Kayamandi, resulting in pressure on the already underdeveloped infrastructure and a deterioration of living and housing conditions. Many people are forced to live without privacy or adequate living conditions that support health and well-being.

4.3 Socio-demographic Conditions

4.3.1 Ethnic Diversity and Cultural Heritage

Kayamandi has a diverse ethnic and cultural composition. The residents mainly belong to Xhosa, Tswana and Cape Coloured ethnic groups, and include a handful of European descendants and immigrants from other African countries such as Lesotho, Somalia, Nigeria or Ethiopia. However, the majority of residents belong to ethnic clans of the Xhosa. The main language spoken in Kayamandi is isiXhosa. The second most common language is Afrikaans, which does not only link Kayamandi residents with the Afrikaans culture in Stellenbosch, but is also a precondition for occupation arrangements in town. Despite the fact that every ethnical group can freely practice its rituals, traditions, religions, and languages since the abolition of Apartheid, migration from rural areas to the semi-rural area of Kayamandi causes cultural transition. Cultural transition inevitably results in a mixture of rural-traditional and urban-western value systems and life styles that may have far-reaching consequences during verbal or physical conflict between residents of formal and informal areas.

4.3.2 Age Structure

According to a survey by the University of Stellenbosch in 2001, the Kayamandi population consists of 51% women and 49% men. The population is characterised by a youthful age structure. In 2001, about one third (33.9%) of the population was between 0 and 15 years of age. More than half (55.6%) of the population was younger than 25 and nearly 70% younger than 30 years of age. Only 2.8% were 60 years and older. The mean age of the residents was 23 years (University of Stellenbosch, 2001). These figures indicate that older role models and mentors of the youth are virtually absent in Kayamandi (Barnes, 2002a).

4.3.3 Marital Status and Family Units

A survey by the University of Stellenbosch in 2001 revealed that 50% of the population between 16 years and older were single and had never been married. During the survey 42.3% stated that they were married and 4.5% reported that they lived with a single partner (University of Stellenbosch, 2001). The rest reported to be divorced, widowed, or separated from their partner. In contrast to the data on marital status it was found that about 13% of the adult (older than 17 years) population of Kayamandi were single parents, the majority (73.3%) of whom between 20 and 34 years of age. A large proportion of this group (28.7%) formed a household with one or more single parents.

The same survey found that 57.5% of the interviewed women, 12 years and older, had borne a child. More than one third of this group of women (34.5%) had one child, 47% had two or three children and 18.3% had more than four children (University of Stellenbosch, 2001). Furthermore, 42.4% of the women had borne their first child when they were still at school, of which 5.9% testified that they were still in primary school when they had borne their first child. Only 5% of the women were older than 30 years when they first gave birth (University of Stellenbosch, 2001).

In regard to presented data, it can be argued that there are three prevalent types of family units in Kayamandi (their frequency not confirmed). The first identified type of family unit is the nuclear family unit that consists of parents and children. The second most common unit is a single parent family unit that consists mainly of mothers, with one or more children. According to Barbarin and Richter (2001) the main factors that contribute to single parent family units could be childbearing outside of marriage, as well as divorce and separation. The third prevalent type of family unit is a multi-adult, multi-generation living unit or rather an urbanised version of the rural extended family based on clan and kinship networks (Barbarin & Richter, 2001), with limited living space. This type of family unit is characterised by instability caused by migration processes during which members move in and out of these units and therefore permanently change the composition.

In regard to the previous statement, migration also creates instable living conditions and family structures in situations where children do not always migrate with their parents, where they arrive at a later stage or where they lodge with kin or friends after their parents have moved somewhere else (PGWC, 2001). The 2001 US survey revealed that in Kayamandi 4.4% of all children 17 years and younger were living in households that did not include their biological parents. The majority of absent parents (57.1%) resided in the Eastern Cape, while 11.4% were untraceable and a further 11.4% deceased. The majority (97%) of these children with absent parents were related to the nuclear family occupying the residential unit (University of Stellenbosch, 2001). The typical rural and traditional African extended family unit is assumed not to be represented in Kayamandi due to the absence of older generations. The existing data did not point out the existence of so-called child-headed households or guardian family units.

4.3.4 Employment Status and Income Level

In 2001, taking into account the not economically active housewives, the unemployment rate in Kayamandi was estimated at 34% (University of Stellenbosch, 2001). In South Africa, the official unemployment rate in February 2000 was 27% (Lehohla, 2000). The unemployment rate in Kayamandi was therefore higher than the national average. The survey also showed that the majority of the men (67%) and only half the women (49%) in Kayamandi were employed at the time (University of Stellenbosch, 2001).

This inequality in terms of employment might lead to another social problem, namely a large number of women raising their children alone (single-headed households) and without proper income. It is likely that job opportunities are rare, especially for poor, unskilled and uneducated women (Campbell, 2003), a situation that further contributes to poverty in these households. In addition, the highest unemployment rate is reported amongst the 15-29 age group, namely 36.4% (University of Stellenbosch, 2001). This is a possible indicator for a high unemployment rate especially among younger population segments in Kayamandi.

Most of the residents who had an occupation were employed in Stellenbosch, on surrounding farms or in Cape Town. Three quarters of the economically active people were employed full-time. More than 10% worked part time, e.g. three days a week, 6% were self-employed, e.g. as street traders, and 8% were seasonal workers (University of Stellenbosch, 2001).[11] Most people were employed in the service sector (30.3%); general labour (11.3%) and artisan work (9.5%) (University of Stellenbosch, 2001). Occupations in the service sector were cleaning personnel, waiters/waitresses, cooks, garage guards, gardeners or tradesmen working as building workers, assistant plumbers, assistant electricians, and carpet cleaners.

In correspondence with the unskilled jobs, the above mentioned occupations were linked to low monthly incomes. The migration report by the Provincial Government of the Western Cape (PGWC) of 1996 revealed that on a national scale 26% and on a provincial scale 18.4% of employees earned less than R500/month (PGWC, 2001). The following statistics on the actual income distribution in Kayamandi have not been verified. The income distribution report by the US in 2001 showed that 8.7% of the economically active persons earned less than R500 per month.[12] More than half of the employed (56.5%) had more than R500 and less than R1 500 available per month. Only 34.8% of the employed had R1 500 per month or more at their disposal (University of Stellenbosch, 2001). Barnes (2002a) reported in their survey of 2002 that 49% of the households reported an income of less than R500 per month, while 37% reported total earnings of between R500 and R1 000 per month. The Development Action Group revealed that the poorest in the community live especially in informal settlements, and that 59% of this group earn less than R800 per month (Development Action Group, 2002).

Looking at income levels, the income of employed residents is considered generally low with a higher risk of poverty in the female group. One half of the employed women earn R1 000 per month or less as opposed to only 27% of the men. The income of women is considerably lower than the monthly earnings of men (University of Stellenbosch, 2001). Welfare transfers, such as pensions and disability grants, function as important components of household incomes particularly for the very poor (Leibbrandt, Woolard, & Bohrat, 2000 in Natrass, 2003). However, those grants that contribute to the insurances of basic needs seem to be badly distributed in Kayamandi. Only 2.1% of the population received state grants and 1% Child Support Grants. Only a small percentage (0.8%) of the 2.8% of pensioners in

---

11   During the picking season there is an additional influx of people into both communities to take advantage of the additional seasonal employment opportunities offered by the fruit farming industry (Skinner, 2000).

12   "...a family is classified as poor if its total income is less than $1 per day for each member of the household. This is the minimum amount of money economists estimate is needed to feed one person. ...In South Africa, households whose total monthly income falls below the fortieth percentile (R301) are said to be living in moderate poverty....as many as 52 per cent of Africans...are moderately poor." (Barbarin & Richter, 2001)

Kayamandi (people older than 60 years) receives Old Age Grant. Despite the high rate of single parent family units in Kayamandi, only 2.4% of single parents apply for maintenance.

4.3.5 Housing Conditions

Kayamandi can be divided into formal and informal zones. About two thirds (University of Stellenbosch, 2001) to more than three quarters of the housing units have an informal character (Barnes, 2002b). Housing in formal areas has a formal and semi-formal character. Formal units include detached houses (Figure 4.3), hostels[13] and flats/townhouses.

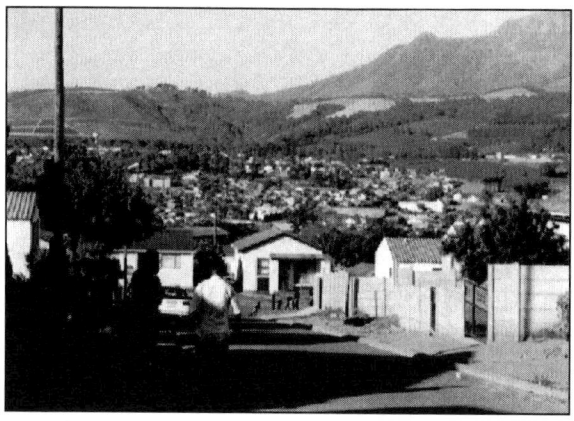

Figure 4.3. Formal Housing (Detached Houses) (Bicher, 2005).

Semi-formal housing units have Wendy houses (prefabricated cottages) in their backyards or backyard shacks as an extension to the main house on the plot. Housing in informal areas is predominantly composed of squatter dwellings (Figure 4.4) with an average of 5x5 metres of floor space (PTT, 2004). The informal dwellings or shacks are constructed entirely or partially of wood, corrugated iron, plastic and other low-cost building material (Development Action Group, 2002). According to the US survey (2001), about 11.2% of the living units had one room and about 60% had two or three rooms (University of Stellenbosch, 2001).

---

13 Up to 20 families live in the hostels, with 6 square meters available per family. Two toilets per hostel, and no bathroom facilities, make a private and hygienic life impossible (PTT, 2004).

Water and sanitation provision are sensitive issues in Kayamandi. According to Barnes (2002b) 12% of the interviewed people said that they had toilets outside, but directly next to the house, whilst the majority of households (64%) used communal facilities some distance from the dwellings. A total of 6.4% reported that there was no toilet available within walking distance (Barnes, 2002b). In general, it seems that only those people living in brick and detached houses have a toilet inside the house (18%) (Barnes, 2002b). People living in informal settlements use public taps for drinking and washing.

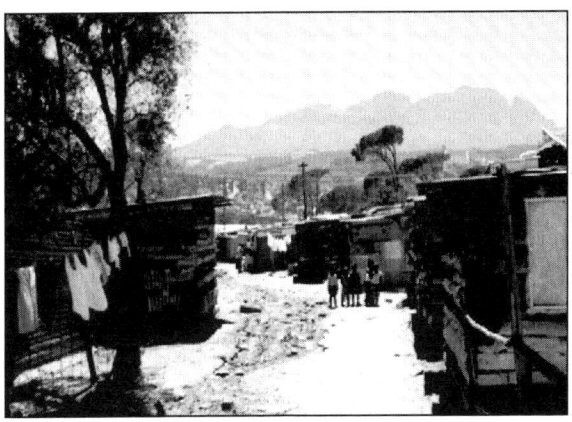

Figure 4.4. Informal Housing (Shacks) (Bicher, 2005).

The Reconstruction and Development Project (RDP), the governmental programme for housing and development in disadvantaged communities, has improved the infrastructure of Kayamandi since 1994. However, most of the residents have been on the waiting list since 1993 (Development Action Group, 2002) and according to the Pilot Project in Southern Africa (2004), 2 300 formal living units would be needed in Kayamandi (Erhard, 2000) to improve living and sanitation conditions for its inhabitants and to help contain overcrowding.

4.4 Health Status of the Population

High poverty levels and hazardous living conditions (e.g. insufficient sewerage system, unsatisfactory water and refuse removal in informal settlements) can contribute to a high prevalence of disease, e.g. tuberculosis, diarrhoea, and malnutrition among a population within a certain living area. The following paragraph describes the prevailing health conditions of children in particular living in this area, and the consequences for their physical and mental health development.

4.4.1 Incidence of Disease

Since 2000, a departmental community health team from the University of Stellenbosch has tested the water quality of the Plankenbrug River every six weeks. The Plankenbrug River runs through Stellenbosch, around the dense settlement of Kayamandi and joins the Eerste River on the outskirts of town (Barnes, 2002a). The tests exposed dangerously high levels of faecal contamination in the river below Kayamandi. For example, in February 2003 a test for *Faecal Coliforms,* taken from a section of the river that runs above Kayamandi, found 329 *Faecal Coliforms* per 100 ml.

At the testing point below Kayamandi the water was contaminated with 12 860 000 *Faecal Coliforms* per 100 ml (Barnes, 2002a). The test detected several bacteria (*B-haemolytic Streptococcus Group A, A-haemolytic Streptococcus*) that can cause severe diseases[14], serious infections in humans, a high fatality rate or serious impairment. So-called 'flesh eating' bacteria that cause infections of the upper respiratory tract (e.g. throat infections and cardiac conditions when the organisms settle on the valves) and rheumatic fever (*Streptococcus faecalis* and *Streptococcus spp, Enterococcus faecalis*) were also detected. Finally, bacteria (e.g. *Staphylococcus species; Enterobacter spp, Klebsiella species; Citrobacter spp; Proteus mirabilis* and *P vulgaris*) that cause skin infections, wound infections, septicaemia, heart disease, arthritis, pneumonia, violent nausea, vomiting and diarrhoea were found (Yeld, 2004; Thom, 2002).

According to Barnes (2002b)[15] this contamination arises mainly from human faeces, waste water and solid waste disposed into the sewerage systems or from some areas in the township that lack sewerage systems. The team of researchers warns that the faecal contamination constitutes a health hazard and that infectious diseases will arise from contaminated

---

14 The organisms were identified at Tygerberg Hospital's Department of Medical Microbiology. Only bacteria were screened – the lack of funds made testing for viruses or fungi impossible (Yeld, 2004).
15 For human use, drinking water should contain **no** *E.coli* organisms. For irrigation purposes, the level should not rise above 2 000 organisms per 100 ml water. Detected *E.coli* organisms at the testing point below Kayamandi were 4 560 000 per 100 ml water (Barnes, 2002a).

surroundings, which will in turn affect all persons coming into contact with the water. In short, the results of tested bacteria indicate a high level of a multitude of diseases within the population of Kayamandi, and intestine infections are most probably widespread.

4.4.2 Diarrhoea and Sanitation Models

The lack of sanitation models in Kayamandi, together with other factors, contributes to a high prevalence of diarrhoea. The sewerage system was originally designed for 5 000 residents in an area where presently more than 28 000 people live. The Stellenbosch Municipality Development Plan of 2001 estimated that one latrine serves 75 people (PTT, 2004). However, the inadequate provision of toilet and washing facilities is only one factor for the endangered health status of humans in this area. Another factor is the inadequate and delayed maintenance of existing facilities, resulting in broken toilets or overflowed drains that in turn increase the pressure on remaining facilities (Barnes, 2002a).

The waste management is provided by the Municipality of Stellenbosch on a regular basis, once a week for formal areas and irregularly for informal areas. Residents from some of the informal densely populated housing areas complain that waste is left for days in the streets where it attract large amounts of insects and stray dogs that tear open the plastic bags. The littered streets often serve as playground for children (Barnes, 2002b).

Diarrhoea is directly related to a lack of access to clean water and appropriate sanitation, and is considered one of the main causes of infant mortality in developing countries (WC Stellenbosch Municipality, 2003). The statistics of the Kayamandi Community Day Care Clinic indicate that, from January to December 2003, only 156 children were treated for severe diarrhoea (WC Stellenbosch Municipality, 2003). However, there are indicators for a much higher rate of children with diarrhoea than reflected in the statistics. In their survey of July 2001 Barnes (2002b) reported that 13% of residents (without making references to the age of respondents) reported one or more cases of diarrhoea. This was at the height of winter, with food spoilage at a low level due to the cold (Barnes, 2002b).

To conclude, sanitation is considered poor due to overcrowding and overstrained toilet and sewerage systems. In addition, the cycle for the transmission of infectious diseases such as diarrhoea is fatal when combined with widespread poverty that accommodates lower resistance to infectious diseases as a result of malnutrition.

4.4.3 Malnutrition among Children

Apart from sanitation, inadequate food distribution within poor communities is an additional health hazard, especially for the youngest and weakest of society, the children. The National Department of Health estimates that 14 million (approximately 30%) of the South African population experience food insecurity. Within this context, children, especially those in rural and semi-urban areas, are the most vulnerable to malnutrition (Mvulane, 2003). The National Food Consumption Survey (NFCS) of 1999 (Labadarios, 2000), which examined the dietary intake of 2 894 South African children aged 1-9 years, reported that approximately one in five children (21.6%) aged 1-9 years of age in South Africa are stunted (Turcotte, 2003), i.e. a form of malnutrition. Turcotte (2003) examined the nutritional status of children younger than five years in a 24-hour recall survey in Kayamandi. The most significant finding in his analysis was the 24% prevalence of stunting in the sample. This is slightly higher than the national prevalence (21.6%). The 3.4% prevalence of malnourishment in Kayamandi was lower than the national prevalence of 10.3% (Turcotte, 2003). These findings show that stunting is the predominant manifestation of malnutrition in Kayamandi.

Children who suffer from stunting (including growth retardation as a result of poor diets and/or recurring infections) tend to have more frequent episodes of severe diarrhoea and are more susceptible to infectious diseases such as malaria, meningitis and pneumonia (Steyn & Labadarios, 2002). Mvulane (2003) states that the health implications of malnutrition range from intrauterine brain damage and growth failure and reduced physical and mental capacity in childhood, to an increased risk of developing diet-related non-communicable diseases later in life. There is also strong evidence that an impaired growth is associated with a delayed mental development, poor school performance, and reduced intellectual capacity (De Onis & Blössner, 2003 in Turcotte, 2003). Studies have indicated that any form of malnutrition contributes to a significant reduction in lifetime earnings which, is likely to perpetuate inequities in health and other dimensions of household welfare in the future (Zere & McIntyre, 2003).

4.4.4 Undetected Disease Prevalence – HIV and TB

The following section gives a brief overview of the statistically registered Tuberculosis and STIs, specifically the incidences of HIV, among the Kayamandi population tested at the Kayamandi Community Clinic. In 2003, 290 cases were reported of patients being infected with Tuberculosis (WC Stellenbosch Municipality, 2004); 73 of the TB patients tested HIV-positive

(WC Stellenbosch Municipality, 2003). In total, 1 012 patients were registered as newly-infected with a STI of which 260 were newly-tested HIV-positive (WC Stellenbosch Municipality, 2003). In comparison, the HIV prevalence in the Western Cape Province in the same year was estimated to be 13.1% (National Department of Health, 2004c) with an increasing tendency.

Members of the National Department of Health in Stellenbosch and nurses at the Kayamandi Community Clinic confirmed that the actual numbers are considerably higher than statistics reflect. The National Department of Health could not, however, provide clear statistics on the actual prevalence of disease in Kayamandi because of the dual health system in Stellenbosch on the one hand and the anonymity of patients in statistics on the other. The other reason for possibly ambiguous statistics is the fact that a much larger number of people have never been tested for TB or HIV. They intentionally accept being untested and untreated to avoid the stigma surrounding AIDS or TB. In this way, both epidemics become additional burdens of fear that worsen existing deprivations of people that live in poor and unhealthy conditions.

In regard to HIV, several risk factors contribute to its transmission and subsequent high prevalence within Kayamandi. Only one selected factor shall be outlined at this point: Widespread sexually related risky behavioural patterns contributing to the transmission of STIs, including HIV. In his research during 2000, Skinner tried to better understand HIV-related behaviour in youth in two case study communities. One of the survey communities was Kayamandi. Using results from his qualitative methods only, Skinner found that although knowledge on HIV/AIDS was good, knowledge on STIs was poor, with high levels of denial and rejection of safer sex practices. He concluded that the ideology of male dominance was probably the central major problem blocking behavioural change and reinforcing the norm of multiple partners. In relation to this finding, he also established that direct or implied monogamy was not considered a possibility by the respondents. When asked about the use of condoms, women also answered they would be scared to request men to use a condom and all respondents stated that condoms were very seldom used since they spoil sex, show a lack of trust or, on a more sinister basis, are seen as a sign that the person has a STI or AIDS.

Skinner argues there is a great fear of being exposed as an STI or AIDS patient. This fear therefore limits access to treatment, especially at the clinic, which is located inside the community and thus highly visible (Skinner, 2000). In short, there seems to be highly complex and risky sexual morals in Kayamandi, which support the transmission and non-treatment of all STIs and the refusal (or oppression) of safer sexual practices. It can therefore be assumed these sex-related norms and behaviours are handed over from older generations to younger generations, putting the latter at risk of becoming infected, e.g. with HIV.

4.5　Crime Rate

Gathering data about the crime rate in Kayamandi turned out to be extremely difficult. With permission from the South African Police in Stellenbosch information was gathered from the Crime Information Analysis Centre in Stellenbosch (CIAC) and the Business Intelligence Menu (2004). Field interviews and field observations contributed to the description of actual crime distribution in Kayamandi.

The CIAC (2004) testifies that crimes in the residential area of Kayamandi are mainly contact crimes such as murder, rape, assaults and robberies (including attempted robberies) against individuals. The majority of these crimes are liquor-related and occur at weekends in dense informal settlement areas (Business Intelligence Menu, 2004). Domestic violence, rape and sexual abuse of children are contact crimes that tremendously influence the mental and physical safety of women and children in their living areas, as illustrated in paragraph 4.5.1. The second most recurrent crimes are property-related crimes such as burglaries, motor vehicle theft and theft of objects from vehicles.

4.5.1　Crime against Women and Children

Three main forms of violence, namely domestic violence, rape and sexual abuse of children are discussed below. These forms of violence are not only assumed to have an impact on the general health of women and children, but are also risk factors contributing to the increasing prevalence of HIV in South Africa (known as the 'Twin Epidemic').

Domestic Violence

From September 2002 until August 2004, 28 cases of domestic violence were reported. The majority of the cases occurred in squatter areas in Kayamandi. The most frequent forms of violence were kicks, strikes, omit, and abusive language and the use of sharp objects. Victims were mainly women and children (Business Intelligence Menu, 2004). Five cases of physical child abuse were connected to domestic violence (kicks, strikes) and neglected/illegal treatment of children (0-18 years) (Business Intelligence Menu, 2004).

Rape and Child Sexual Abuse

From April 2002 until March 2003, 52 425 cases of rape and attempted rape were reported to the South African Police nationally (Rape Crisis, 2005). In Kayamandi, 33 cases of rape by strangers were reported from September 2002 until August 2004. These incidences mainly occurred in densely populated and informal areas and/or in areas adjacent to the police station. All victims were female and forced to have sexual intercourse concomitant with physical violence (they were held down) or other objects (including guns). The mean age of rape survivors was between 12 and 30 years (Business Intelligence Menu, 2004).[16]

According to the national statistics at the time, girls under 18 were particularly vulnerable to rape, constituting approximately 40% of reported rape and attempted rape cases nationally, with 12 to 17 year-olds reflecting the highest rape ratio per 100 000 of the female population (Human Rights Watch, 2004b). In their book *Sexual Abuse of Young Children in Southern Africa* Richter, Dawes, and Higson Smith (2004) support the findings, that approximately 15% of all rapes involved children under 12 years and that 41% of cases involved children 18 years or younger. In Kayamandi eight cases (24% of all rape cases) of child sexual abuse (0-18 years) were registered from September 2002 until August 2004. In four of all cases (12%) the victims were between 9 and 12 years of age (Business Intelligence Menu, 2004). This means, the results on child rape in Kayamandi are somewhat different from national findings. Thus, available statistics should be interpreted with care since they only include rape by strangers; international scientific results in this field conclude that most incidences of sexual abuse occur by someone known to the child (Richter et al., 2004).

As so far as the results show, violence against women and children in Kayamandi most often occurred in three informal settlement areas and dense squatter areas. These areas are characterised by a high poverty rate whilst a multitude of social and health problems go unpunished and unnoticed. Thus, those findings support the assumption that the statistics on domestic violence, rape and sexual abuse of children do not reflect the actual situation in Kayamandi.

---

16 The statistics only include rape between two strangers. Rape in a relationship, rape of men, oral rape and rape with objects are excluded from these statistics (Rape Crisis, 2005).

4.5.2 Indications for High Crime Dispersal

In general, reporting of all crimes to the police is low in South Africa. The reporting of rape as a highly feared and stigmatised crime is particularly low. Rape Crisis (2005) assumes that only one out of 20 cases of rape and/or sexual abuse, including sexual abuse of children, is reported to the South African Police. Reasons why people do not report crime to the police are manifold and include social and cultural factors, e.g., financial dependence of women on their husbands and/or stigmatisation of rape victims and/or people living with perpetrators.

According to CIAC information, most crimes occur overt weekends and at night. People state that during these periods a state of emergency dominates the atmosphere in Kayamandi with little police supervision, especially at night. Residents, especially women, try not to leave their houses or walk around the area at night since the narrow and dark pathways between shacks are where sex-related attacks happen. This situation is life-threatening to women and a limitation to their personal freedom and safety.

Although, there is a small police station in Kayamandi, which is supervised by two police officers inside the station and two on motorised patrol, most of the residents reported that they were not aware of the police station or preferred to address the police station in Cloetesville. Despite this lack of information, the reality is that the South African Police do not have a good reputation within South African society due to their involvement in torture and violence against civilians during Apartheid as well as recent incidences of corruption in the police system. In addition, race-consciousness is still very apparent in South Africa. Police officers in Stellenbosch belong mainly to the coloured and white communities and the trust of the black community in police officers in town is therefore low.

As a result of historic events and the reasons mentioned above, the South African society in general, and the Kayamandi community in particular, operates by two judicial systems: One system executes official law and order; the other its own moral and vigilante judicial system that punishes crime without using government institutions. The latter is present mainly in townships and rural areas.

4.6 Educational Status of the Population

The educational level of the Kayamandi population is considered to be extremely low and the number of persons leaving school with a proper qualification is unsatisfactory. In 2001, a survey by the University of Stellenbosch asked persons about their highest level of education. Two percent (2%) had never participated in any formal education; 20.2% had completed a primary school education (Grade 7/Standard 5). A high drop-out rate is prevalent at high-school level, with only 14% of the people interviewed completing Grade 12 (Standard 10). Only 1.9% studied at university and obtained a degree/postgraduate degree (University of Stellenbosch, 2001).

The low level of education can partly be attributed to educational restrictions imposed on the black population during Apartheid, when black people attended poorly-equipped schools often with teachers who receive a minimum on up to date educational training. At that time, the goal of the educational system was to educate black people for occupations in low qualified jobs. Presently in South Africa the social and financial status of the individual defines his/her access to high-quality educational institutions (see also 4.6.2). More recent statistics on the educational level of the population in Kayamandi are not yet available.

4.7 Existing Infrastructure

In comparison with the town of Stellenbosch, the infrastructure of Kayamandi is considered insufficient as health care, social services, educational institutions and municipal services are underrepresented compared with the number of residents. An independent study by Dennerlein and Adami (2004) on a new town planning concept for Kayamandi portrayed the large discrepancy between existing and required public and social facilities. A new concept is needed to fulfil internationally standardised measures for town (-ship) structures (Dennerlein & Adami, 2004).

4.7.1 Health Sector

Two different medical or health systems are present in Kayamandi. The first is based on a western approach represented by a community clinic and one private doctor. The other medical system is represented by traditional medical approaches as practised by traditional healers (diviners, herbalists, and faith healers). People in Kayamandi tend to use both medical spheres in the belief that there should be a balance between the mental/physical being, the environment, and the spiritual world (ancestor belief).

The Community Clinic, prescribing western medicine, provides primary care services to 4 000 patients per month. Eleven nurses, health counsellors and health promoters work at the clinic. The nurses provide primary health care services including a cure service (children and adults), immunisation services, antenatal services, family planning services, TB treatment and counselling, and care for chronically ill patients (high blood pressure, epilepsy, diabetes, asthma). Special health programmes include the Mother-to-Child-Transmission-Programme, PEM-Scheme-Programme (food supplement to HIV-positive mothers and their babies as well as malnourished children), a Counselling Service (STIs, TB), a Health Promotion Service that teaches oral hygiene at primary schools and a Sex Awareness Programme at high-school level for which the schools have to apply. The study on town planning came to the conclusion that at least five primary care clinics and one hospital (secondary health care) have to be established in Kayamandi to cover the health requirements.

4.7.2 Educational Sector – The Case of Ikaya Primary School

The overcrowded educational institutions in Kayamandi present a problem. Only one primary and one secondary school offer primary education for children and youth until the age of 18. The Development Action Group (2002) estimated that most school children who live in Kayamandi attend schools within walking distance, e.g. Ikaya Primary School and Kayamandi High School. A few children attend schools in Cloetesville and Stellenbosch or commute by train to schools in Paarl and Cape Town (Development Action Group, 2002). The Ikaya Primary School (translated as 'nice school'), the only primary school in Kayamandi, primarily accommodates children from disadvantaged black population strata within the community. In 2004, 1 700 learners and 33 teachers (including one principal, two deputy principals and five Head of Departments (HODs)) were registered at the school. There are some 45 to 60 learners per class. This means a teacher-learner ratio of 1 to 52, if one includes the principal and the two deputy principals in this calculation.

The Ikaya Primary School opened in 1995 as a public school and is located on the east side of the township in a former industrial area. The school building is built in a Spartan fashion with two elongated buildings surrounding a courtyard paved in concrete (Figure 4.5). The school is surrounded by a high wire-netting fence with an automatically operated iron gate as the main entrance. The learners are accommodated in 32 classrooms in two brick buildings and three prefabricated buildings. The classrooms all have a similar size, height and number of windows. The classrooms are poorly equipped and many classes are short of chairs and tables. The school does not have a playground, a gym, science laboratories, a school hall or a library.[17]

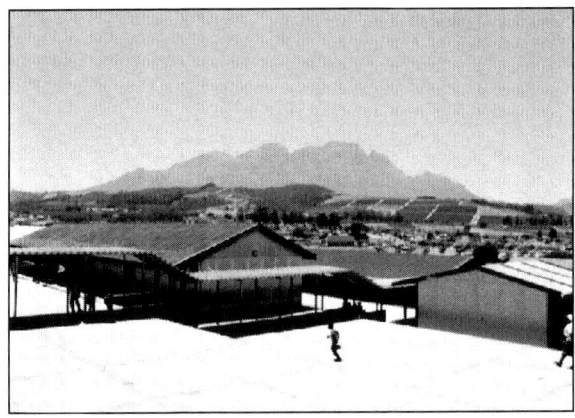

Figure 4.5. School Building – Ikaya Primary School (Bicher, 2005).

The sanitation can be described as critical, overburdened, and most often not in working condition. Vandalism, break-ins and violent arguments between learners are the most frequent forms of crime. Vandalism is directed at school facilities (windows) and furnishing. The school fence is destroyed on a regular basis by neighbouring residents looking for a short-cut between living areas. This in turn creates a security risk. Break-ins involve the theft of test results, video equipment and computers. Violent arguments occur mostly among learners in higher grades. Therefore, the school atmosphere can be described as authoritarian. Corporal punishment by teachers usually involves beating on hands and backs with a stick. To sum up, Ikaya Primary School is an overcrowded learning environment with individuals of diverse social, health and psychological backgrounds, most often overburdened by adults and teachers.

Future plans of the Department of Education to improve the educational system in Kayamandi include a restructuring of the complete school system. A School for further Education and Training that would accommodate Grades 10 to 12 is currently being built. Kayamandi High School will

---

17   Since the middle of 2005, the school has been part of the EQUIP programme, a business-based organization managed by the National Business Initiative (NBI). This initiative, in cooperation and in accordance with the needs of the specific school, implements sports and leisure time activities on the schoolyard.

become the secondary school accommodating Grades 7 to 9. The primary school will accommodate all children from Grades 1 to 6.

Considering actual school attendance, it is unclear whether restructuring will improve the educational infrastructure. According to the US survey from April to May 2001 23.6% of the total population were between 5 and 14 years old. This figure more or less coincides with the figure of 22% (of children between the age of 5 and 14 years) as reflected in the national census of 2001 (Statistics South Africa, 2001). With reference to information from school clinics in Stellenbosch, approximately 900 learners attend schools outside Kayamandi in Cloetesville, Idasvalley, the surrounding areas of Stellenbosch and private schools. Of the 28 000 people living in this township, 6 608 children possibly at primary school age, with only 1 700 learners registered at the primary school. The resulting question should be: How many children in Kayamandi do actually not attend school at all?

Dennerlein and Adami (2004) estimated that at least eight primary schools and five secondary schools would be needed to meet the actual requirement of basic education in Kayamandi. Another demand is the establishment of a centre for illiterate adults and children with learning problems. Due to the low educational level illiteracy is expected to be high, especially within the adult population born during Apartheid and among those that have migrated from rural areas with lesser access to educational facilities.

4.7.3 Public Institutions

The public institutions in Kayamandi include a small council office, a recently opened public library and a police station. Younger children use mainly the library and its green area to do their homework or to spend their spare time. To satisfy the demand, however, two more libraries are needed (Dennerlein & Adami, 2004). A post office was recently opened under supervision of a non-governmental organization (NGO). A taxi rank is located adjacent to the police station, with a highly frequented crossroads at the main entrance of Kayamandi. This area is considered dangerous and risky for pedestrians. What is needed, at least, is a restructuring of the entrance to Kayamandi and the erection of a bus station (Dennerlein & Adami, 2004).

4.7.4 Social Service Sector

The following governmental and non-governmental social services targeting different groups are represented in Kayamandi: The *Child Welfare*

Organization is a non-governmental organization that promotes, protects and enhances the safety, well-being and healthy development of children (Child Welfare South Africa, 2005). The Kayamandi Child Welfare Office employs two social workers who are responsible for 28 000 inhabitants. The office has a high staff turnover because of low income, high work load and low levels of qualification. And apart from Child Welfare, no other professional social service organization in Kayamandi works exclusively with children of primary school age or younger, and the demand is indeed great.

The *Ikamva Lehtu Centre* (translated as 'our future') incorporates both a youth centre and an AIDS Awareness Resource Centre where older youth, especially male youth meet to play pool, billiard or table tennis, and where they are peer educated on HIV/AIDS. The centre cooperates mainly with the secondary school in Kayamandi. One manager and two assistants are employed. According to Dennerlein and Adami (2004). *Prochorus*, a religious non-governmental organization, offers programmes in emergency relief, feeding with Skim, school fee sponsorships by foreign donors for poor children, job creation and a street kids programme. Nine people are employed at Prochorus.

In addition, individuals or donators from overseas contribute to increase services. One example is the established NGO *Bridge the Divide – Greater Stellenbosch Development Trust* that runs a new project for after-school care and job recreation. After-school care is extremely important for the protection of children while their parents are at work. Another very impressive initiative by an unemployed lady known only as Maria is a day-care centre that accommodates up to 150 children a day. This woman convinced the Stellenbosch Municipality to allow her to use the town hall in Kayamandi (built in 2003, and rarely used) for the day-care centre on a rental basis.

The demand on the social service sectors is great in the presence of a widely overburdened community by extreme poverty and uncontrolled influx. For example, to fulfil standards on a stable social service structure at least five more youth centres are needed to meet the demand. Other urgently needed social services are an alcohol prevention centre, since alcohol addiction among the adult population is high and causes numerous problems that affect family life (e.g. domestic violence) and child health (e.g. link between malnutrition and alcohol consumption of parents); a family crisis centre; an AIDS hospice and a rape and violence crisis centre.

4.7.5 *Informal Business Sector*

Approximately half of the population of Kayamandi is not employed in the formal sector and try to make a living through participation in the economically vital informal sector (PTT, 2004). In the year 2000, Kayamandi accommodated 179 informal businesses including 72 spaza shops (small shop), 42 fruit and vegetable shops, 29 shebeens (informal pubs in private homes), fifteen barbers and hairdressers, nine butchers, seven street-sellers and five repairmen. In addition, there were beer brewers, milk-sellers, herbalists, healers, builders and photographers (Erhard, 2000).

Two thirds of the informal business sector operates from huts within the informal settlement areas. Because the big market centres are located exclusively in Stellenbosch and usually close at 8 pm, most spaza shops trade between 6 am and 10 pm and cater for workers on their way to work or returning after a long working day (Erhard, 2000). Because of the absence of shopping centres in Kayamandi, the majority of residents do their main shopping in central Stellenbosch. The central mode of transport is the taxi, with one-way tickets costing R6 per person. Kayamandi is in urgent need of a market place where sellers can work in suitable facilities and where the products on offer can be quality controlled. Building such shopping areas also means improving the sellers' professional qualifications and expanding their businesses.

A tourism centre for overseas visitors is presently being built at the entrance to Kayamandi. The ethics involved in the exposure of poor living conditions to affluence is questionable. In addition, it can be assumed that a conflict-stricken community will become more unstable and divided: On the one hand those groups that will make a living out of tourists and tourist tours through the area, and on the other hand those that will be excluded from the new market and be left feeling caged (see also Campbell, 2003).

4.7.6 Community, Recreational, and Religious Sector

Kayamandi has no assembly points, market places or small parks for recreational purposes. Particularly important for the improvement of the infrastructure is a place where small businesses can settle. The architects Dennerlein and Adami (2004) suggest that at least six urban squares and public spaces, three park recreational areas, two sports fields and five playgrounds have to be included in a discussion of a new township structure.

The infrastructure of the religious sector in Kayamandi is well established, with approximately 50 church buildings which include both formal houses and shacks. Several religions e.g. Christian churches and traditional African Christian churches are represented.

4.8 Conclusion

In January 2002 South African officials signed the Johannesburg Declaration on Health and Sustainable Development. The declaration calls on health issues or determinants that affect health which can only be solved by national and international cooperation:

> Paragraph 19: We emphasize that many of the key determinants of health and disease – as well as the solutions – lie outside the direct control of the health sector, in sectors concerned with environment, water and sanitation, agriculture, education, finance, employment, industry, mining, urban and rural livelihoods, trade, tourism, transport, energy and housing. We draw attention to the fact that health issues are frequently inadequately considered when development decisions are made. We reaffirm that addressing the underlying determinants of health is key to ensuring ecologically sustainable development and sustained health improvements in the long term, whilst further recognising that much progress has been made in forging closer links between health and other sectors. (WHO et al., 2002)

Despite the South African agreement to this international legislation, it needs to be realised that South Africa remains a country characterised by dramatic social inequalities (Campbell, 2003) reflected in a community such as Kayamandi. The impact Apartheid had on the material level is worst in socially-disadvantaged communities where it affected housing, income, access to resources, educational opportunities, access to employment, lifestyle, access to leadership positions, and the right to practice one's own culture, amongst others (Skinner, 2000). Nowadays, with legal political representatives of the community in the town councils, only hesitant actions are taken towards building a healthy community.

Kayamandi is a concentration of the poorest strata of the population of Stellenbosch. The township comprises more than 28 000 residents living on 7.5 ha[18], with a migration flow of 150 new people every month. An extension of the area is planned but the process is slow. More than two thirds of the settlement area consists of informal housing units such as shacks. The risks to individuals living in the township are diverse, in particular the environmental conditions and the physical layout of the area that cause a series of health risk factors. The township lacks a well-planned architectural structure, e.g. streets,

---

18 In 2005, the town council of Stellenbosch bought more land to the northern upper side of Kayamandi. It has not yet been developed.

open spaces, sports ground and playgrounds. The chaotic and unplanned structure prevents not only a supportive community life but generates disciplinary and social issues. The densely populated informal settlement areas and the lack of sewerage systems and controlled electricity systems cause risks to human life. Child safety involves traffic and hygienic living conditions; dense living environments pose special risks to their health. Basic requirements like access to water, shelter, knowledge, health care, employment and other productive resources directly influence the risk that individuals and households run of being threatened by poverty (PGWC, 2001).

The households in Kayamandi most vulnerable to poverty, insecurity of tenure and inadequate living conditions are those in informal settlement areas that are characterised by single-parent (mostly female) family units with children, high unemployment rates and an average monthly income of less than R1 500 (Development Action Group, 2002). To meet basic needs, e.g. food, clothing and housing, the average Kayamandi household (consisting of three persons[19] and earning R1 000 per month) has to make do with R11 per day. Poverty is a pronounced problem for households headed by single females with children of primary school age. While unemployment is over-proportionally prevalent in young people, who often have minimal life and work ambitions due to their limited education, most employed residents work as unskilled workers in low-wage jobs. In other words, wide segments of the population living in Kayamandi are especially vulnerable to extreme poverty, since a low or irregular income contributes to malnutrition and starvation.

As chapter 4 clearly indicates, health, social and environmental hazards are widespread, increasing the number of factors that negatively influence the physical health and mental status of each individual in the case study community. These findings should be considered in recommending the need of health-promoting intervention working with different target groups and incorporates a magnitude of health topics in the community of Kayamandi.

---

19 In 27% of the households there are two and more people, and in more than half of the households (53.5%) there are three and more persons dependent on one income (University of Stellenbosch, 2001).

CHAPTER FIVE

Research in the Conditions of a Developing Country – Aims and Challenges

5.1 Introduction

South Africa is classified as a middle-income country with one of the highest GINI indexes in the world and an alpha coefficient of 0.59, second in the world after Brazil (World Bank, 2003). These statistics reflect a society that is deeply divided into lower and upper social strata. For this reason, it can be assumed that any study undertaken under such social conditions is also exposed to a variety of risk factors that might affect its validity and reliability. Therefore, to do justice to such risk factors in terms of accountable research, chapter 5 starts by describing factors on the macro-economic, working environment, social and personal level which have an intrinsic influence on the working conditions for researchers in a developing world environment.

The foundation of the evaluation of the specifically designed school-based life skills programme on AIDS and sex education form the aims and objectives which are depicted in detail. Because the study presented was organised in a semi-urban location in South Africa, it was necessary to determine a comparable community to meet control measures. The selection procedures of the particular communities, i.e. Kayamandi and Crossroads, are described in detail; both are situated in the Western Cape Province of South Africa. These communities are the locations of the two primary schools participating in the study. On the aforementioned issue of conducting research in a developing country, chapter 5 outlines the difficulties and obstacles experienced during this study and its endeavours to meet the demands of national health research standards. Therefore, the chapter concludes with a portrayal of the reality of actual research in a disadvantaged setting such as the Kayamandi community.

5.2 Psychosocial Research in the Conditions of a Developing World

Research, including research in the fields of psychology and health in low- and middle-income countries is often criticised for (1) focusing on insignificant problems rather than on significant psychiatric problems, (2) being donor-driven and that their priorities are set by external donor agencies, (3) the quality of research is generally lower, and (4) the information generated not being documented well enough to be used for other sectors of society (Alem & Kebede, 2003). However, it needs to be taken into consideration that conducting research in developing countries demands from researchers to work in often extremely difficult working conditions. Alem and Kebede (2003) list four categories of challenges: (1) the macro-economic environment, (2) the working environment, (3) personal factors, and (4) the intrinsic nature of psychiatric research.

The *macro-economic environment* includes the social, economic, and political environment which is influenced by natural and human disasters like civil war, high rates of violence or international economic recession creating instabilities for research (Alem & Kebede, 2003). Another factor is that research generally has little social appreciation in countries where 70% of the population are illiterate or where more than 50% live in poverty. Thus, researchers are often in a position to apply for funding from the public sector whereby the donor can initially dictate the research objectives of the investigation (Alem & Kebede, 2003). This becomes especially problematic if the studies and interventions are not relevant to local situations or are linked up with cultural sensitivities (De Jesus Mari, Lozano, & Duley, 1997). Another consequence of private sponsoring is that long-term field studies and pretests are often inappropriately focused on research schedules because of limited funds.

The *work environment* or infrastructure is often characterised by inadequate budgets and equipment, and a lack of technicians and support staff. An underdeveloped infrastructure results in limited access to up-to-date journals and books for literature reviews. Other major challenges are national and institutional research protocol review and approval mechanisms which are slow, causing delays and frustration for donors and researchers. The limited number of skilled researchers and specialists in developing countries does not only reduce the quantity and quality of research but also affects the range of explicit meetings and exchange processes between researchers in the field (Alem & Kebede, 2003).

On the *individual/personal level* the level of income of researchers and support staff plays an important role. Low budgets prevent appropriate staff training on the planning and implementation of research projects (Alem & Kebede, 2003). According to De Jesus Mari et al. (1997), only 5% of global research funds are devoted to research on the developing world's health problems (Commission on Health Research for Development, 1990), although the middle- and low-income countries bear the greatest burden of health hazards and thus have the greatest need for research.

Lastly, the absence of a register system for sampling processes and the fact that western *psychiatric instruments* are directly translated into local languages have a tremendous effect on the validity of the research results (Alem & Kebede, 2003). Furthermore, as Alem and Kebede (2003) state, the usefulness of instruments and the resulting effects on the participating and often illiterate communities are not appropriately tested. Consequently, any approaches tested in western countries may need to be adjusted or modified to different cultural (Institute of Psychiatry, 2004) and social settings.

Thus, researchers who work in a developing world situation are often exposed to a variety of influences from social, economic, and personal realities, e.g. limited access to information and material, as well as financial, strategic and infrastructural constraints (Saxena & Poter, 2004). It can finally be assumed that where such negative influences exist, they can, to a certain extent, limit the outcome of any study undertaken in such environments and, consequently, make it very difficult for this group of researchers to meet the standardised demands on accountable psychosocial research.

5.3   Aims, Objectives, and Ethics of the Study

The aim of the study is to evaluate the effects of the applied life skills programme on AIDS and sex education to encourage psychological and social competencies among pre-adolescent children (10-11 years of age). By gaining knowledge and testing new skills, the objective is to position them so that they can cope with prevalent life tasks and enhance the development of health behaviour. Furthermore, the pre-adolescent age group was selected, as this period constitutes the time between childhood and the onset of puberty, and is the developmental phase in which sexual socialisation and the development of personality shape the value system and behaviour of an individual (Oerter, 1995b). Consequently, the study proposes that children should receive health and sex education before their own value system and health behaviour is fully developed and before they become sexually active, in order to avoid the contraction of an HIV infection later in life. Therefore, four specific research objectives arise from this aim:

(1) To analyse psychological variables which are considered to sustain the development of positive mental health enhancing protective behaviour within individuals;
(2) To evaluate the efficacy of the implementation procedures and methods;
(3) To examine the quality of personal relations among the participants and health promotion trainers, contributing to a class and learning atmosphere that enhances mental health; and
(4) To analyse the proximal and distal domains in which the intervention takes place, and which are assumed to entail risks that influence the development of health behaviour of the participating individuals outside of the intervention.

Besides the scientific knowledge gained, this study attempts to be effective in other ways. The study has two long-term expectations: first, the intervention should result in the full implementation of an effective life skills programme on AIDS and sex education for Grade 4 at the school surveyed, and second, the intervention should become part of community-based projects as the only project that primarily focuses on health promotion among pre-adolescents. The duration of research covered the time from September 2002 until August 2004 and was divided into five phases, outlined in table 5.1.

The study was approved by the human ethics committee of the University of Stellenbosch (Department of Psychology) and the Departments of Education in Paarl and Cape Town. The required consent was also provided by the school principals at the Ikaya Primary and Nomlinganiselo Primary School, learners in the selected classes and their parents and/or guardians. Regular meetings were held with school psychologists at the School Clinics in Stellenbosch.

Table 5.1.
Duration of Research from 2002 until 2004 and Content of Research.

Phase	Time	Content
First	September 2002 – January 2003	Negotiation of access at community and school level
		Field Study I
		Selection and training of two health promotion trainers
	October 2003	Casual observations in Grade 4 classes at Ikaya Primary School
Second	January 2003 – February 2003	Application for research at provincial level
		Phase of re-testing the quantitative instrument
		Parent meetings
Third	February 2003	Pretest with control and intervention group
	March 2003 – July 2003	Intervention I
		Interim parent meeting
		Participant observations I
	July 2003	Posttest with intervention and control group
		Post parent meeting
		AIDS workshop for mothers
Fourth	September 2003 – November 2003	Parent meeting
		Intervention II
		Participant observations II
	November 2003	Follow-up test 1
	November 2003 – December 2003	Field study II
Fifth	January until August 2004	Field study III
		Participant observations III (Grade 5)
	April 2004	Follow-up test 2
	August 2004	Opinion poll

5.4 The Procedures of Selecting Communities and Primary Schools

As explained in the previous paragraph, the survey was predominantly conducted with pre-adolescents between 10 and 11 years of age. The primary school learners attend the Ikaya Primary School in Kayamandi (intervention group) and the Nomlinganiselo Primary School (control group) in Crossroads at Grade 4 level. These primary schools, located in two exclusively disadvantaged communities – Kayamandi (Stellenbosch) and Crossroads (Cape Town), – therefore represent the lowest strata of South African society. The majority of the participants were Xhosa; the remaining participants were of Sotho, Zulu or Swazi descent. The main language spoken was isiXhosa.

The participating primary schools were selected based on a range of functional criteria and organizational conditions which are listed below.

The selected communities had to:
 (1) Be within an hour's drive from Cape Town,
 (2) Have existed for at least 30 years, in order for a community culture to have developed,
 (3) Have a majority of residents belonging to the Xhosa ethnic group, and
 (4) Have some internal civil structures to facilitate access and an intervention at a later stage (this applied only to Kayamandi) (see also Skinner, 2000).

The selected schools had to:
 (1) Have been long-established primary schools,
 (2) Have two classes similar in cultural, language, age and gender composition,
 (3) Allow a selection of samples by class membership, and
 (4) Have no existing or ongoing AIDS educational programme.

To maintain the listed selection criteria it was, in fact, unlikely that any community and its local primary school would have been able to fully meet these requirements. After careful consideration, and in order to maintain the local separation of intervention and control group design, communities and schools, the communities of Kayamandi and Crossroads and their primary schools were selected as they fulfilled most of the functional criteria. The limitations of the selected schools are considered and discussed in the following section.

5.4.1 A Brief Comparison of the Selected Communities

Kayamandi and Crossroads are extremely disadvantaged long-established black South African communities in the Cape Metropolitan catchments area and home to a variety of civil structures (e.g. social, political). Crossroads is located in an urban area situated in the Cape Metropolitan surrounded by townships such as Khayelitsha, Nyanga, Philippi, New Crossroads and KTC.[20] Kayamandi is situated in a semi-urban area in which the main part of the study was conducted.

The majority of the residents in both communities belong to the Xhosa ethnic group and originate from the Eastern Cape Province and from areas like the Transkei and Ciskei. Both communities are affected by urbanisation processes. The gradual migration within the Cape Metropolitan Area or between the Eastern and Western Cape Province lead to the instability of family structures in both communities. The most prevalent family systems are urban-extended, single-headed, nuclear, foster parent or legal guardian (including child-headed) family units. Foster parents or legal guardians who take care of children are more prevalent in Crossroads than in Kayamandi.

Both communities are characterised by overcrowding, poor living conditions (more than 50% informal housing like squatters), a high unemployment rate or low-income groups, a high level of illiteracy, frequent violence and the lack of recreational facilities. Gang-related crimes are more prevalent in Crossroads than in Kayamandi. As Crossroads is part of the Nyanga/Crossroads Development Plan, and has a far more diverse and developed infrastructure than Kayamandi, the differences between an urban and semi-urban infrastructure, including access to information on AIDS, were considered during the data analysis.

5.4.2 The Selected Primary Schools

As outlined in the previous paragraphs, Ikaya Primary School in Kayamandi and Nomlinganiselo Primary School in Crossroads constitute the two case study schools in this study. Both schools are long-established primary schools located close to the children's places of residence. The surroundings of the schools are dirty and fail to provide adequate safe playgrounds for the children. After-school care is not available in either school. The school buildings consist of two long red brick buildings with additional prefabricated classrooms surrounded by wire-netted fence.

---

20 Meaning of KTC is not known.

The majority of children in both schools belong to the Xhosa ethnic group. The vernacular is isiXhosa; with the second most frequent language either being Afrikaans or English, depending on the teachers' language skills. Both schools had a similar age and gender composition at the pretest of the survey. The majority of children at Nomlinganiselo Primary School were born in the Cape Metropolitan Area or have moved from within the Western Cape Province to Crossroads in recent years. At Ikaya Primary School, the classes mainly consist of learners who have migrated to the Kayamandi community from the Eastern Cape Province in recent years or were born in the Kayamandi community. This means that the groups differ with regard to their migration patterns. While the children in the control group migrate mainly within the municipal or Western Cape area, the children in the intervention group migrate mainly across provincial borders – from a rural and impoverished province to a semi-urban area in a better-developed province.

Nomlinganiselo Primary School accommodates children from the KTC, Nyanga and Crossroads areas. Throughout the survey Nomlinganiselo Primary School was subjected to extensive restructuring processes by the Western Cape Department of Education with a limited number of classes and learners by January 2004 as a result. The school's physical infrastructure was improved during the period of survey, and although the school personnel structure underwent several changes, the quality management seemed to be guaranteed throughout.

Ikaya Primary School is the only primary school and, therefore, mainly serves the Kayamandi area. The school had experienced tremendous problems in preparation for the implementation of Curriculum 2005 and consequently lagged behind in the reformation processes coordinated by the Western Cape Department of Education. In addition, Ikaya Primary School experienced a change in management during the last phase of the intervention, as evident in the school atmosphere that was characterised by a power struggle on management level. Apart from poor equipment, a shortage in staff and the high workload of staff members, this lack of leadership led to an inability to act and to fulfil their duties on behalf of teachers and learners.

The following problems at schools were listed by the two class teachers who attended the survey:

(1) Low payment of school fees;
(2) Perceived absence of parents in their children's educational process;
(3) High numbers of learners with reading and writing problems;
(4) Shortage of books and teaching material (worse at Ikaya Primary School);

(5) Practice of corporal punishment as disciplinary method;
(6) Crimes like theft and vandalism, (alcohol abuse, drug abuse, e.g. dagga/mandrax, and sodomy between school children were reported only at Nomlinganiselo Primary School).

Neither school taught the governmentally prescribed life skills programme on AIDS and sex education before/during the Intervention I. Although elements of AIDS education were evident in the living environment of both samples, this education was directed towards secondary school children and did not directly affect the participating primary school learners.

5.5 Negotiation Access for Psychosocial Research in a Semi-urban Setting in South Africa

When doing psychosocial research that examines human beings, specific negotiation procedures and consideration are indicated, especially when the study is undertaken in a developing world context. This is of special importance when the researcher has a first-world background and has been socialised in a different culture. As De Jesus Mari et al. (1997) state, studies and interventions should not only be relevant to local situations, but must also consider cultural sensitivities and include a learning process from community to research level. Such a long-term negotiation process is considered to be extremely relevant to gain a better understanding of the environmental and cultural factors influencing the psychological development of the participants. The following section outlines the specific procedures safeguarding appropriate legal, ethic and cultural steps throughout the evaluation process at provincial, community, school, and personal level in the case study community of Kayamandi.

5.5.1 Approval for Research at Provincial Level

Application forms for gaining permission to carry out the survey at Ikaya and Nomlinganiselo Primary Schools were submitted to the Western Cape Department of Education (Education Research) in Cape Town and the Department of Education in Paarl. Before submission, permission was asked from the case study schools (Ikaya and Nomlinganiselo Primary Schools), Stellenbosch AIDS Action (SAA), Stellenbosch Child Welfare Organization, and the Departments of Social Work and Psychology at the University of Stellenbosch. The University of Stellenbosch (Department of Psychology) provided local supervision over the entire period of the evaluation.

In the middle of January 2003, the departments gave permission for this survey without any delay. The attached conditions included, among others, ethical considerations, final reporting to the Western Cape Department of Education, half-yearly oral reports to the School Clinics in Stellenbosch, and reporting of cases of child abuse in the intervention group to the institutions responsible.

5.5.2 Negotiation Procedures at Community Level

Negotiations were conducted with several governmental and non-governmental institutions and organizations within the Kayamandi community and in Stellenbosch five months before the intervention took place. These experts served as gatekeepers since access to the community would not have been possible without their permission. One objective was to spread the vision of the pilot study and to establish a network of safety and support for conducting the pilot project with important people (stakeholders) within the Kayamandi community. In addition, meetings with stakeholders in the community were also seen as an appropriate cultural behaviour in accordance with the valid code of respect. The showing of respect, as part of the hierarchal system, between one person (older, male or an insider) functioning as an authority and another person (younger, female, or an outsider) asking and following advice, was a fundamental cornerstone in the carrying out of the survey.

Negotiation was also used to discuss with stakeholders the prevailing cultural-sensitive norms and values important in the design of research methods and implementation of the intervention. It became clear that in Kayamandi the fear and stigma surrounding AIDS were significant, with a strong taboo on talking about sex. Therefore, experts recommended that questions directly related to sexual attitudes or behaviour be avoided in the survey because of the youth of the participants, the cultural norms concerning sex and AIDS, and the diffusion of family life. It was feared that if intervention included sensitive issues, organizations and people in the community would refuse to support the intervention. The advice from the experts was thus a definite consideration in the administering of the quantitative instrument (questionnaire). They also demanded that the original proposal, written in and for a European context, be completely revised for the prevailing research conditions. The final version of the proposal was a result of the interaction with local experts and a learning process on the researcher's side. This phase finally formed the foundation of a supportive cooperation between the researcher and local experts throughout the duration of the research.

5.5.3 Negotiation Procedures at School Level

Special negotiation procedures were also undertaken at the Ikaya Primary School in particular. The researcher made personal contact with the principal prior to the intervention in September 2001. In September 2002, she presented the programme to the school staff. Regular information sessions with the principal and Grade 4 teachers were held during breaks, before the implementation of the life skills programme on AIDS and sex education. This phase also included casual observations in Grade 4 classes at Ikaya Primary School to select one class for the intervention. Aspects for observation included class composition (age, gender), verification of marks, teaching methods and classroom atmosphere (Appendix A). Four Grade 4 classes were observed (one teacher refused to allow a researcher in class). The results revealed that class composition and the verification of marks were similar in the observed classes. However, class atmosphere was strongly dependent on the character and professionalism of the teacher.

The second objective of class observations was to find one class teacher willing to participate in the intervention, because the Stellenbosch School Clinics requested that a local class teacher be involved. The institution hoped that through this course of action teachers at the school would later be more willing to implement the life skills programme on AIDS and sex education at Ikaya Primary School, which had failed in the past. Although all the teachers were asked about their willingness to participate in the survey, only one teacher clearly expressed interest in participating with her class in the intervention. This teacher was also the one who had reached the best marks in the assessment of classroom atmosphere. In the end, all Grade 4 class teachers gave permission to this specific teacher to take part in the intervention with her class. This consent was of special importance for the later acceptance and support of the intervention in the school environment, the reason being that all future personal interactions will take place in a highly hierarchical system (e.g. school).

The negotiation process at Ikaya Primary School was finalised in a meeting with the principal, the deputy principal and one class teacher of the chosen Grade 4 class. During the meeting, the following arrangements for the project were made: the intervention was integrated into the timetable as part of the life orientation curriculum, one classroom was made available, and one class teacher joined the sessions as support teacher on a regular basis.

5.5.4 Negotiations with Parents

In order to safeguard ethic codes, the first parent meeting was held after receiving permission from the various departments and organizations. Several parent meetings were held during and after the interventions. The first parent meeting was attended by all the people directly involved (health promotion trainers, researcher, class teacher), the upper management of the school (principal) and the manager of the cooperating NGO in Kayamandi, and had three goals.

Firstly, for HPTs and evaluator informed parents on the content of and need for health and sex education, the magnitude of the project and its positive outcomes for the children, school and community. Secondly, that parents should feel part of the project and therefore become part of the educational process and take responsibility right from the beginning. Thirdly, to give parents the impression that the people involved provided a safe and personal framework for their children. In the end, all participating legal guardians gave a signed permission for their children. Due to the high illiteracy rate[21] among parents, older children, neighbours or friends signed on their behalf.

Finally, two pre-parent meetings were held because the number of participating parents fluctuated between ten to fifteen parents per meeting in a class of 45 learners. There were several obstacles to reach the parents or legal guardians of the sampled children. Besides the fact that many parents seem to have a complicated, reluctant, or even disinterested attitude towards the school and its events, and therefore avoid any presence at school, many of them were suddenly concerned that they would have to pay additional school fees for their children's participation in the programme. Knowing the difficult financial situation of the parents and their understandable feeling of embarrassment, parents were additionally informed by letter inviting them to attend a personal parents' meeting where they were informed that the programme would be free and voluntary. Many parents signed the agreement papers without taking part in any parent meeting.

Contact with Nomlinganiselo Primary School was established in November 2002. Because of the sensitive nature of research, it was difficult to make contact with a school willing to support the survey. Similar to the finding at Ikaya Primary School, the personal relationship with the class teacher formed the basis for a trustful partnership between the school and the

---

21 According to the World Bank (2001), the average illiteracy rate in South Africa in 1999 was 15% of the total population.

research team, which made the survey possible. The contact teacher at Nomlinganiselo Primary School informed the parents of the children in her class and requested their consent in a parent meeting.

5.6 Unanticipated Events – Resulting Limitations

As explained at the beginning of chapter 5, a study in this context is often limited by the macro-economic and working environment, together with personal and psychological factors. The survey was conducted in four research phases between September 2002 and August 2004. Specific and unplanned events, which had a significant impact on the survey as a whole, are outlined in this section.

5.6.1 First Phase – Armed Robbery

After an official meeting at Nomlinganiselo Primary School, the research team and the contact teacher experienced an armed robbery on the schoolyard that was witnessed by learners, teachers and neighbours. It is very much likely that children of the control group observed the armed robbery too, which might have influenced their attendance in the survey in a non-predictable way. In addition, the contact teacher was severely traumatised and had a nervous breakdown that forced her to resign from her job in the following weeks. Despite the fact that this teacher was prevented from applying as a support person, another teacher took over her position in the following months. Subsequent visits to this school were made under police protection, whilst contact with the school was organised by fax or telephone. Apart from the first-hand trauma experienced by the project team, this incident caused a delay of two to three weeks in the research schedule due to a loss of official documents and agreements.

5.6.2 Second Phase – Tight Research Schedule

In February 2003, the pretesting of the quantitative instrument, the questionnaire, was undertaken at Ikaya Primary School in Kayamandi. As stated at the beginning of the chapter, it was not possible to find appropriate psychological instruments that had already been standardised in the South African context, applied to pre-adolescents and translated into a specific language such as isiXhosa. Apart from the absent standardised quantitative measures for children, the time for the pretest was too tightly determined to claim validity. A number of unplanned conditions and events resulted in the inappropriate procedure: the complete revision of the research proposal resulting in a late application for research due to limited staff and financial conditions of the research project, the long and unplanned negotiation process on community and school level and, finally, the armed robbery.

5.6.3 Third Phase – Restructuring Processes at Nomlinganiselo Primary School

The management changes and restructuring processes (*"Curriculum 2005"*) in both schools were assumed to cause a slow and continual sampling drift at the case study schools. Finally, these expected changes affected mainly the control group. During the posttest in August 2003, Nomlinganiselo Primary School experienced a restructuring process during which the number of learners, classes, and teachers were reduced, and a new principal took over who had to be newly-informed about the research matter. At the same time, the school took part in a national programme on "safe schools" whereby the safety standards were extended, e.g. the installation of a barbed wire fence and personnel responsible for managing the gate. During that time, the school seemed to have changed its school and learning atmosphere from being rather integrated in the community to being more secluded. The principal and participating class teacher of the control group explained that armed robberies had happened several times at the school, increasingly on days when teachers received their salary. During the follow-up test 2 in May 2004 safety procedures were again reduced, and again the school and its individuals experienced a time of change.

5.6.4 Fourth Phase – Changes in Research Design and Staff

South Africa is a country undergoing transformation and reformation processes, which are undoubtedly needed. However, unannounced changes can have far-reaching implications especially for research surveys. In this case they affected the research design, and therefore the complete outcome study.

Firstly, in September, the Nomlinganiselo Primary School implemented the governmental life skills programme on HIV/AIDS without notifying the research team. After ethical considerations, it was decided not to intervene in this process, even though the Departments of Education in Paarl and Cape Town had given their permission assuring that the original structure would be preserved. To safeguard the survey, it was finally decided to convert the control group to a quasi-control group.

Secondly, Intervention II, functioning as a booster session, was undertaken at Ikaya Primary School from September until November 2003. During this phase, one health promotion trainer had to leave the project as she was pregnant. This then meant a change in the team's composition: a new volunteer had to be introduced, and the team had to adapt its working procedures in the late stages of the survey. It is therefore believed that this change in staff influenced the quality of the sessions in Intervention II and resulted in a changed learning atmosphere in the intervention group.

5.7 Conclusion

In conclusion, the predominant challenges for the survey presented were detrimental on: (1) macro-economic working conditions (i.e. limited funding and schedule restrictions), (2) restricted access to psychometric measures for this specific group of samples, and (3) unanticipated events such as an armed robbery or the control group having to be converted into a quasi-experimental group because of administrative confusion.

Apart from these aforementioned obstacles which the survey experienced, the cornerstones of the research could be safeguarded. First of all, access was obtained to two comparable primary schools which were courageous enough to participate in this study with a sensitive cultural nature. Even parents, often illiterate and with a lack of knowledge about the content of the programme, allowed their children to attend an AIDS and sex education programme. Also local experts were won to support the survey by being entitled to have a say on research content and methodology.

In other words, with regard to the sensitive nature of this assessment study, the specific ethical procedures were not only followed to protect the rights and privacy of every participating individual, but also formed a safety net for a survey which is exposed to many influencing factors on a personal, social (incl. cultural) as well as research level. Although, the described events and conditions had a tremendous influence on the validity and reliability of this study, the following chapter 6 describes how methodical procedures were applied to control such influences.

CHAPTER SIX
Methodology of the Study

6.1 Introduction

The following description of the research design, and its underlying methodology, provides details about the quantitative, quantitative-qualitative and purely qualitative research instruments including relevant sampling, data collection procedures, techniques of data analysis, as well as any limitations. This variety of methods was used to gain an extensive result and to cover a detailed view of the setting in which the intervention was undertaken. In this study, eight major instruments are introduced to gather research data for the presented study:

(1) Evaluation of needs: field interviews;
(2) Process evaluation: documentation of the intervention; learners' reports, reports by health promotion trainers, and participant observation by learners of the intervention group;
(3) Outcome evaluation: questionnaire and opinion poll.

The data collection instruments are used to (1) characterise the intervention and its implementation, (2) identify its effects on the individual and interpersonal level, and (3) identify factors and conditions that might influence the intervention.

6.2 Methods of the Needs Analysis

Knowing that the development of individuals' health behaviour and the environmental risks and resources that influence health-related behaviour share a deep interconnectedness, the aim of these methods was, first of all, to explore the social conditions for the mental and physical development of children in Kayamandi outside the intervention undertaken. The accompanying underlying objectives were to detect factors affecting the research and, consequently, its outcomes. Methods used for the needs analysis were an extensive literature review, supplemented with regular field trips, as well as the qualitative instrument of field interviews evaluating the proximal and distal context in which not only the children progressed, but the intervention also took place.

6.2.1 Sampling

Field interviews were done with experts and stakeholders from governmental and non-governmental organizations from March 2004 until June 2004. The samples were selected after a long personal negotiation process to build trust (see chapter 5, par. 5.2) and should therefore have an increased validity and reliability of the data. The participating interviewees were selected using the following three functional criteria:

(1) The interviewee works for a health, educational, social, governmental or non-governmental institution that works with/for children in Kayamandi.
(2) The interviewee has a leading role in his/her institution/organization.
(3) The interviewee agrees with the field interviewee design.

In the end, nine people agreed to participate in the interview sessions: from the non-governmental religious and public sector ($N=2$), the governmental and health sector ($N=3$), and governmental educational sector ($N=4$). Contact with church leaders or party members could not be established over the research period and the support by social workers from Child Welfare was unsatisfactory due to staff change or refusal. Child Welfare was therefore not included in the interview list.

6.2.2 Description of the Instrument

The half-structured interview was framed by an introductory guide in the form of a questionnaire, so as to build a framework for the interview sessions. In other words, the questionnaire formed the basis for the interview sessions, in which further probing by the interviewer was possible (Appendix B). The half-structured interviews and also the questionnaire included 14 items on cultural, socio-economic, family, health, and educational conditions in the target group's living environment. The items were the same for all respondents. The questions for interviewees were:

(1) Which factors influence children in their mental and physical development process from childhood to adolescence in Kayamandi?
(2) What kind of positive and negative factors support or hinder children in developing a strong mental and physical growth in Kayamandi?
(3) What role do the educational systems play in the mental development of children in Kayamandi?
(4) What role do the families play in the mental development of children in Kayamandi?
(5) How can a one-year life skills programme influence children in their mental and physical development?

6.2.3 Data Collection Procedure

The outline of the field interviews was specifically designed and interviews were organised in six phases (Table 6.1). In phase one, the interviewer introduced herself, the research purpose and the content of the interview session. Afterwards the interviewee was asked to introduce himself/herself and the institution to which he/she belonged. During interviews the interviewer constantly made field notes and re-read the field notes to the interviewee if a statement was unclear. The first session ended with the handing over of the questionnaire and allowing the interviewee to clarify any remaining questions.

The second phase took place one week later. The purpose of the second interview session was to collect the questionnaire; questions were asked which followed the structure of the questionnaire on the living conditions for children in Kayamandi. The interim phase was used to complete the interview design. The questionnaire was transcribed digitally, answers were pre-analysed and questions were formulated to expand the interviewees' statements in the third interview phase. The formulated questions on the interviewees' statements were used during phase three and the interviewee was asked to clarify any remaining questions or comments. The last session ended with handing over the copy of the questionnaire to the interviewed person; a copy was signed by the interviewee for the interviewer, and a note of thanks by the interviewer.

Table 6.1.
Design of Field Interviews illustrated with its Six Phases.

Design	Data collection	Data collection	Data analysis – Interim	Data collection	Data analysis
Interview procedure	Introduction of research purpose and researcher	Asking questions relating to living conditions for children in the community/ field	Transcription of QN papers	Asking questions from the QN	Transcription of additional comments
		Questions relating to work and institution		Clarification of equivocal answers or prevention of cultural or linguistic misunderstandings and unclear points	Comparison of results from interviews and QN papers
				Additional comments by interviewee	Final analysis
Questionnaire (QN)	Handing over QN papers	Collection of QN papers	First analysis of interviewees' answers	Handing over copies of QN paper to interviewees	Final analysis
Time	30 minutes	45 minutes		60 minutes	
Duration (in weeks)	1		1 to 2		4

There were four reasons for using a three-fold interview design. First, it was needed to limit misunderstandings in the communication process between the interviewee and interviewer as a second language (English) was used in the interviews, and thus to increase the validity of the gathered data. Second, it was extremely important to clarify statements and to expand thoughts of the interviewees' who were repeatedly questioned over a period of two weeks. Thus, the design supports a stable process of communication in which the interviewee has time to reconsider statements and turn them into culturally understandable patterns, and/or allow the interviewee to add statements which were lost in the (sometimes interrupted) interview atmosphere. In other words, this specific interview design should also rectify the limitations resulting from the specific interview situations in the field. For example, the interviews were mainly held at the institutional office during working hours where there were interruptions by the telephone or people walking in and out the office. Only two interviews were held on private property at times convenient for the interviewees.

6.2.4 Data Analysis

The analysis included two phases. In the first phase, each interview was read carefully and was analysed independently in order to make sure that the contextual factors were noted, 1) to make sure that the meaning is clear, 2) to identify and extract key themes and 3) to identify quotes. Quotes that were illustrative of themes were also highlighted at this point. In the second phase of the analysis, the interviews were re-read and the categories examined across all the interviews to look for both shared and divergent understanding of factors influencing child development. All the interviews were read through one final time to check that no information had been ignored and to make sure the categories drawn up were representative of the data and that statements had not been influenced in one way or the other. Every detail of information had to be taken into account and adjustments made to the analysis. The final result included the dominant themes as well as the variations that were found on these themes (see also Skinner, 2000). Some of the quotes may appear confusing due to poor sentence construction or a lack of vocabulary. In some of the quotes additional editing notes were implemented with careful consideration not to change the content of the statement. Due to small number of interviewed people and their well-known status in the community, the applied coding system using letters as identification instruments neither refers to the interviewees' institution nor their gender.

6.2.5 Limitations and Strategies to Guarantee Data Correctness

The main limitation of the interview procedures is the fact that the interviews were not tape-recorded. The decision not to use tapes was made after the interviewer realised that interviewees felt threatened and did not give open answers in the presence of evidence like taping. Incidentally, Morrell (2001) also reported on this same issue in his qualitative survey on corporal punishment in South African schools. He stated the sensitivity of the subject was acknowledged and the interviews were not tape-recorded in order to ensure anonymity. The interviewer in the present survey also presumed that the interviewees would give more socially accepted answers and statements with taping than without. It can possibly also be supposed that the half-structured interview sessions without taping created a more relaxed interview situation. To limit the loss of information notes were taken from memory during and immediately after the interview session; in addition the interviewees were asked to check the transcribed statements. Finally, seven of nine interviewees participated in all three sessions and only two did not go through the three-phase procedure.

As already outlined in the previous paragraph, another limitation during interview sessions was interruptions, especially within the school environment. These could only be reduced, but not totally avoided by the interview design. As an example: based on African culture doors were usually left open during the interviews. Closed doors are defined as impolite and imply talking behind someone's back. The open door policy also prevented any rumour being spread about intimate relationships between researcher and interviewee (if one was male and the other female): thus avoiding any possibly ensuing uncomfortable situation for both interview partners.

6.3 Methods of the Process Evaluation

For the process evaluation five instruments were utilised. One purely qualitative method included project documentation. The reports by health promotion trainers and learners, as well as the participant observations with four learners of the intervention group can be described as a mixture of qualitative-quantitative methods.

6.3.1 Documenting the Intervention

The aim of the documentation of the programme was to monitor and evaluate the aims of the project in terms of validity and to reflect on the actual events during the intervention. It exemplifies first and foremost the intervention sessions for the later analysis of the implementation process. A diary was used during the team meetings for notes on lessons content and methods and relevant events, special incidents and observational findings. The documentation was also done in comparison with session planning and team reporting after each session and at the end of Intervention I. The design of the programme documentation included four phases: pre-documentation, data collection, post-documentation, and final documentation. The data analysis was done by reporting, screening and analysing the data.

6.3.2 Reports by Health Promotion Trainers

In the knowledge that both health promotion trainers were non-professional educators, the decision was made to do a quality evaluation of their teaching. At first glance the report by the HPTs, given after each session, assessed their self-confidence and evaluated their assessment of the suitability of the teaching methods used during the session, using a short formula. The sessions were assessed using a 5-point rating scale (from 1=excellent to 5=bad). Additional descriptive comments were possible (Appendix C). Results of the reports were discussed two days after the session in every follow-up meeting that functioned as supervision for HPTs. All data were computed into a Microsoft Excel 2003 database, double checked, and analysed. The gathered quantitative data were analysed using the calculation of mean.

Additional comments by HPTs followed the analysis of interviews already reviewed in the analysis of the field interviews (see chapter 6, par. 2.4). In short, the qualitative results were proofed separately, later checked for similarities and discrepancies between HPTs and combined descriptively at the end of the process. The booster session (Intervention II) was not analysed because in the middle of Intervention II a change of staff took place, which is thought to have influenced the quality of the sessions (e.g. learning atmosphere) and consequently the derived data.

6.3.3 Learners' Report

Participants of the intervention group were asked to assess their attitude towards each session once a week. This method was intended to examine the children's emotional well-being and their general attitude to the topic, lesson methods, classmates (same and other gender) and HPTs as well as the acceptance of the intervention model. The method was similar to an election process: 'One vote for one voice'. Only children from the intervention group were involved in the learners' reports.

Description of the Instrument

The instrument was created in the form of two yellow posters. The first poster contained a table with two columns ("I like"; "I do not like"). The rows assessed the attitude towards trainers, relations to boys and girls, relevant topics, used methods, and the confidence sentence as an ice-breaker entry at every lesson. The second poster was to evaluate the general emotional attitude towards the lesson in the form of statements ("I have fun", "I feel ok", and "I am bored"). The simple design of the instrument was considered to be suitable to the expected low level of literacy within the intervention group and their young age.

Data Collection Procedure and Analysis of Data

The data collection took place two days after every intervention session (every Friday morning). At the beginning of the reporting, only children who had attended the previous session were asked to take part in the report. The posters were attached to the black board in the classroom and then each child received seven stickers in the form of dots. Boys received green and girls orange dots. Two learners posted their dots on the posters at the same time, while the researcher controlled the evaluation process to avoid wrong or double markings by learners. The data were entered into the Microsoft Excel 2003 database and double-checked. The first two report results were excluded from the analysis because of pretesting considerations and the newly introduced instrument. The data were analysed in terms of the general attitude towards the outlined sessions, including feelings of comfort towards applied methods and existing working relations with the same and the other gender, as well as teaching staff. The data were specifically viewed for gender differences over time. All results were measured by additive calculation and multiplied by 100 to show the percentage of positive and negative attitudes for each category.

Limitations

Because the sessions took place in the afternoon, the concentration of the children and their participation in an additional 90-minute workshop was expected to be low after a long school day. Thus, it was decided to do the reporting session on another school day; possibly on a Friday morning. To allow for memory-lapses, the two-day period between the specific session and the corresponding report of the learners was considered a limitation on the collected data. In addition, even though the researcher observed the data collection procedure, especially over the first testing phases, wrong markings were set. The first two reporting sessions were consequently deleted from the analysis. It was also assumed that over time a generally constant (and positive) attitude to and opinion of the programme and its content developed among participants, which might be reflected in the data (grouping).

6.3.4 Participant Observations

The participant observations refer to the development of social behaviour of four children (age range 9-12 years) attending the intervention group over a period of one year. Although the instrument comprised almost all the different types of behaviour of the specific participants, it also drew inference from the intervention group on a deputy level. The method of participant observations was used to collect comprehensive additional process data that provided evidence for social learning from a model (intervention) (Bandura, 1986). In addition, the observations provided information about personal (development of the individual over time) and interpersonal (interaction and communication with other classmates) factors and the environmental context (classroom). This means, the participant observation allowed the evaluation of the development of the individual in his/her social and physical environment.

Each session content was defined as an 'event' in which the participant's activity, time management and resource expenditure was observed. To ensure representation, participants were randomly chosen and in relatively equal gender (two girls, two boys), without having any knowledge of the participants' background, personality or school performance. The observation was done at the same place, day, time, and situation (during sessions) to avoid changes in the observational situation and setting.

Description of the Instrument

For measuring behaviour, a coding system was used that applied social behaviour as the independent variable. The dependent variables were (1) general attitude with three dimensions, (2) nonverbal expression with five dimensions, (3) acts of communication with four dimensions, and (4) social interaction/communication with six dimensions. The self-administered category and coding system was organised in homogenous and independent 'relational' and four 'consequence' categories. All presented categories were grouped in opposite dimensions to control the observer's responses, for example friendly – unfriendly.

The relational category included details on age, name, class, setting, topic, activity, and the position of the participant in the classroom. Narrative descriptions of additionally observed events and the communication and interaction ability of the focus child were recorded in field notes (Appendix D). The consequence categories included details on general attitude, nonverbal body language, acts of communication, and social interaction. The general attitude category measured the level of comfort that the focus child expressed in the specific educational situation (method and lesson content). The child's general attitude towards the lesson content was divided into three categories: willing, undecided, negative.

The body language observed signs, actions, and reactions in facial and bodily expressions including arms, hands, legs, and body posture. Acts of communication (spoken language) observed the actual utterances (voice tone) generated by a child, for example expression of words and way of communication with other learners or trainers or teachers during the intervention sessions. The observation focused on the sound of voice and the resulting speaking ability of the focus child. The content of the conversation did not form part of the observation. The social interaction category (i.e. interaction with other learners/teachers or trainers) mainly observed gestures or performances of the subject as well as a child's failure and/or success to interact with interlocutors. This category seemed to be extremely important to observe general behaviour towards others in connection with the participant's ability to express his/her opinion in the interaction with other learners and/or a teacher or trainer.

The categories were measured by frequency dimensions in a 7-point rating scale (1=never to 7=all the time). The rating scale was used to complement direct observations and to help the observers to detect (Pellegrini, Symons, & Hoch, 2004) how often certain behaviour or sets of behaviour occurred.

Data Collection Procedure

Observation took place during Intervention I (March 2003 to June 2003) for four-and-a-half months and Intervention II (October 2003 to November 2003) for one-and-a-half months. Two observers noted down the observation of participants in the classroom setting. The observers were not directly involved in the learning sessions. Special rules and time frames for the observation and reporting procedures were established. At the beginning of each session the exact time, place, seating position of each participant, and content of lesson with method were described. After a silent agreement between the observers, a 15-minute observation was done, during which each observer made field notes with interpretations and notes on the phenomena (Pellegrini et al., 2004). One observer measured time and finished the observation session with a nonverbal sign to the second observer. At the end, the observers coded the observed behaviour in the checklist separately from each other. A new observation started after each observer had finished the recording procedure. To avoid observer fatigue, only two participants were observed per week and session.

Data Analysis

For the purpose of analysis, the data gathered were analysed using predominantly qualitative description. The analysis was executed in three steps: (1) computerising and reporting of the checklist for each participant, (2) discussion of the similarities and differences and transformation of the results and (3) a final report on each participant about the observation findings.

Analysis of Instrument

The reliability of the checklist is judged in terms of consistency. Intra-observer reliability was assured by the involvement of consistent observer(s) who had a sound knowledge of the instrument. The definition of categories and coding was continuously repeated. In accordance with the statement above, two observers scored the same session live and at exactly the same time. One external observer was chosen to avoid interobserver biases.

The observer reliability, specified as interobserver reliability, was analysed by Kendall's Tau B and Pearson Correlation. The interobserver agreement was statistically measured by Kappa and was tested in a repeated reliability test of a sample of observations through immediate comparison sessions after the observations (Pellegrini et al., 2004). In short, while the interobserver reliability merely marks the similarity of ratings, the interobserver agreement reflects the exact agreement between observers. The interobserver reliability measured higher than the interobserver agreement. Although a significance in interobserver reliability was found, the degree of interobserver agreement was predominantly unsatisfactory (exactable are Kappa $\leq .75$) (Table 6.2). Only the Observation Phase II (O2) values show adequate results for both interobserver reliability and interobserver agreement.

Table 6.2.
Interobserver Reliability measured by Kendall's Tau B and Pearson Correlation and Interobserver Agreement measured by Kappa.

Phase (t)	Observation session	Interobserver reliability		Interobserver agreement
		Kendall's Tau B	Pearson correlation	Kappa
1	1	.45	.52	.05
1	2	.65	.73	.31
1	3	.63	.73	.26
1	4	.50	.61	.24
1	5	.55	.61	.32
1	6	.85	.96	a)
2	1	.76	.42	.90
2	2	.71	.43	.86

Note. t = testing point. a) = Kappa could not be measured.

As the statistical analysis of the data shows, there were significant limitations to the reliability of the used instruments. Some limitations effecting validity and reliability are outlined in the following paragraphs.

Limitations and Strategies to Guarantee Data Correctness

Factors affecting validity can be the detection of being observed and observer bias. The detection of being observed was prevented by the observer being present during the entire session and distracting attention by looking around the whole class. In order to avoid observer bias and to increase objectivity different strategies were used: (1) the second observer was an external person who was unaware of the research hypotheses or group assignments; (2)

neither of the observers were informed about the profiles of the participants (social background, learning achievements, and characteristics); (3) interdependence was produced by immediately re-checking the results after the observations. However, two observers observed the same participants over a long period and therefore an increase in expectations and knowledge about the participants and a correspondent loss of objectivity could be noticed, which most probably influenced the derived data.

The poor visibility of the participants in the crowded and sometimes even dark classroom made it difficult for one or both observers to consistently observe the participants. Corresponding comments were made in the checklist and were considered in the analysis. Another limitation affecting reliability and validity was reactivity. The observers were noticed as special guests by the class and participants during the sessions. In addition, one explanation for the recurrence of reactivity could be that the observers were not part of the ethnic group that was being observed. It is assumed that reactivity played a role especially at the beginning of Observation Phase I. There were attempts to reduce this limitation by visiting the class before observation sessions took place. However, only one observer was present and known to the intervention group before the start of Intervention I. The external observer paid a first visit to the observation setting only one week before the first observation phase started. It is clear that this was insufficient time to reduce reactivity right from the start of Observation Phase I.

Furthermore, a third observation phase followed the completion of Intervention I and II. These sessions were held during normal school lessons. Limitations were due to (1) observed violence and corporal punishment in the participants' classes, which was assumed to influence the participants' social behaviour and observers' judgement; (2) the frequent absence of teachers resulting in the cancellation of several observation sessions; and (3) teachers who felt forced to hold the lesson because the observers were present and waiting in their class. As the limitations of the sessions were considerable and therefore uncontrollable, it was decided to cancel Observation Phase III.

6.4   Methods of the Outcome Evaluation

The outcome evaluation used two methods, one purely qualitative (questionnaire) and one consisting of qualitative and quantitative methods (opinion poll).

6.4.1 Questionnaire

The quantitative evaluation of the life skills programme employed a quasi-experimental design with an intervention group (IG) and control group (CG) using a self-administered questionnaire. The duration of the quantitative evaluation comprised the period from March 2003 until April 2004. The time between pre- and posttest was four-and-a-half months, between post- and follow-up test 1 five months and between follow-up tests 1 and 2 another four-and-a-half months (Table 6.3).

Table 6.3.
Factorial Analysis with repeated Testing with Intervention Group (IG) and Control Group (CG).

	t1		t2		t3		t4
Intervention group (IG)	Pretest N=41	(X) I	Post-test N=41	(X) II	Follow-up test 1 N=41		Follow-up test 2 N=41
Control group (CG)	Pretest N=39		Pretest N=39	(Y) I	Post-test N=39	(Y) II	Follow-up test1 N=39
Period (months)	0		4 ½		5		4 ½

The long period between pretest and follow-up test 2 was chosen in order to provide results on the existing knowledge and individual psychological development of participants regarding the sustainability of the intervention results. The intervention group received a non-governmental school-based life skills programme on AIDS education (X) at Ikaya Primary School in Kayamandi (Stellenbosch) with two independently working health promotion trainers. During Intervention (X) I, which constituted the real intervention, learners received 16 sessions of 90 minutes each. Intervention (X) II had the character of a booster session to deepen the knowledge and skills from Intervention (X) I, with four sessions of 90 minutes each.

The control group at Nomlinganiselo Primary School in Crossroads (Cape Town) did not receive any intervention during the pre- and posttest period. During follow-up tests 1 and 2, the control group received the governmental life skills programme on AIDS (Y) (without prior notification of the researcher) under guidance of the Grade 4 class teachers and changed its character to a quasi-control group. This change was neither foreseeable nor preventable and resulted in a research design in which the control group underwent two pretests. Both intervention are indicated as (Y) I and (Y) II.

Variables and Hypotheses

The following section explains the variables in conjunction with the research hypotheses. However, before explaining these interdependencies, a brief introduction on the research model will be provided. The used variables reflect the theoretical construct of the Social Cognitive Theory (Bandura, 1986); the applicability of this construct in this research context is critically analysed in chapter 2. The independent variable is the intervention itself (instead of behaviour). The reason for this is that health behaviour is assumed to be only just developing in pre-adolescence and therefore cannot yet be detected at this stage. The dependent variables are the cognitive variable (knowledge of HIV/AIDS), psychological variables (self-esteem, self-efficacy) and social variables (inter-gender communication, social responsibility) and had to test the psychological and cognitive development of the participants of the intervention on the individual and interpersonal level.

Knowledge of HIV/AIDS, the first dependent variable, included providing information about HIV/AIDS. This information raised awareness and formed the fundamental basis for an adequate response to the health threat by HIV and AIDS. The hypothesis was that learners in the intervention group had developed a higher knowledge of HIV and AIDS than the control group. Global self-esteem, the second dependent variable, is considered a multidimensional construct, consisting of affective, cognitive, motivational and behavioural domains. Rosenberg, Schoenbach, and Schooler, 1995 claims that global self-esteem is defined as the attitude towards an object (the Self) (see also Zanobini & Carmen, 2002). It is assumed that a person with high self-esteem will show a higher competence to make protective decisions in difficult life situations. Bandura (1977) defines self-efficacy, the third dependent variable, as the judgement of one's capability to accomplish a certain level of performance. He states that perceived self-efficacy is a significant determinant of performance that operates partially independently of the underlying skills (Bandura, 1986). Schwarzer (1992) adds that individuals create and develop self-efficacy beliefs that become instrumental to the goals they pursue and to the control they are able to exercise over their environments. It was assumed that learners in the intervention group had higher levels of self-efficacy and, thus, displayed higher competence in protective behaviour.

The fourth dependent variable is gender communication. This variable denotes the learners' ability to positively interact with others, their ability to take the perspectives of others into consideration as well as the degree of acceptance they gain from others. In other words, it assesses the social relationship qualities of girls and boys. It was assumed that girls and boys in the intervention group will show better inter-gender communication which makes it possible to talk about taboos and complicated issues with the other sex and to facilitate a common decision-making process, which will also protect the other sex in future intimate relationships. The study was designed to examine the learners' willingness and commitment to carry out tasks that are assigned to them by their teachers and their parents, including homework and other tasks. This entailed the learners' responsibility to abide by the rules and regulations of the school and/or home. The behaviour regarding social responsibility, the fifth dependent variable of the study, also expressed the value and attitude system towards socially relevant and problematic issues like HIV-infection. Thus, the study analysed whether the learners in the intervention group showed a higher level of social responsibility than the control group.

In summary, in terms of the variables it was expected that individual self-esteem, self-efficacy, inter-gender communication, social responsibility, and knowledge about HIV and AIDS would increase from pretest to posttest and it is assumed that those results can be sustained over the follow-up test 1 and 2. Although all hypotheses are related to the non-governmental intervention (X), the presentation of the results explores the effects of the governmental intervention (Y), too.

Sampling

A total number of 80 Grade 4 level children were involved in the quantitative instrument, the questionnaire. Forty-one children belonged to the intervention group (Ikaya Primary School) and 39 children belonged to the control group (Nomlinganiselo Primary School). The gender distribution was balanced, with 40 girls and 40 boys in total. The age in the groups ranged from 8 to 14 years. More than three quarters of the participants (77.5%) were 9 to 11 years old; five children (6.3%) were eight and 11 children (13.8%) were 12 years and older. All the participants were from an African/black background. The ethnic distribution among learners was predominantly Xhosa; a small number were Tswana or Sotho.

Description of the Instrument

The open and closed questionnaire was employed to gather data from the children in pre-, post- and two follow-up tests. Because no standardised tests for this specific age group (pre-adolescents) and language (isiXhosa) were available at the start of the survey in South Africa, most of the variables were self-constructed (social responsibility, knowledge 1, knowledge 2) and partly made use of existing scales (Self-Esteem scale by Du Bois et al. [1996]; Self-Efficacy by Schwarzer [1996]; and Gender Communication by Hudson [1992]). Only the self-esteem scale had already been translated into isiXhosa, but had never been used for pre-adolescents.

The questionnaire is composed of three parts that deal with local and other factors that are presumed to be important for the development of healthy and protective behaviour in the individual and towards others (Appendix E). Part A consists of three open items on age, gender and grade, and one closed item on the family background. The question on family background, "With whom are you living now?" has twelve possible answers (e.g. mother, father, grandparents). In Part B, the items are constructed on the basis of theoretical as well as empirical grounds that may be used to identify psychological development in individuals that might protect them from HIV infection later in life. The items for self-esteem (Part B) were adapted from Du Bois et al. (1996) for assessing multiple domains of self-esteem in young adolescents; the items for self-efficacy (Part B) were taken from the Schwarzer self-efficacy scale (Schwarzer, 1996).[22] The items for inter-gender communication were taken from the index of peer relations (IPR) (Hudson, 1992). These items were redrafted for the particular context and age group. The social responsibility items were developed by the researcher and had to be tested in this context. Finally, five variables for self-esteem, eight variables for self-efficacy, six variables for inter-gender communication and five variables for social responsibility were used. In the second part, the study uses a 3-point rating scale of "I agree", "I disagree" and "I am not sure". Thus, a high score (3) in a particular measure represented a higher degree of that behaviour or entity; a low score (1) presented a lower degree of that behaviour or entity. Missing or false values were scored with 0. In order to guard the results against possible bias due to the response style, items were negatively worded and the score was changed respectively. The value of the scale was standardised on the 3-point rating scale in which the additive scores were divided through the number of items for the specific variable.

---

22 At the beginning of the study only the self-efficacy scale for adults was accessible to the researcher.

Part C contains all items on knowledge of HIV/AIDS. The researcher formulated most of the items herself because the available questionnaires had not been used for pre-adolescents before. The researcher combined items from different questionnaires used in South Africa (Boshoff, Pretorius, & Ungerer, 1993; Valois & Kammermann, 1984; Everett, 1995). In addition, the items had to be formulated in a way that the young age of the participants and their general low literacy level regarding medical knowledge were accommodated. The items were orientated on the construct 'dangerous or non-dangerous'. The response format in part three consists of two scales on knowledge of HIV/AIDS. Knowledge scale 1 recorded general knowledge on HIV/AIDS. This scale used 16 items, for example "What does AIDS mean?", "What does safer sex mean?", "Where does the HI-Virus come from?" Knowledge scale 2 used 10 items on HIV transmission and protection, and asked questions such as "How can someone become infected with the HI-Virus?", "What kinds of body fluids transmit the HI-Virus?", "What protects you from the HI-Virus?" The response format in part three used "Yes", "No" and "Not Sure" options and therefore used a 2-point scale. A score of 1 is assigned for right answers and 0 for wrong, including missing and false answers. This means the right answers were counted and divided by the number of questions, and multiplied by 100 to get the percentage of right answers.

Considerations about the Language Applied

The items and questions were originally written in English, and then translated into isiXhosa. The questionnaire for the present study was translated by an independent translator of the Human Science Research Council whose first language is isiXhosa. The translation back into English was done by another person whose first language is isiXhosa. This translation was compared with the original version, and any discrepancies were resolved by negotiation between the two translators. Although the translated version of the questionnaire was tested in a pilot study, it cannot claim validity because of a too small number of samples participating. As the Du Bois self-esteem scale had already been used in South Africa and translated into isiXhosa (Wild, Flisher, Bhana, & Lombard, 2002), it was revised for this specific age group.

Data Collection Procedure

Both groups underwent the questionnaire sessions within the same school week. The questionnaire was administered in isiXhosa in a classroom situation under supervision of two trained research assistants, the class teacher, and the research manager. First, the intervention and control groups were identified; names were listed and coded to ensure data protection and anonymity. A specific data collection procedure was employed to motivate learners and ensure the correctness of the data collection. The procedure was as follows: (1) introduction of the research team and the purpose of the visit; (2) explanation of the code of ethics (every answer is voluntary and treated in confidence); (3) handing out of a questionnaire and pencil for each learner; (4) separating learners with reading and writing problems (identified by the class teacher, supervised by one research assistant); (5) slow reading of the questionnaire by either the class teacher or one research assistant and (6) slow reading of each item twice; (7) questions on the definitions of words during the reading; (8) the researcher checking the correctness of the procedure; and (9) ending of session with the distribution of food and drinks to the learners. At the beginning of the first session, the trainers explained two items and answer schemata. Many children used the opportunity to ask questions to ensure the correctness of their answers. A complete redesign was undertaken to avoid strenuous learning processes during follow-up test 1.

Data Analysis and Analysis of Instrument

The final categories for the analysis of the family background were entered into the Microsoft Excel 2003 database. Six categories were administered: (1) urban-extended (multigenerational including children, parents and grandparents), (2) nuclear (biological parents and children), 3) single-headed (one biological parent and children), (4) nuclear and stepparents (one biological parent, stepparent and children), (5) extended and stepparents (multigenerational, biological parent with one stepparent), and (6) special (legal guardians) family systems. The psychological and cognitive variables were computed using the Statistical Package for Social Sciences (SPSS 11.5 for Windows). Some cases were deleted from the database: being absent (including migration), reading and writing problems, mental disability, and refusal.

The data gathered from the questionnaires were analysed using means, factor analysis and exploratory data analysis. Factor analysis was used to determine the reliability and validity of the instrument, that is, the questionnaire. Between both scales there exists a slight correlative connection ($r=.32$; $p<.01$). Starting point of the realised scale formation on the constructs was an item analysis of the pretest results. Interestingly, regarding the psychological variables, items with negative wording on self-esteem (e.g. "I sometimes think I am a failure" or "I often feel ashamed of myself"), communication between genders (e.g. "The boys in my class do not seem to even notice me" or "The boys in my class seem to look down on me"), and social responsibility (e.g. "I do not care about what other people think about what I do" or "I do not feel responsible for whatever I do in my life") could not be implemented in the scales because of an absent selectivity. The reason for this could be problems of the samples to understand the items. According to the educational personnel at the case study schools, children at that age do not use negative statements in their native language isiXhosa. Those items had to be excluded from the analysis and consequently caused a loss of information. Table 6.4 shows the internal consistency and the range of the selectivity of the scales after the item analysis.

Table 6.4.
Data Analysis of Questionnaire by Cronbach Alpha, Number of Items, and Selectivity of Scales.

Variables	Cronbach's alpha	No. of items	Range of selectivity	
			Min	Max
Self-esteem	.61	5	.29	.46
Self-efficacy	.65	8	.22	.52
Gender communication	.66	6	.31	.62
Social responsibility	.64	5	.34	.46
Knowledge 1	.81	16	.25	.55
Knowledge 2	.72	10	.23	.50

The effects of the intervention were measured by factorial ANOVA to discover significances, the analysis of mean and the analysis of variances and error; the Greenhouse-Geisser was used to correct the degree of freedom for the assessment of critical coincidence of the F-Values. A Scheffétest was applied for the comparison of pairs (measurement by hand in accordance with Bortz, 1999). Finally, a McNemartest was used to carry out a full exploration of the examination between pretest and all following three-test phases on both knowledge scales.

Limitations and Strategies to Guarantee Data Correctness

Two limitations were regarded as the most limiting to the validity and reliability of the survey. First, at the time of the administering of the questionnaire no standardised tests were available for this age and language group or the research rationale in South Africa. The result was that a self-administered questionnaire had to be developed that consisted of different items from different scales. To reach reliability of this instrument it would have been appropriate to do an extensive pretest with the instrument. However, and this is the second most affecting limitation, the pretest turned out to be inappropriate due to constraints in timetables mainly effected by unanticipated events (see chapter 5, par. 6.2).

Further limitations for this instrument have been the identification of the real ages of learners, among others. Many learners gave a different birth date than was written in the school register. Teachers provided the following explanations: (1) parents did not inform their children about their birth dates because of their own illiteracy, (2) some learners did not have birth certificates because they were born at private homes in rural areas away from public clinics or administration centres, and (3) because of the extreme poverty in many families special dates such as a birthday are not celebrated. In the end, the analysis of age groups was measured on the basis of listed birth dates in the school register. In addition, despite a system of verification of marks to identify learners with learning problems, the procedure could not identify such cases because of confusing school marks in the registers, as was the case at Ikaya Primary School.

Consequently, it can also be assumed that learners who had reading and writing problems were not identified. Both teachers explained that because of the high learner-teacher ratio many learners with learning problems were undetected. The teachers did, however, indicate those learners with reading and writing problems who were known to them and who were then excluded from the analysis.

The period between pretest and the second follow-up test amounted to 12 months during which learners underwent extensive biological and psychological changes from pre-adolescence to adolescence. These developments were taken into consideration in the analysis by writing the measured differences between means from test phase I to test phase IV. It was also assumed that learners underwent a learning process in answering the test items. This learning process could possibly influence test results; consequently, a new design of the questionnaire containing the same items was designed for test phase III.

There possibly existed additional learning input on HIV/AIDS. Media campaigns on HIV/AIDS, discussions with other people and learners about HIV/AIDS or about the life skills programme at school or at home may have had an influence on learners' knowledge. It was established that no other planned and direct intervention took place in the living environment of the children in either of the groups before intervention.

Furthermore, research results in general are assumed to be strongly influenced by the social environment, for example parents and school authorities that in turn influence the development of health and social behaviour outside of the intervention. Initial attempts to understand these influences were made in an extensive field study, field interviews and the literature review. Because of financial and time constraints interviews with the strongest pillars of socialisation for pre-adolescent children, namely their parents, could not be undertaken and is considered a further limitation.

6.4.2 Opinion Poll among the Intervention Group

The aim of the opinion poll was to examine children's long-term general attitude towards the implemented life skills programme on HIV/AIDS and sex education and their physical environment. The survey was done in August 2004, five months after follow-up test 2 and eight months after the end of Intervention II. Only learners from the intervention group who attended five different Grade 5 classes at Ikaya Primary School at the time, and who were specifically concentrated for this survey, took part in the poll.

Description of the Instrument

The opinion poll had the character of a voluntary activity session which used three methods to gain results: individual decision-making, brainstorming, and group work. During individual decision-making children were asked to assess their living environment ("What is Kayamandi like?"), express their attitude towards the life skills programme on HIV/AIDS and sex education ("Did you like or did you not like the life skills programme?") and if they would recommend the programme to other learners ("Do you think other children should receive the same life skills programme?"). These questions were answered by standing next to the appropriate opinion pinned on the black board. Participants were also asked to express what they think is ugly and/or beautiful in their community using the brainstorming method by which every learner was asked to give two answers. The final group work in mixed gender was aimed at clarifying questions ("What made you happy/sad in the life skills programme?"). The methods were used one after another; specific time frames were set to guarantee a flow of activities. The gathered quantitative and qualitative data were counted by two research assistants, immediately documented, computerised, and finally analysed.

6.5 Conclusion

The chapter 6 illustrated how the research topic was translated into specific research aims and its measurable pendants within a quasi-experimental design. In order to guarantee a strong instrument design, the combination of qualitative and quantitative instruments was used to maximise validity. The applied research instruments provided information on the development of individual learners, as well as possible intervening factors from their environment. Additional issues such as cultural implications were taken into consideration. The research scheme was designed to collect comprehensive data that provides information about the research questions from different perspectives. The validity of data was proved by a clear explanation of the phenomena and by the control of all possible biases that may have falsified the research finding.

CHAPTER SEVEN

The Child Mind Project – Implementation Process

7.1 Introduction

Faced with an omnipresent AIDS pandemic in South Africa the National Integrated Plan (NIP) envisages, as one of its key strategies, the introduction of a formal life skills programme in schools to prevent the further spread of HIV in the South African society (NDOH, 2001). The first priority is set on the fact that life skills programmes have to teach "qualities that are necessary to empower individuals and their communities to cope and engage successfully with life and its challenges in South African society" (De Jong, Ganie, Naidoo, & Prinsloo, 1994; Vergnani, Flisher, Lazarus, Reddy, & James, 1998, p. 52).

In relation to HIV preventive approaches with children such programmes should focus on the strengthening of individual and interpersonal skills and talents that result in risk-free behavioural intentions and in protective behaviour later (Pinquart & Silbereisen, 2004). It is therefore assumed that these programmes should reach children and youth before they have established behavioural patterns that place them at risk in terms of mental and physical well-being (WHO, 1992b; Vergnani et al., 1998).

Chapter 7 presents the evaluation results of the implementation process of the non-governmental school-based life skills programme on AIDS and sex education – called the *Child Mind Project* (CMP). The CMP is outlined as a preventive school-based learning intervention performed in cooperation between two non-governmental institutions working in the field of health promotion and a governmental public school. The implementation procedures of the programme are explained, together with programme planning and strategy development, performance within a classroom setting, and developed concepts, messages and materials. Chapter 7 concludes by paying attention to specific influences and obstacles confronting this health enhancing programme and its effective implementation in an impoverished setting like Kayamandi.

7.2 Background of the Study

In 2001, the later researcher-in-chief[23], independently contacted several stakeholders within the community in order to initiate and support the implementation and evaluation of a school-based life skills programme on HIV/AIDS at the primary school in the local township. The formulated research proposal was subsequently presented to several non-governmental and governmental organizations in Stellenbosch, e.g. Stellenbosch AIDS Action, the Ikaya Primary School, the school clinics, the Child Welfare Organization, the Department of Social Work, and the Department of Psychology at the University of Stellenbosch.

The Ikaya Primary School was especially keen on participating, because they felt incapable of implementing the governmental programme and, consequently, of fulfilling the governmental guidelines. Two things should be mentioned at this point: firstly, at the time of the preparations for the pilot study the governmental programme was still in its publishing process; secondly, although ten teachers at Ikaya Primary School received training on the governmental programme in August 2002, the Stellenbosch School Clinics stated that the teachers refused to teach this programme at their school (Stellenbosch School Clinics, 2002).

Finally, all the contacted institutions cautiously undertook to participate in the study. As agreed with the SAA and this particular primary school, the next step was for the evaluator to apply for overseas funding and for research permission from the Western Cape Department of Education in Cape Town and Paarl.

Once all pre-preparations, the allocation of funding and the establishment of a coordination structure had been concluded, the pilot study started in August 2002 as a cooperative initiative between two South African non-governmental organizations, Ikamva Lethu Centre and Joy for Life[24], and the governmental educational institution, Ikaya Primary School that supported the implementation of the programme. On the basis of the manual designed by the PPASA[25], a new learning manual was developed that followed

---

23 For the purpose of comprehension it was decided not to use a personal form in this paragraph. However, to prevent any confusion, the author of this book is the same as the evaluator-in-chief.

24 Joy for Life became a second partner in the course of the intervention because the Ikamva Lethu Centre became embroiled in restructuring processes (reaching independence from SAA) and financial instabilities towards the end of the pilot phase.

25 The same manual formed the basis of the later revised governmental Life Skills and HIV/AIDS Education programme, taking into consideration materials from Soul City published by the Western Cape Department of Education in 2002 (2002a, b, c).

specific learning conditions, individuals' learning capabilities and demands during the pilot study. The project's name, *"Child Mind Project"*, is based on suggestions made by children in the intervention group at the end of the first intervention in August 2003. With the death of one of the health promotion trainers at the end of the pilot study, there was no time to prepare a new health promotion trainer for the project. Another problem arose from the funding side. With the instable structural frame of the Child Mind Project and the fragmentary personnel situation, sustainable funding could not be acquired. In August 2004, the cooperation partners decided not to sustain the project over the period of the pilot study.

7.3 Coordination Structures and Community-wide Implementation Procedures

The structure of the pilot study can be divided into two columns (research and project) with six levels regarding funding, the tertiary institutions involved in Germany and South Africa, South African governmental and non-governmental organizations, and the project team (Figure 7.1, see also Table 7.1).

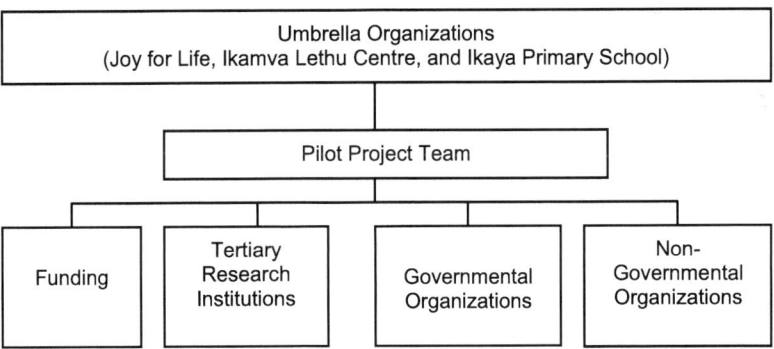

Figure 7.1. Project Structure of the Child Mind Project illustrating its six Levels.

The tertiary institutions involved were the German University of Leipzig (2002-2004), the Free University of Berlin (2004-2006), and the Department of Psychology at the University of Stellenbosch, South Africa (2002-2006), in particular. The South African and German tertiary educational institutions supervised the evaluation of the pilot study and were involved in the cooperation agreements.

The research was funded by the DAAD (2002-2003) and the RLS (2003-2005). The German developmental aid policy NGO SODI and private sponsors provided funding for the project side. The project had a total budget of R12, 387.42 and mainly consisted of the expenses for health promotion trainers.

Two South African non-governmental organizations assumed the role as project partners and legal guardians of the CMP. The first project partner, Ikamva Lethu Centre, is based within the Kayamandi community. At the beginning of the pilot study, this organization used to be part of the SAAC and became an organization under Section 21 in 2003. The Ikamva Lethu Centre is both a youth centre and AIDS awareness centre that offers peer educational training. This organization offered support in negotiating the project with several stakeholders in religious and cultural groups, and took over responsibility for the project within the community to safeguard the project and its staff members who were living in the community. In addition, the Ikamva Lethu Centre also offered its hall for the Drama on Abuse session and equipment for sports activities. Joy for Life, the second partner, is a long-established and experienced day-care and educational centre that encourages people infected with or affected by HIV/AIDS to live positively. The organization also offers AIDS awareness workshops for adults at corporate, governmental and non-governmental institutions. Although the organization is based in Cape Town, it played a crucial role in the project supervision, fundraising support, workshops for staff and teaching materials. The organization also held a Mothers' Workshop on HIV/AIDS for mothers of the intervention group in August 2003; as the main role models for children, mothers were addressed on healthy living with or in the presence of HIV/AIDS.

The Ikaya Primary School, despite having extremely limited resources, acted as third partner and provided the platform for the CMP. The school management integrated the project in its weekly schedule, and provided the infrastructure (e.g. classroom, electricity), teaching materials (e.g. copies, television, video recorder) and personnel support (e.g. participating class teacher, official participation in parent meetings).

The project team consisted of two health promotion trainers who ran the sessions, one (voluntary) class teacher, one research assistant who supported participant observations and the researcher-in-chief, being responsible for the project management and evaluation of this study.

The protection of appropriate ethics and cultural values, as well as additional support in case study work and outdoor workshops throughout the evaluation process was ensured by constant contact and meetings with local experts from educational, health, welfare, religious-based and public organizations within the Kayamandi community.

For protective and strengthening matters a network with several stakeholders was established to ensure that a wide range of resources could be allocated. Networking with community stakeholders and services within the target community and the school setting was of special importance to mobilise people in charge of and experts in children's needs and demands (see chapter 5, par. 5.2). For this reason, the project was expected to become more popular and consequently more manifest and sustainable in the pool of other welfare and health approaches within the community after the pilot study. Finally, the project mobilised and made use of resources from seven non-governmental and governmental institutions.

The *Ikamva Lethu* Centre and *Ikaya Primary School* were immediate partners of the CMP in its physical surrounding. The *Kayamandi Community Clinic* supported the project team in providing information on health, guiding a trip to the Community Clinic and supervising – in cooperation with the school and project team – cases of ill-treatment and other health problems surfacing in the intervention group (e.g. the epileptic fits of one learner).

With regard to instructions by the National Department of Education to report every case of abuse to the existing child welfare system, contact was established with social workers of the *Child Welfare Organization* in Kayamandi and the head office in Stellenbosch, although this organization ought to have supervised the project team in the management of potential social cases (neglect and sexual abuse) within the intervention group during intervention.

The *Drama Group*, consisting of young actors from the community, organised a play on abusive situations linked to the lessons on sexual abuse. In addition, *Prochorus*, a religious-based NGO, organised field trips for the project manager, thereby providing useful grounds for discussion on the existing social and political atmosphere in the community and relations to officials in Stellenbosch. Finally, the *Kayamandi Community Alliance*, as the link between all organizations, functioned as a source of information on the political and social developments within the community.

Table 7.1.
Organizational Structure of the Child Mind Project.

Country	Level	Research			Project		
	Funding	DAAD (2002-2003)	RLS (2003-2005)		SODI (2002-2004)		Private Donors (2003-2004)
Germany			*Supervision*				
	Tertiary Institutions	University of Leipzig (2002-2004)	Free University of Berlin (2004-2005)				
			Affiliation				
	Tertiary Institutions	University of Stellenbosch (2002-2004)	HSRC (2002)				
		Permission	*Reporting*		*Social*	*Health*	*Education*
South Africa	Governmental Organizations	Dept. of Education	School Clinics		Child Welfare	Community Clinic	Ikaya Primary School
		Health	*Education*	*Welfare*	*Adult/AIDS*	*Youth/AIDS*	*Theatre*
	Non-governmental Organizations	Social Work/Religion		Public Organizations	Joy for Life	Ikamva Lethu Centre	Drama Group
South Africa Germany Austria	Child Mind Project Participants	Observer		Evaluator/ Coordinator		Trainers & Class Teacher	Children & Parents

144

7.4 The Learning Programme

As explained in the previous paragraph, the first step to realise a life skills programme that emphasises sensitive issues such as HIV/AIDS and sex, was to specifically focus on strong and supportive project implementation within its closer social context. Such a focus ensured to safeguard the holistic, cooperative and inclusive approach which is multidisciplinary, intersectional and community-based (Magome et al., 1997/1998). The second step was the realisation of a practical and sustainable project character that pays special attention to the cultural background and the developmental stage of the participants (Magome et al., 1997/1998). Thus, the evaluated programme and its sessions and content were specifically designed for learners in the pre-adolescent stage (10-11 years) attending an impoverished public primary school in Kayamandi.

7.4.1 The Underlying Pedagogical Concept

The aims of the Child Mind Project were mutually agreed with national guidelines for life skills programmes on AIDS of the National Department of Education (2000). More specifically, the high-ranking aims of the life skills programme on AIDS and sex education or any other programme are to:

(1) Promote and develop positive values and attitudes so that [participants] understand and accept themselves as unique and worthwhile human beings,
(2) Help [participants] to understand, acquire and practise relevant basic life skills and to display attitudes and values that improve relationships in the family, group and community,
(3) Practise life skills and support decision-making skills with particular emphasis on assertiveness with regard to sexual issues and general life situations,
(4) Develop necessary knowledge regarding HIV/AIDS,
(5) Develop acceptance of different lifestyles and opinions and stimulate respectful behaviour towards different people and to hold personal beliefs and values in demonstrating values and respect for human rights as reflected in *Ubuntu*,
(6) Support children's rights and their knowledge of child protection agencies,

(7) Develop responsible and accountable behaviour and healthy lifestyles within the participating individual, and
(8) Encourage learners to evaluate and participate in activities that demonstrate effective human movement and development (PPASA, 1997; Magome et al., 1997/1998).

In summary, the individuals participating in a life skills programme are supposed to develop a life construct based on positive self-esteem, participation and individual opinions that enhance health-promoting behaviour. This also means that acquired cognitive, emotional and social competencies and skills be converted into active behaviour (Jerusalem, 2002b) that aims at the development of sound and positive mental health (Elias & Weissberg, 2000). Therefore, the CMP programme contains three main components: the development of the values and attitudes of the participating individual (e.g. self-efficacy), the transfer of knowledge on health (e.g. HIV/AIDS) and the development of competencies (e.g. social responsibility) (Figure 7.2).

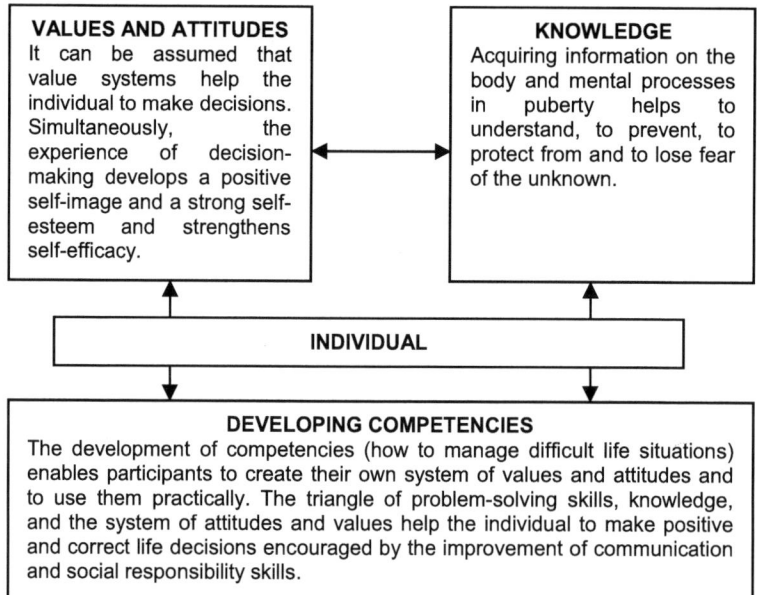

Figure 7.2. Three Basic Components of the Presented Life Skills Programme on AIDS and Sex Education (see also PPASA, 1997).

To deepen this construct, the main emphasis of the CMP is not only to give information on ways of transmission of and protection against the infection with HIV, for example. In the centre of the intervention stands the conveying of competencies for the development of the personality of the individual (e.g. self-esteem and self-efficacy) and an increase in the belief in one's own competencies and decision-making skills (e.g. non-violent interaction and communication about taboo topics such as AIDS and sex between boys and girls). The assumption is that the acquisition of such competencies will finally result in the development of protective sexual behaviour later in life.

7.4.2 *Intervention Phases and Topics Covered*

The learning programme was carried out in two intervention phases: The first intervention was the real programme and the second had the character of a booster tool to deepen the knowledge and skills participants had acquired in Intervention I. The first intervention phase took place from March 2003 until July 2003 and included sixteen sessions on eight topics to change individuals' perspectives from individual to group level and finally to community and cultural level. The second intervention phase contained topics on self-esteem, HIV/AIDS, sexual abuse, and death. The programme was taught one period (time slot in class schedule) a week on a voluntary basis. It was allocated on the timetable, according to the policy indicated in the Interim Curriculum (NDOE, 1997). To ensure meaningful discussions and understanding of the topic, each lesson in the classroom of the intervention group lasted 90 minutes.

The learning programme deals with a wide variety of topics, which are assumed to support the development of skills, and supports the coping mechanisms for developmental tasks and the necessary competencies. Several methods and topics were revised during the preparation of the sessions to make them more appropriate for the age of the participants and the learning and social conditions at the Ikaya Primary School.

Self-esteem was taught to develop confidence, assertiveness and a realistic self-concept in the learner. This also went hand in hand with creating motivation for making life decisions and providing the individual with coping strategies for difficult life situations. Lesson content included the identification and building of healthy bodies and healthy minds (Table 7.2).

The topic *Relationships to Family and Friends* taught different kinds of family systems, friendships and lifestyles that exist in South Africa. Ubuntu was introduced as a principle to respect other people. Children should learn how to relate to other people within their families, classrooms and communities by caring for others, sharing with others, cooperating with others, having compassion for others, acting with honesty, justice and fairness and be hospitable to others (PPASA, 1997). Related issues like peer pressure and the difference between love and sex were also introduced during these sessions (Table 7.3).

Sessions on *Understanding my body* explained the physical (internal and external organs, sexual intercourse) and mental development from childhood to puberty in relation to feelings, and the well-being of body and soul. In-between these sessions an extra outdoor event took place to the Kayamandi Community Clinic. The tour was guided and lectured by the manager of the Clinic (Table 7.4) with the goal to introduce this medical institution and its staff to the children and to make them feel more comfortable with it in case they needed medical support or advice.

Topic four: *Keeping my body safe and healthy*, involved a health promoting session on hygiene to protect the body against any kind of disease caused by germs and bacteria, and sexually transmitted infections (HIV/AIDS was not specifically outlined at this point). General information on risks of and protection against infections was given and risk awareness was encouraged. In the same session a picnic was held in the classroom where several kinds of food (e.g. fruits, vegetables, dairy products, bread) were introduced as inexpensive alternative protection of the immune system (e.g. garlic, carrots), and as part of a healthy nutrition and lifestyle (Table 7.5).

The session on *HIV and AIDS* defined the disease and explained its transmission as well as available protection. The explanation of sexual intercourse and later of the transmission and prevention of HIV/AIDS included the A(bstinence), B(e faithful), C(ondoms) and D(elay sexual debut) strategy as part of a free decision-making process of the individual (Table 7.6). The lessons also dealt with contraceptive methods, such as the use of male and female condoms and the antipregnancy pill. The objectives were to reduce fear and to empower the children to deal with the disease in everyday situations. Contraceptive methods such as condoms were introduced and explained; this was against the recommendation of the original manual (PPASA, 1997), which only introduces condoms in Grade 6. The decision to implement the condom distribution in this session was made after many learners requested information on these questions in the secret box. The questions proved that there was a great need for information on contraceptive and protective methods. Social aspects of the disease, such as stigmatising HIV-positive people were talked about in groups. The learners had to decide whether an HIV-positive child should be allowed to attend their school. This task and its results are outlined in more detail in chapter 9.

The session on *Abuse* covered any kind of (emotional, physical, sexual) abuse and aimed to improve the understanding of wanted and unwanted physical contact and the resistance to outside pressure to have sex. However, special attention was paid to sexual abuse due to the high number of child sexual abuse in South Africa according to official statistics (see also Human Rights Watch, 2004c). Behavioural guidelines and contact numbers were given to the children so that they knew where to find help (Table 7.7). In this regard, a local drama group invited the intervention group at the Ikamva Lethu Centre to attend a play on physical and sexual abuse stories of children, which the actors defined as typical for the location.

The session on *Caring for an ill person* was introduced in terms of hygiene, nutrition and responsibilities, and explained standard procedures when taking care of a sick person at home (home-based care) (Table 7.8). In addition, information on and skills of first aid and hygiene were conveyed. The last topic, *Dealing with Death* was introduced together with the previous topic and discussed rituals and beliefs in death and stages of grief, which were illustrated as part of the life circle (Table 7.9).

Table 7.2.
Topic One – Self-Esteem with Lesson Goal and applied Methods.

Session	Method
\multicolumn{2}{c}{**Topic One**}
\multicolumn{2}{c}{Self-esteem – Understanding myself (healthy bodies, healthy minds)}
1	Black board teaching/explanation; Group work in mixed gender: Art/drawing a "Treasure Map"
2	Explanation on Code of Conduct; Group work in mixed gender: Art/drawing a "Treasure Map"; Homework: "Facts-about-my-body-table"
3	Performance/presentation of group results; Explanation: "Healthy bodies, healthy minds"/Discussion on healthy Lifestyle; Motivation activity: "Confidence Sentence"
16 (Booster)	Individual work: Personal "Body Map"; Presentation/performance of results; Discussion on self-esteem
Goal	Identifying and building a positive body image; finding a personal "confidence sentence"

Table 7.3.
Topic Two – Relationships with Family and Friends with Lesson Goal and applied Methods.

	Topic Two
	My relationship with family, friends and the community
Session	**Method**
4	Motivation game/Fun; Explanation: "We are all part of a family" (different types of families that exist in SA); Group discussion: "Different Family Types"; Collage/Art: "My family?"
5	Motivation/Music: "Tree Song"; Decision-making: Collage displayed next to the correct family type; Discussion on friendship; Individual work: friendship web
6	Discussion: Results of friendship web; Brainstorming: "What else do you want to do in the life skills programme?"; Homework: Create a "Friendship card"
Goal	Definition of types of families and friendships

Table 7.4.
Topic Three – Understanding my Body with Lesson Goal and applied Methods.

	Topic Three
	Understanding my body
Session	**Method**
7	Introduction: Secret box; Explanation: "Understanding my body"; Group work in mixed gender: Physical and mental changes from childhood to puberty; Performance/presentation of group results
8	Division of class into two groups according to their gender; Explanation of internal and external organs, including reproductive organs; Individual work: Filling in copies with names and functions of body parts; Fun: Naming some embarrassing slang or silly names for the body parts or organs
9 (Outdoor Trip)	Division of class into two groups according to their gender; Explanation: Sex education (slowly and sensitively); Explanation/story telling on sexual intercourse; Game/relaxation: soccer for boys and netball for girls Introduction to the Kayamandi Community Clinic; Explanation of the functions of the clinic, rooms, and responsibilities of staff
Goal	Examination of external changes from birth to puberty; Explanation of functions of the main body parts (internal/external); sexual intercourse and pregnancy

Table 7.5.
Topic Four – Health and Hygiene with Lesson Goal and applied Methods.

	Topic Four Keeping my body safe and healthy
Session	**Method**
10	Explanation: "Keeping you healthy"; function of the body defences/immune systems and hygiene; Food event/experimental learning: healthy food and its functions
Goal	Making responsible choices and taking responsibility for one's own health; understanding the body's defences or immune-system; prevention of the spread of diseases by germs and bacteria

Table 7.6.
Topic Five – HIV/AIDS with Lesson Goal and applied Methods.

	Topic Five HIV/AIDS in my world
Session	**Method**
11	Explanation of HIV/AIDS: Definition, ways of transmission and protection, living with HIV and healthy lifestyle; Protection methods (condom distribution) and presentation of several contraceptives (functions)
12	Group work (seven groups of same and mixed gender, on voluntary basis): Decide whether a HIV-positive child can attend their school if they were the principal; Presentation/performance of results; Explanation: Human Rights and law in the South African Constitution for people living with HIV
17 (Booster)	Group work in mixed gender: Answering questions on the definition of HIV/AIDS, transmission of and protection against HIV, testing; Presentation of results by learners; Explanation by HPTs
Goal	Definition of HIV/AIDS; transmission of and prevention against HIV/AIDS; Prevention of discrimination against people infected with HIV (Human Rights Aspect)

Table 7.7.
Topic Six – Sexual Abuse with Lesson Goal and applied Methods.

	Topic Six
	Sexual abuse – Keeping safe from unwanted touch
Session	**Method**
13	The class was seated like in a theatre to watch the video (mixed gender); Explanation: Abuse of bad, confusing and good touch; Video: "Good and bad touches"; Card game: "touch" and "feeling" cards; Music/song: "That is nobody's body than mine" from the video with the learners
14 (Outdoor Trip)	The class was seated like in a theatre to watch the play (mixed gender); Drama play: Drama on physical and sexual abuse; Discussion of drama: What kinds of abuse exist (including sexual abuse)?; Who are abusers?/Who gets abused?; Explanation: Good and bad touches and feelings; Individual work/card game: Revision and "touch" and "feeling" cards; Explanation: Safety rules, behavioural procedures if abuse happens, and Help lines (no. Child Help Line)
18 (Booster)	Music: "Tree Song"; Explanation (Repetition): Abuse; Individual work: Personal "Action Plan"; Music: "That is my body"
Goal	Definition of (sexual) abuse; reviewing good and bad touches compared to related feelings; action plan (recognise, report, respond) against sexual abuse

Table 7.8.
Topic Seven – Caring for an ill Person with Lesson Goal and applied Methods.

	Topic Seven
	Caring for an ill person
Session	**Method**
15	Explanation: Caring for someone (needs of a sick person, daily schedule, hygiene); Group work in mixed gender/experimental learning: Wound treatment; Role play by trainers: Visit at the doctor (explanations, instructions)
	Presentation/demonstration: Treatment of diarrhoea (mixture)
Goal	Caring for an ill person (needs, feeling of comfort) and planning a routine; hygiene – special topic: diarrhoea and making a simple oral anti-dehydration mixture

Table 7.9.
Topic Eight – Coping with Death with Lesson Goal and applied Methods.

	Topic Eight When someone I love dies
Session	**Method**
16	Discussion: cycles of grief
19 (Booster)	Explanation: stages of grief; Discussion: different cultural beliefs in death and funeral traditions; Art: Drawing a memory card; Music/relaxation: "Tree Song"
Goal	Discussion on the circle of life from birth to death and different ways to mourn for somebody

The final event in the Intervention I phase was a day trip with the class to the Two Oceans Aquarium in Cape Town in August 2003. The class was informed one week before the excursion. The first goal of the class trip was to signal appreciation to the participating children for attending the project and secondly, to demonstrate the success of the project in equipping children with skills to adjust to new demands and behavioural patterns within a new setting.

In summary, because the main goals of the CMP was to build the foundation for the acquisition of appropriate and correct knowledge on HIV/AIDS, to encourage positive mental responses and resilience among individuals, and to develop protective health behaviours, it foremost incorporated a positive and encouraging life philosophy reflected in the variety of topics and teaching methods.

7.4.3 *Presentation Methods and applied Language*

As Bandura (1986, p. 21) states, human functioning is explained as a model of triadic reciprocity in which behaviour, cognitive and other personal factors, and environmental events all operate as interacting determinants. Human nature is characterised by a vast potentiality that can be fashioned by direct and observational experience into a variety of forms within biological limits. Thus, any intervention, learning model as Bandura calls it, must put special emphasis on its framework and methodology using mainly participatory and experiential methods to allow participants to observe and, at best, to test modelled behaviour for their own use.

In the CMP consequently, special emphasis was given to the application of a vast variety of teaching methods during sessions which allowed participants not only to acquire new knowledge but also to observe action or to apply skills. The following methods were used: frontal teaching, individual work, group work, open discussion, brainstorming, physical activities, drama, and outdoor trips.

Frontal teaching or black board teaching was applied when new topics and content were introduced or repeated to the learners to embed new knowledge, to deepen general knowledge and to dispose of false knowledge or misunderstandings. Every lesson started with a revision of the previous lesson and its content, which gave the HPT's not only the chance to conduct the class but also to summarise for learners the learning result. This method in turn required from learners the ability to listen and concentrate. However, as Bandura (1986) also found, the children achieved significant gains in knowledge when instruction was interspersed with the demonstration of the principles, whereas they learned little when the same information was presented through verbal instruction alone. The decentralised methods in particular paid attention to the demand that new knowledge and skills are best acquired with participatory and active methods. Active learning approaches, on the one hand, are seen as the most effective way in which young people can learn health-related and social skills, and on the other hand, offer the opportunity to organise difficult sessions with more enjoyment and comfort to enlarge the emotional status of the participants.

The first active method, the *individual work* method was thought to be relevant when learners needed to assimilate the learned knowledge and interlink it with their personal belief system. This method was usually linked with artistic methods. Art (e.g. collage) and music (e.g. a song about abuse or the tree song) played a significant role in sessions on self-esteem, relationships or death in families. The method of *open discussion* was mainly used when an interaction between health promotion trainers and learners had to be encouraged. Open discussions especially, strived to develop the expression of an individual opinion, a positive self-esteem and the ability to participate in the context of a problem.

Group work, the third participatory method, was a particularly important method by which learners had the opportunity to discover the practical aspects of the information they were given. Group work is regarded as important for the development of identification, empathy and solidarity for one's own and the other gender and it should therefore encourage the skills for non-violent inter-gender communication and common decision-making processes. This method was also considered to encourage learners with low self-confidence to speak, open up, and get involved in discussion in smaller groups. In mixed gender group activities, learners mostly chose their group themselves. The use of gender specific group work came into effect in the session on sex education to create a more intimate atmosphere. At the end of each group work session, groups had to elect one learner who presented and/or performed the results to the class, which was supposed to encourage this specific learner's confidence and increase his/her language skills.

Another participatory method, *brainstorming*, was used when children had to make decisions with the whole class on, for instance, the type of outdoor trip or the name of the project. *Physical activities* (e.g. games, sports, plays) were used to encourage individual expression and relaxation and/or to reduce stress, for example during sex education; sport (soccer and netball) was used after the first session on sex education. The *drama on abuse*, as another important active method, was important to communicate real life situations in a playful manner so that learners could observe and feel free and safe to openly ask questions about such a sensitive and often shameful issue.

Outdoor trips, the last method, were seen as practicable to introduce the living environment into the educational setting of the children; a visit to the community clinic, for instance, made the organizations more familiar to their community. Another outdoor trip was made to the Two Oceans Aquarium in Cape Town. The goal of this method was to allow the practising of recently acquired skills and competencies and the probation within a real life setting. The learners thus had the opportunity to feel part of a new experience outside their familial, school or community setting, and were encouraged to handle new demands successfully in the application of their newly learned skills.

Finally, a very important factor to consider when applying educational programmes is that of language application. As the National Department of Education's Language-in-Education Policy suggests, learners should learn more than one language and use the language that they best understand as the language of learning and teaching (1996). In agreement with the school management and parents the sessions in the life skills programme on HIV/AIDS were taught in isiXhosa and English and used educational material designed in both languages. The first language of the participants, isiXhosa, was used in most of the culture related sessions about friends and families or the death of loved ones. English became relevant during sessions on cultural taboo issues such as sex, HIV/AIDS, physical development during puberty and sexual abuse. In this respect, English functioned as a bridge between taboo and accepted cultural topics.

7.4.4 Educational Material and Supplementary Teaching Material

Teaching materials were mainly used and/or copied from the PPASA manual (1997). Supplementary teaching material and additional information were taken from several sources: Joy for Life (2003), Educational Support Services Trust for the Department of Justice and Constitutional Development

(2003), National Department of Health (2000), Soul City (unknown), Quaker Peace Centre (1999; 2002), Western Cape Department of Education (2002a, b, c), the National Film Board of Canada (Foon et al., 1984), and the German life skills and health promotion projects at schools by the German Bundeszentrale für gesundheitliche Aufklärung (Bzga).

7.4.5 Programme Performance – Creating a Safe Classroom

Specific instruments like the *code of conduct* or the *secret box* and a clearly defined temporal framework and embedding rituals were designed to create a supportive teaching environment and to encourage trust between the HPTs (role models) and the children. The code of conduct was compiled to create a place of emotional (Lourens, 2004) and physical safety during the sessions. Because personal standards of conduct provide a further source of motivation (Bandura, 1986), it is believed that the atmosphere had to be one of social appreciation and rewarding behavioural consequences without aversive actions or punishment. Consequently, it was of special importance to create an encouraging learning environment with HPTs as living models for participants to increase their observational learning and make the model more likely to produce good results (Bandura, 1986).

The code of conduct contributed to symbolising a living democracy with participation, representation, rights and duties for every individual involved. Eleven rules and regulations were presented as a valid and fixed behavioural guideline for every person present during the session (learners, trainers, class teacher and observers). In general, the rules, for example "We give everyone a chance to speak" or "We do not laugh about people" were also intended to ensure that trainers and learners did not use psychological or physical violence (e.g. "We do not use violence – here or outside the workshop – including hitting and being horrible to people") to provide a guideline on how to solve problems within the classroom (Appendix F). The code of conduct was compiled according to the Peace Education Programme by the Quaker Peace Centre (2002) and the Primary School Kit of the United Nations (1995). The Commitments and Rules were printed on an A4 poster and made visible on the information board in the classroom.

The outcome was regarded as positive; only two disciplinary incidents occurred during Intervention I and II. In one session, two boys were jumping on the tables and fighting. While the rest of the class reacted with disregard and surprise, a reprimand from the trainer's side was enough to manage the situation. The other incident occurred during Intervention II. The participating teacher intervened once with corporal punishment (beating on hands) without intervention from the trainers. At this point it becomes clear, that behavioural patterns for the management of difficult situations are still in use in day-to-day school life unless they are prevented by long-term training on problem solving skills within classroom settings.

The secret box was introduced as an instrument to ask questions which the children did not want to ask trainers directly or in the presence of other learners; the box thus functioned as a mouthpiece. Although the box was located in the classroom, every question or comment was treated with confidence and only the health promotion trainers were allowed to open the box.

A special framework for each session was compiled with an *entry* and *exit* ritual. This framework was intended to ensure continuity and reliability of the project team as well as the time frame within a school day, given the often unpredictable time management and presence of school teaching personnel. The sessions were opened with a *confidence sentence*, implemented in session three on self-esteem. The sentence read: "There is no one else like me. I will become the best I can be in life because I am ..." The learners had to find an appropriate adjective that described them best. The end of every session was symbolised by the handing over of an apple. This action was meant to encourage a positive group dynamic among the members of the class to encourage patience and self-organization without using violence. For example, at the beginning of Intervention I the children fought for their position in the row to receive an apple. Weeks later the ritual became common place and the children calmed down. Through this procedure the children should have learnt, first and foremost, that they were all treated equally. Everyone thus received an apple as a symbol of equality.

7.5 Involvement of Health Promotion Trainers, the Class Teacher and Parents

The goal of every single instrument in creating a safe and encouraging atmosphere during sessions was to produce trust between the learners, the involved class teacher and the health promotion trainers, and to encourage a protective and empowering teaching atmosphere. For this reason, specific learning programmes for HPTs, as well as information and involvement initiatives for the class teacher and parents were implemented to ensure the safety of the programme and to safeguard the aims of the health promoting initiative within the class room, school and private sphere of the participating children. The following paragraphs describe the specific initiatives adapted to the needs of the different stakeholders and/or guardians.

7.5.1 The Health Promotion Trainers – Training and Preparation of Lessons

Two young unemployed women from the case study community were selected and trained as health promotion trainers in this specific life skills training on AIDS and sex education. One HPT had worked as a trained voluntary AIDS counsellor at the Kayamandi Community Clinic and the second HPT had received training in child development and protection from the Eye on Child Project at the Child Welfare Organization in Kayamandi. The intention of this course of action was to empower especially young people *from* the community to give them further training and to put them in a position to be role models *in* their community.

The preparation phase of trainers and lessons covered the time from October 2002 until February 2003. This phase was divided into three parts: (1) workshops on the manual and related literature, (2) weekly meetings where the topics were discussed and questions about the topics were answered, and (3) final lesson planning, which was done one month before the intervention. Preparation of lessons was organised in two-weekly team meetings for two hours each. These sessions had the character of a workshop in which the content of the topics were discussed, literature was allocated to trainers to keep a stable and continuing training, and daily information between the coordinator and health promotion trainers were exchanged. Problems with single learners, disciplinary issues, learners' reactions and social, educational or health problems were debated in the follow-up sessions. The follow-up session took place immediately after the end of each lesson. Due to the non-pedagogical professional background of the health promotion trainers, effort was made to ensure a high quality of teaching style, accuracy of the taught knowledge and the constant progress of the programme. The meetings therefore functioned as a supervision of the ability and emotional state (e.g. building self-confidence) of the health promotion trainers.

The sessions were conducted by two female health promotion trainers, firstly because the HPTs could support each other during the sessions with regard to knowledge, teaching skills and conflict management in the classroom setting. This constellation put them in a position to support each other, which should encourage a further learning process on teaching qualifications and confidence. Another advantage was meant to be that teamwork made the classroom arrangement easier and allowed working in (gender-specific) groups. Furthermore, the HPTs could work with either girls or boys, according to their specific preferences. The mutual sympathy between the HPTs over the course of the intervention was proved as a precondition for working together as a team.

Additional training for the HPTs was particularly applied during the school holidays. The trainers attended workshops organised by the Planned Parenthood Association of South Africa (HIV/AIDS Advanced Training: Training-Of-Trainers), Brahma Kumaris – World Spiritual University (Living Value Workshop) and Joy for Life (Living positively with HIV/AIDS). The trainers were also encouraged to visit the intervention group during normal lessons and to observe the children's behaviour outside the intervention. The objective of such visits was to establish personal contact with teachers because health promotion trainers were expected to slowly take over responsibility for and ownership of the programme in phases following the pilot study.

7.5.2 *Involvement of the Class Teacher*

One class teacher was invited to attend the sessions so that her involvement ensured a flow of information from project team level to school management level in order to make project management easier. The other objective, similar to the request from the Stellenbosch School Clinics, was to identify a supporter of the CMP who was able to sustain the coordination of the programme at the school after the pilot study. Regular meetings took place between the team and the class teacher during which agreements were reached on ways to assist learners with social problems, parent meetings and meetings with management staff of the school were organised, or applied teaching style and methods were discussed.

7.5.3 *Parents' Collaboration*

In the National Department of Education's Public School Policy of 1996, the relationship between parents and school is defined by a set of rights and responsibilities. In that respect, the school has the responsibility to inform parents about their child's learning process or new learning activities and, whilst the parents have to liaise with school staff and have to monitor their child's educational process.[26] The pilot study as a learning activity on school property had to involve parents in four ways to safeguard the ethic codes.

---

26 The policy also requests parents to support the school in disciplinary matters without clearly defining the content and procedure for this. This point becomes extremely relevant in paragraph 7.5.3.

Firstly, more than five parent meetings were held before, during and after Intervention I and II. This was of special importance to encourage the acceptance of the project and to guarantee the protection of the health promotion trainers who lived in the community. For instance, the interim meeting took place after the sex education session to double-check with parents whether the children and the parents as their legal guardians felt comfortable with the methods used. More than half of the parents and the school governing body joined the last parent meeting where children presented their knowledge on healthy food and wound treatment and received their award.

Secondly, the meetings guaranteed a flow of information from project to parents and allowed parents to ensure that the programme content was appropriate to their educational, cultural and religious convictions for their child. During meetings parents confirmed that they checked their children's homework and acquired new knowledge from children. This leads to the assumption that the communication between parents and children was encouraged during the pilot study.

Thirdly, parents were put in the position of informed advisers, where informative material or advice was given to them in terms of child care, protection and medical support. All information and correspondence were provided in isiXhosa. Furthermore, a Mothers' Workshop was organised by Joy for Life because women tended to be quiet in parent meetings where men were also present. Therefore the project team decided to offer a workshop on HIV/AIDS for mothers, sisters or female legal guardians whose children were part of the intervention group. The goal of this workshop was to establish a personal and direct contact between the mothers or legal female guardians and trainers and, by setting them on an equal footing, to gain some more knowledge about their children.

Lastly, parents were invited to meetings at school on case work, for example sexual abuse or medical problems of children. It was always made clear that the parents were fully in charge of their children's education; they were offered support in the hope that they would feel less dominated by officials from the school or the pilot project team.

7.6   Special Influences and Events during the Pilot Study

The following describes specific influences and events which occurred during the pilot study. Such influences, specifically on sexual and physical abuse, are assumed to not only have a tremendous effect on the emotional and physical developmental process of children growing up with those experiences but also a great influence on the outcome of health promoting initiatives in terms of their health enhancing goals.

7.6.1 Outcomes of the Secret Box

The work of the project team was not only limited to the implementation and realisation of the project. Much effort had to be put into case work in the intervention group. As explained in paragraph 7.4.5, the secret box was applied as a mouthpiece for those learners who were too shy or ashamed to ask specific questions in the presence of other classmates. However, during the process of the intervention, the secret box became not only a highly respected and frequently used instrument of learners who felt a need to ask (intimate or forbidden) questions but also to receive help in regard to family problems or personally experienced abuse.

The notes in the box can be divided into five categories: (1) pregnancy, (2) sex, (3) HIV/AIDS, (4) notes of thanks, and (5) letters explaining problematic situations within the children's families and life. Questions from categories (1) to (3) were answered without mentioning the name of the learner in front of the class during the relevant sessions; most of these letters were signed with the learner's name even though HPTs had made it clear that questions could be asked anonymously. Notes of thanks (4) and letters explaining problematic situations (5) were answered with a letter to the specific learner inviting him/her to speak with the project team.

7.6.2 Cases of Sexual Abuse in the Intervention Group

Six letters contained issues related to physical, mental and sexual abuse, or described situations of neglect, caused by the separation from parents, and poverty in the immediate family. All cases were first discussed in the project team and specific decisions were made to ensure confidentiality of information. Learners who had asked for help received a letter that invited them to speak to the members of the project team if they still wished to be supported. If a learner decided to speak and permission was given to carry on with the case work, the class teacher became involved in the case work. At this point one case shall serve as an example of what turned out to be the most problematic to handle.

One girl wrote the following letter after the session on abuse:

> Misi, Uncle let us think that he will send us, me, P... and N..., to the shop, but instead he locks us up into room. He says to us we must give him that. I ask him what that is and I would say no. I do not want to. The others will do the same, too. I say I tell dad or scream he'll say, he is not afraid of him or mom. When I scream, he says shut up. When we opened the door, I got out the others followed me. When he says, we must come back or he says I'll give you money. I'll say, I don't want this money on anytime of him for that matter. The others don't say anything. They listen to me. (NM, female, 10 years old)

In the same week, the participating class teacher reported that two girls had come and reported a case of child sexual abuse to her. After receiving the letter and information, the team and class teacher invited the girls to a meeting. In the meeting the girls described an attempted sexual abuse. They stated that a third female cousin living in the same household was affected by the attack as well.

At that critical point, following regulations from the Department of Education and the School Clinics, the principal was informed about the case and was asked for advice. One day later, one of the mothers was invited to a meeting at the school. With her permission the principal, the class teacher and the project manager joined the meeting. The encounter also revealed that the attempted rape turned out to be a performed rape. The mother was apparently extremely overwhelmed by the situation and explained that the present sexual abuse was possibly done by her own 19-year-old brother. She also stated that one of the girls had already been raped by an old man (uncle) when she was eight years old. The mother reported that the girl had never been sent to a doctor but she had examined her daughter to see if she was still a virgin. The family background can be defined as extremely impoverished. Only the father had a part-time job financing his two children, the mother, his sister-in-law and his brother-in-law. The mother explained further that she had been asking for help at the local Child Welfare Office a few months before the last event, but social workers had sent her to the police station without any support. Mrs. M. confirmed that she knew of the abuse because the last time the girls had reported the new incident to her was three days before the girls decided to report the case to the class teacher and the project team.

During this meeting the principal tried to report the case to the social workers at the Child Welfare Office and the Community Clinic. However, as it was Friday afternoon and just before a one-week school holiday neither institution was available. Consequently, the result of the meeting was that the principal would contact the manager of the Stellenbosch Child Welfare Organization after the school holidays. Mrs. M. stated that she would consult the social workers as well as the Community Clinic with her daughter for an examination. She also said that it would be of great help if the uncle was forced to leave the home. A new meeting was scheduled for after the school holidays. After the school holidays the situation was as follows (without external professional intervention): the family system, assumingly the male head of the family, had decided to send one of the girls to the Eastern Cape Province; the two others still lived with their family in Kayamandi. The abuser was sent to an unknown place to live with other kinship.

With regard to this situation the project team decided to report the case and to send copies of the written report to the Child Welfare Office. In the meeting with one of the social workers it was confirmed that the mother had reported the case to them in April 2003. They had sent her to the police and the local clinic. One year later in August 2004, the project manager asked the same social workers about the case. They could not find the report files. As a result of this meeting, the project manager had a personal meeting with the Child Welfare manager in Stellenbosch who was surprised to hear about this case.

The final outcome of the case was disappointing. This case of child sexual abuse had never been reported to the police. The separation of the two girls, who were close friends, can be regarded as a secondary trauma. None of the three children have received any psychological or medical supervision at any time. The parents were left alone in their search for help, without adequate support by official institutions. The perpetrator was never charged for his illegal action and now lives in an unknown place; most probably with access to other children. Finally, the girl who was brave enough to report the case disappeared with her father from Kayamandi in January 2006. Her present location is unknown. In the end, the process came to a complete standstill; all attempts to support the girls, including those of the CMP team, failed.[27]

7.6.3 Corporal Punishment as a Pedagogical Approach at Ikaya Primary School

This paragraph describes two incidences of observed corporal punishment at Ikaya Primary School performed by a teacher and a father. One incident

---

27 This particular case can be compared to many similar stories reported in Richter et al. (2004).

occurred when the two observers entered the classroom for an observation session. Ten learners (boys and girls who attended the intervention group) were standing at the front of the class and were being beaten on their hands with an orange stick by their female teacher. The moment she noticed the visitors, she stopped the beating and all the learners went back to their chairs (Lindner & Otto, 2004). The second incident was observed on another observation day in front of the classroom. A young girl from Grade 4 ran past the observers, followed by three other children and a man with an orange stick who tried to catch her. When the man got hold of the girl he started to beat her heavily on her whole body. The observers did not intervene because one of the teachers held them back, explaining that this was the girl's father and he had the right to discipline his child. Several children from different classes observed the scene, most of them belonging to classes that were attended by participants for observation. Not one of the present teachers intervened (Lindner & Otto, 2004).

As a consequence, the third observation phase that was scheduled for March 2004 was cancelled because such traumatic experiences are assumed to cause tremendous changes in the social behaviour of the participants, and also reduce the objectivity of observers. However, if the research question for participant observations would have been based on identifying health hazards in the school environment, which assumingly endangered the success of any health-promoting intervention, then it certainly would have been necessary to take those data into consideration. Therefore, in anticipation of the concluding chapter, the recommendation can be made that further evaluation research in this field should consider including the question of health hazards in the school environment as a fundamental part of the research design.

Furthermore, the description of observed scenes of corporal punishment, even on management level, depicts the practised pedagogical approach at the school. The majority of pedagogical approaches and disciplinary methods at the school demonstrate the strong contrast between the authoritarian and rigid approach that is still being practised in the everyday school setting on the one hand, and the applied life skills programme that follows an open and participatory approach on the other. These disciplinary practices are assumed to have indirectly influenced the project in regard to the enhancement of competencies like problem-solving or psychological factors life self-esteem among participants. The observation of physical abuse was reported to the Stellenbosch School Clinics in the half-yearly report sessions.

7.7 Conclusion

Chapter 7 described the implementation process of the CMP. Coordination was based on educational cooperation between the primary school and two non-governmental organizations working in the field of health promotion on AIDS in South Africa, Joy for Life and Ikamva Lethu Centre. Several local institutions supported the CMP with their expertise and helped to implement it in its physical environment, the Kayamandi community. The pedagogical concept of the implemented CMP strictly followed national guidelines for life skills programmes on AIDS of the National Department of Education (2000). Because the goal of the programme was foremost to strengthen and increase the mental development of the participants, it encompassed a magnitude of topics that surrounded the attendees' demands appropriate to their age and intellectual capacity. The participatory and active teaching methods (e.g. group discussion) followed Bandura's Social Cognitive Theory (1986) in order to allow participants to observe and to test modelled behaviour in their own physical and social context. Specific safety measures such as the code of conduct were introduced in the classroom to ensure an atmosphere that encouraged happiness and well-being.

The two health promotion trainers and the class teacher acted as educational personnel of the intervention group. The health promotion trainers were educated in this specific learning programme and teaching methods, whilst the class teacher, also a member of the project team, was responsible for the netting of the project with the school and needed to ensure the appropriateness of teaching procedures. Parents were invited to five parent meetings to inform them on the presently taught topics and to guarantee their full involvement in their child's educational process.

In addition, the CMP was confronted with several abuse cases that happened outside (e.g. child sexual abuse by a relative) and inside (e.g. corporal punishment) of the school environment. These cases are assumed to have had an additional influence on the project's effectiveness by endangering its main goal to empower and enhance mental health within the individuals.

CHAPTER EIGHT
Assessment of the Programme by Health Promotion Trainers and Learners

8.1 Introduction

It is imperative that monitoring and evaluation are an integral part of a pilot study of this nature. Therefore, chapter 8 exclusively analyses the effect of the model (X) by measuring the cognitive and emotional convictions of all participants, in this case, health promotion trainers and learners. All gathered data on the general attitudes of the health promotion trainers and learners towards the learning programme and its elements will be presented in the following paragraphs. Data were taken from three sources: (1) the HPTs' report, (2) project documentation, which includes final reports from both HPTs written after Intervention I, and (3) learners' reports. Consequently, the main focus of the feedback from HPTs and learners is on the evaluation of Intervention I.

The chapter 8 starts with the presentation of the results gathered from the HPTs' report. These results refer to the HPTs' assessment of their self-confidence with regard to their assessment of the suitability of the teaching methods used in the class, within the framework of the session content. The second part of this chapter contains results from learners' reports containing derived data on the general feeling of comfort in the sessions, their acceptance of the outlined methods and their actual attitude towards learning with their own and the other gender and health promotion trainers.

The last part of chapter portrays the results of the participant observations of two boys and two girls of the intervention group regarding their expressed social behaviour during Intervention I and II. These process data can be used as content validity data and explore further the link between the implementation of the programme and children's achievement (Pellegrini et al., 2004). In other words, with regard to the conviction that the programme can only be effective if it is based on the needs and age of this specific group of children, the instrument was meant to derive information from the observed children's attitude towards and reaction to the implemented programme.

8.2 Results of the HPTs' Reports

As explained in chapter 7, the sessions of the Child Mind Project were carried out by two young women from the Kayamandi community. Previously, the one woman (HPT1) was a voluntary counsellor for HIV patients at the Community Clinic and was specialised in the medical field of sexually transmitted infections. The other woman (HPT2) had volunteered to work in the project for child care and protection by the Child Welfare Organization in Stellenbosch. For the reason that both women's professional backgrounds were not based in the education field, they were trained in the programme content and methods in an extensive three-month workshop before the onset of the intervention, and attended additional workshops during and after Intervention I.

Because both HPTs started as intermediate trainers, it was important to examine their self-reported self-confidence to manage sessions and implement newly learned teaching methods in the classroom context. In other words, the assessment of the HPTs' progress in the accumulation of self-confidence could be an indicator of the accumulation of new technical skills, which could finally increase the quality of the sessions over the course of time.

It was therefore necessary to clarify the following questions: firstly, was there an increase in the health promotion trainers' self-confidence in their teaching ability over the course of Intervention I? A strong belief in the own confidence is significant for internalising new knowledge and being able to deal with new challenges. Thus, a high level of confidence was assumed to be related to an increase in the HPTs' self-confidence to utilise new methods, to identify with their position as trainers and to harmonise their relationship within the team, which undoubtedly also had an effect on their relationship with the class. And secondly, whether the HPTs, as experts, regarded the applied methods as appropriate for the taught topic? This question was meant to assess if in the opinion of the HPTs the used methods were able to pass on knowledge and skills to the learners effectively. With regard to the assumed low literacy level of the participants and the disadvantaged educational setting, the methods needed to be implemented in an as easy practicable way as possible. This meant that those methods assumed to have the greatest learning effect on the participants had to be applied.

The following paragraph will start with the description of the health promotion trainers reporting from their subjective perspectives view on the success and difficulties of their work in order to depict the teaching and classroom context. In this way the HPTs also assessed the suitability of the outlined intervention.

8.2.1 Analysis of the Data by the Project Documentation

The following paragraphs utilise the results of the project documentation, including the health promotion trainers' final reports, to clarify the results from the following weekly health promotion trainers' reports. In these reports the health promotion trainers assessed the programme in three ways: (1) the quality of the relations between the HPTs and with learners, (2) the suitability of the applied methods and quality of teaching, and finally (3) the changes in the learners' behaviour as an indicator of successful teaching.

The Quality of Relations in the Classroom Setting

It became already clear during the workshop sessions that the health promotion trainers would act according to their personal abilities, skills and fields of interests in the classroom. They established in the first session a specific working relationship in which HPT1 took over a leading position in the key teaching methods. Health promotion trainer 2, the younger and less experienced trainer, acted as supportive partner in individual tasks and group work, and ensured the learners' attentiveness in the classroom. This work relation was reported to be pleasant for both women. Interacting together in a team was of extreme importance in order to implement the project successfully, and could also have contributed to their being at ease when teaching. It can be assumed that the quality of the established partnership increased the confidence to tackle new tasks and to increase their own skills as health promotion trainers. The spontaneously developed and clearly divided fields of responsibility in the classroom setting established a solid partnership between the HPTs over the course of Intervention I.

The relationship to the children in the intervention group was assessed as positive and functioning on a basis of mutual respect. HPT1 expressed that she was proud that she was not only regarded as an educator but also as a friend. HPT2 described working with learners as 'marvellous' and reported that she was proud to be part of their group as an educator.

Although the children's recognition of their work was sensed, the relationship with the children's parents, in contrast, was described as ambivalent. The greatest criticism by the HPTs was expressed when parent meetings were organised and the majority of parents did not participate in those. For example, in her report, HPT2 regretted that only four parents came to the interim parent meeting whose purpose was to convey information on the sex education session and ensure that both parents and trainers would feel comfortable with the proposed methods used in the session. Even though the absence of parents was also interpreted as a disregard of their work, HPT1 stated conciliatory that, despite the absence of many parents, those who did come to the interim parent meeting said that they were impressed by the work they had done. In her final report to the parents she wrote the following statement: "As the educators we can really make a difference in your child's life" – an expression of her great pride in her own work.

The Suitability of Applied Methods and Quality of Teaching

The following paragraphs describe the HPTs' experiences with the most important teaching methods and explain their assessment of these methods' practicability during the sessions in Intervention I. The data used were again obtained from the project documentation.

Frontal teaching was emphasised by the HPTs' as very important when new topics were introduced or already existing (false) knowledge had to be reshaped in the minds of the participants. *Individual work* was usually combined with art or games. It was stated that to avoid a too demanding situation for children the individual work methods need to be clearly introduced, explained and supervised by educational personnel. For example, during one session each child received two photocopies, each showing a set of cards. The first set of cards displayed different situations where adults interact with children in an unambiguous or ambiguous situation. The other set of cards displayed children's faces expressing various feelings. The two sets of cards had to be matched by the learners, so that each facial expression was matched with the suitable situation. The children needed two sessions with repeated explanation to be able to do this individual work. A male learner (L.) stated: "I am totally confused about all these feelings."

Conducting a *group discussion* was noted as extremely difficult in a class of more than 40 learners of this young age. Firstly, without correct guidance the most confident learners dominated the discussion in the groups, and therefore influenced group results. Secondly, groups should be guided by trainers because learners with such a low level of literacy need support in making written notes for later presentation of group results. However, while learners preferred to present the group results orally at the beginning of Intervention I, HPTs reported that the children's' reading and writing skills improved over the course of time, although their level of literacy was still low. They presented their group results in the form of written notes in English or isiXhosa.

The separation of children in *gender-specific group work* was assessed as important for a comfortable feeling for children during the sessions "Inner and Reproductive Organs" (Session 8) and "What is Sex all about?" (Session 9). The gender separation made it easy for the boys and girls to balance feelings of shame and interest, especially when the learners had questions they preferred to ask to someone of their own gender. Several interesting incidences occurred during these sessions: Some boys touched other boys to see if the organs were in the 'right' place and made fun of it. Girls tended to touch their own bodies and silently asked other girls questions. In regard to the separation of gender inside of one room, it can be concluded from this experience that the first session was extremely important for the learning process of the individual about him- or herself and the other. Subsequent to this experience, games or sport activities were implemented after sessions on very sensitive and taboo issues to allow learners to relax by experiencing physical freedom and enjoyment in the group, for example after the sex education session.

Methods which included art, such as songs were described as especially liked by the learners despite the limited resources of things like colour crayons and pencils. These tasks were easily supervised by the HPTs. The *drama play* on two abusive situations was assessed as extremely impressive for the learners. The drama play was acted out by a group of young actors from the community. It was a method that deeply touched the emotions of the participants and anticipated negative feelings such as personal fear. The HPTs deemed it essential that further similar interventions should also provide the children with emotional aftercare. *Experiential learning*, such as the wound treatment in Session 15 turned out to be very effective in the HPTs' opinion. Learners worked in mixed gender groups and treated someone's fictitious wound. The practical use of this newly learned skill could thus be proven in a real situation. The class teacher had a small wound on her arm on that day. By treating the teacher's wound, one of the girls performed the first aid she had learned – and all the other learners in the classroom could observe this action first hand.

The *self-confidence sentence* was described as playing a big role in improving self-confidence. After Session 2 (*Self-Esteem*) the project team decided to implement the confidence sentence as a constant ritual encouraging confidence. The sentence was meant to be an entrance-ritual to open each session and become a strong incentive to encourage learners to be brave and more confident during the sessions during the course of the programme. Although, HPT1 took over a critical position towards this instrument throughout the Intervention I; in her final report she stated that the children knew the sentence by heart and that they had accepted this ritual at the beginning of each lesson.

Apart from the increase in self-confidence and skills among the HPTs, it was also found that teaching methods like group work or brainstorming were difficult to implement in the classroom. Both HPTs concluded in their reports that more workshops and practice were needed to improve teaching skills and classroom management over time. For example, HPT2 assessed her own professional qualification as often too friendly and said she was afraid of losing control over the class, which she had experienced during the absence of her partner. The loss of control happened during a conflict between two boys, which she felt incapable to solve while being alone in the classroom. The statement expresses, on the one hand, that she obviously enjoyed working as part of a team much more than working as an individual in front of the class and, on the other hand, her great need to improve conflict management skills so as to feel personally safe within the classroom environment and become capable of fulfilling her role as a trainer – even in difficult situations.

Other problematic fields included the tight time schedule, which they felt hindered the effective application of methods. HPT1 mentioned that this problem occurred in the last lesson in particular, where too little time was available to thoroughly cover the topic ("When someone I love dies"). She also suggested that at the end of each session there should be more sport activities, for example soccer or netball.

Perceived Changes in the Children's Behaviour

In their last report for the project documentation the health promotion trainers had to state whether they perceived changes in the children's behaviour as a result of them focussing it from the start of the programme until the end of Intervention I.

In their reports, HPT1 and HPT2 stated that they had noticed a change in the girls' behaviour in particular over the course of Intervention I. They said they had observed that the boys were more self-confident than the girls, who seemed to be shy and less confident at the start of the project. After four sessions the girls seemed to feel free and more confident, because they started to ask more questions during these sessions than ever before. As an impressive example of this, HPT2 reported an incident with one of the youngest girls. HPT2 opened a condom during the session on HIV/AIDS to show it to the class. After the lesson the girl came to her to tell her to wash her hands after touching the condom. HPT1 described it as an 'amazing' story because the child did not only link the knowledge from the previous session on hygiene (Session 10) with sexual health hygiene learned in the session on condom use (Session 11), but also acted as an 'instructor', which is not part of the authoritarian educational system at school.

Both health promotion trainers agreed that discussion (communication) in the class increased with group work. They were also convinced that children enjoyed working with each other more towards the end of Intervention I.

> They could even discuss between one another without being afraid of saying what was on their minds. I do not regret that I enjoyed it because I experienced many things and learned about myself. I just want to say that they took part in everything we ask them. They enjoyed themselves during the lessons. I was impressed when they were playing the doctor dressing a wounded patient. (HPT2)

Both women described these changes observed in the children as the result of their work: The fact that they could see positive changes in the interaction between girls and boys, as well as among them, were regarded as indicative of their success.

8.2.2 Analysis of Data by the HPTs' Report

The following results were gathered from the health promotion trainers' reports, in which the trainers were asked to give their opinion on their assessment of their self-confidence in their position as trainers and the suitability of the applied method within the framework of the topic. The results were assessed on a 5-point scale ranging from 1 (excellent) to 5 (bad).

Assessment of the HPTs' Self-Confidence

Regarding the assessment of the HPTs' self-confidence[28], HPT1 started at a high level (Session 2, $M=2.25$) and maintained this level until Session 9 *(What is Sex all about?)* ($M=2.00$), with a relapse in Session 8 *(Body Changes)* ($M=2.33$). From Session 10 *(Health and Hygiene)* ($M=1.75$) to Session 12 *(HIV/AIDS)* ($M=1.20$) an increase in the assessment level of HPT1's self-confidence is visible. A relapse occurred in the first session (13) on rape and abuse ($M=2.00$), which can be attributed to the new and demanding content of the topic. Her self-confidence increased again in the last two sessions.

Health promotion trainer 2 started off more self-critical in Sessions 2 *(Self-Esteem)* ($M=2.75$) to 5 *(Relationships in Family)* ($M=3.00$). The self-

---

28 Session 1 and 11 are not depicted in the analysis. Session 1 functioned as a pretest of the instrument. There was also no report in session 11 because one of the HPTs was absent due to illness.

assessment level increased in Session 6 *(Friendship)* (M=1.33) and decreased slightly in Session 8 *(Body Changes)* (M=2.00), after which she scored better than 2. In Session 10 *(Keeping the Body safe and healthy)* (M=1.60) and session 12 *(HIV/AIDS)* (M=1.20) the means measured match (or almost match) the means of HPT1 and finally exceeded the self-assessment results of HPT1 up to Session 15 *(Care and Death)* (M=1.00). Finally, HPT2 ends with an excellent (M=1.00) assessment of her self-confidence.

In summary, HPT1 had a high level of self-confidence right from the beginning and more or less maintained this throughout the programme. A factor contributing to this high self-confidence level could be the fact that during Intervention I HPT1 linked the newly acquired knowledge with topics from her previous working field in the clinic. The means indicate that her confidence in her teaching increased with the presentation of known knowledge, for example AIDS prevention (Session 12). HPT2 started at a lower level, which increased over the course of time and even exceeded the level of HPT1 at the end.

Although the derived data can lead to the conclusion that HPT1 has a steady confidence and HPT2 has a growing confidence, the data have to be focussed with care and can be regarded as misleading, because both health promotion trainers assessed their 'professional' confidence as ranging from predominantly excellent (1) to good (2). The derived results can be explained by three reasons. Firstly, an overestimation of their work could be the result of saving face in front of the assessor. Secondly, they assessed their own work as extremely valuable as any kind of self-criticism could be regarded as a personal failure and could lead to the withdrawal from the project. Campbell (2003) found similar results in her qualitative survey with peer educators in the Caltonville Project. Finally, the self-evaluation of one's own confidence is a demanding tool which is influenced by internal, dispositional, as well as external and causal factors that adulterate the scores in self-assessments.

Assessment of the Suitability of the Methods

The results of the scale 'Suitability of Methods' by the HPTs indicate that up to Session 5 *(Friendship)* HPT1 tended to assess methods less critically (M=2.00) than HPT2 (M=2.75).

In Session 6 *(Family and Friendship)*, both trainers changed their assessment of the suitability of the methods (class discussion, brainstorming, individual work): HPT1 took a more critical stand (M=2.00) than HPT2 (M=1.67), while HPT2 also showed a stronger positive trend than HPT1. They held this position until the end of the intervention. Exceptions are

Session 3 *(Self-Esteem)* and Session 10 *(Keeping my Body safe and healthy)*, where both HPTs reached the same mean ($M=2.30$, $M=1.80$) for the methods used (confidence sentence, frontal teaching, and individual work).

With regard to applied methods, HPT1 assessed the suitability of the methods (frontal teaching and discussion in class) most critically in Session 3 *(Self-Esteem)* ($M=2.80$), Session 7 *(Body Changes and Growing-up*; frontal teaching, explanation, mixed group work) ($M=2.27$), and Session 12 *(HIV/AIDS*; frontal teaching, distribution of contraceptives) ($M=2.20$). HPT2 assessed the suitability of the methods in Session 2 *(Self-Esteem)* to 4 *(Relationships and Family)* and scored better than 2 from there on. Both HPTs regarded the methods (drama play and card game) used in Session 14 *(Abuse)* as the most appropriate to lesson content.

On the whole, the results show that both HPTs assessed the method suitability most critically at the beginning of Intervention I. Over the course of time, they rated the methods from excellent to average and unanimously expressed a positive tendency, while the HPT2 is showing a more positive trend than HPT2. In other words, the suitability of the methods was regarded as predominantly appropriate for the content of the various sessions, and therefore both HPTs came to the conclusion that the methods used were suitable for implementation in the programme when working with this specific target group.

The Link between the HPTs' Assessed Self-Confidence and the Suitability of the Applied Methods

In order to understand the link between the HPTs' self-confidence and their assessment of the applied methods it is imperative to present the results of both scales for each HPT at this point of discussion. Figure 8.1 and 8.2 combine all the results and give an indication of the trend set. The presented figures in this paragraph present the means assessed on a 5-point scale ranging from 1 (excellent) to 5 (bad). For a better understanding of the results, the scores on the scale are reversed and specifically explained numbers in the text are bold marked on the graphs.

HPT1 tends to assess herself more positively than the suitability of the applied method most of the time. In order to provide more detailed information on the actual scoring of the methods by HPT1, specific scores are presented. HPT1 assessed most critical session 3 the confidence sentence, showing HPT1's resistance towards the method. Furthermore, frontal teaching (score 4) and group work (score 3) in Session 7 and decision-making in mixed groups (score 4) in Session 12 were also assessed by her as being most inappropriate. This means, the negative scores point to two methods, namely frontal teaching and group work, and one newly implemented method ('decision making') which can be assumed to be the most difficult to apply in a classroom setting. In all three sessions HPT1's critical analysis could be regarded as an indication of extreme responsibility and, to a certain extent, a feeling of overload during these sessions, because she bore the greatest responsibility for teaching and discussions (Figure 8.1).

In figure 8.2 HPT2 shows an almost matching assessment of herself and the suitability of the methods with a positive trend over the course of Intervention I. A minimal difference occurs in Session 8 *(Inner and Reproductive Organs)* where she assesses the method activity more positively (M=1.33) than her own preparation to carry out the method (M=2.00) in the classroom setting.

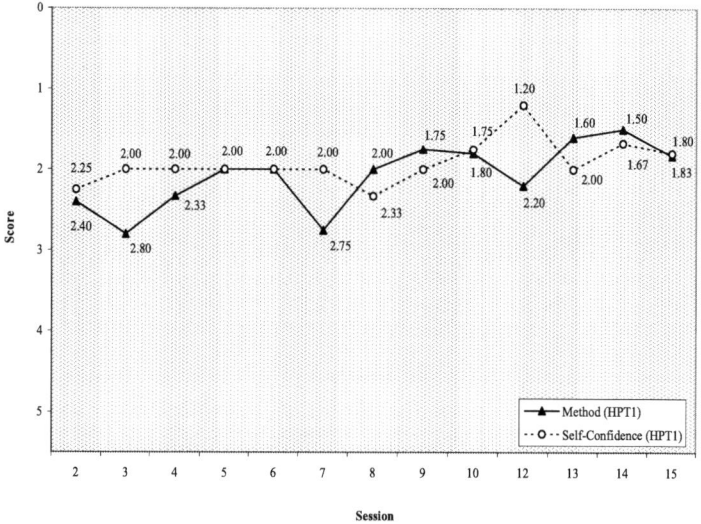

Figure 8.1. Comparison between Results of Self-Assessment and Method by Health Promotion Trainer 1 (HPT1).

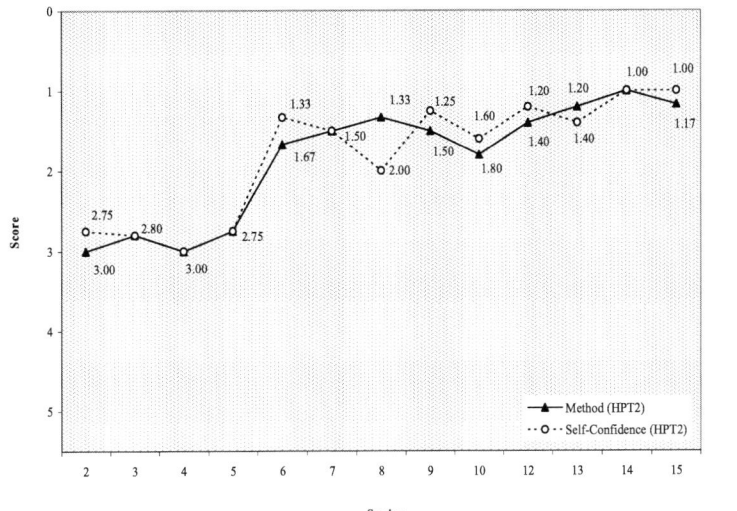

Figure 8.2. Comparison between Results of Self-Assessment and Method by Health Promotion Trainer 2 (HPT2).

In summary, both HPTs maintained a constant or slowly increasing level of self-confidence and assessment of the suitability of the teaching methods in the classroom setting over the course of time. The gained results predominantly reflect that both HPTs assessed the suitability of the applied method in a similar fashion to their own self-confidence to carry out the method in the classroom. The strongest discrepancies between both scales by HPT1 and HPT2 appear in Sessions 3 *(Self-Esteem)*, 7 *(Body Changes and Growing-up)* and 12 *(HIV/AIDS)*. The results of HPT1 indicate that she took a critical stand against the methods used more often and assessed her own confidence in a more positive way than the methods. These results signify her more responsible position in the sessions and her greater responsibility to implement methods effectively. The results also indicate a stronger 'learning course' for HPT2 than for HPT1. HPT2's more positive results could be a result of the partnership existing in the education sessions – she had a supportive and self-confident partner with whom she implemented methods during these sessions.

8.3 Results of Learners' Reports

The following results are taken from the weekly learners' report that examined the learners' attitudes towards the programme (see chapter 6, par. 3.3). The gathered data are analysed in regard to the learners' general attitude towards the evaluated programme, their feeling comfortable with the programme content and the used methods, their acceptance of the HPTs, and their feeling comfortable about being in a learning situation with learners from the same and other gender. The quality of the relations, which should be based on fairness, mutual respect, understanding and trust, should therefore support the acquisition of knowledge and new competencies. It is thus believed that the quality of comfort is seen as an integral part of an emotional construct that enhances the quality of perception and therefore frames the learning process during the intervention sessions on the individual level.

8.3.1 Learners' General Attitude towards the Life Skills Programme

The number of participating learners ranged from 35 to 45. The learners' general attitude in thirteen sessions during Intervention I is divided into three categories: (1) fun, (2) ok, and (3) boring. More than 90% of the girls expressed that they had had 'fun' and only a minority, 9% of the girls, reported they had felt 'ok' during Intervention I (Figure 8.3).

Almost two thirds of the boys expressed that they had had 'fun' (61%) or felt 'ok' (9%) while almost one third of the boys (30%) expressed that they had been bored during the sessions in Intervention I (Figure 8.4). The results thus reveal a strong discrepancy between female and male attendees' attitude towards the programme. While, the general attitude of female attendees tended to be similar, their male counterparts expressed a more critical point of view during the complete Intervention I.

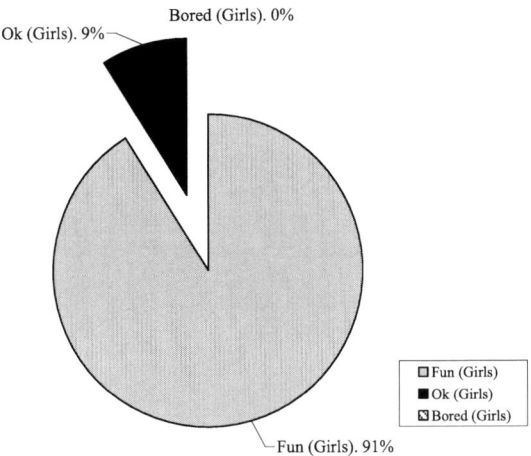

Figure 8.3. Girls' General Attitude towards the Life Skills Programme during Intervention I.

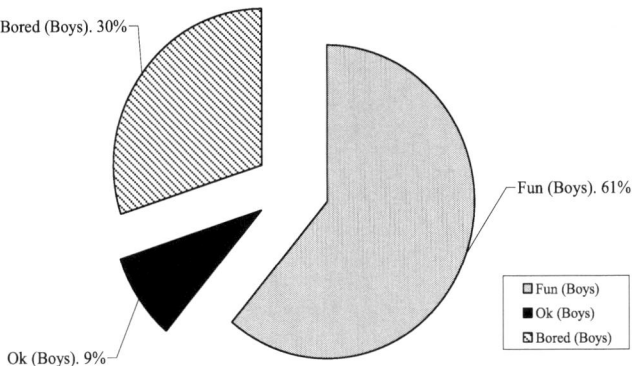

Figure 8.4. Boys' General Attitude towards the Life Skills Programme during Intervention I.

Several conclusions for the presented gender differences in attitude towards the programme can be made. First, girls expressed not only a more balanced attitude towards the programme but they also had a greater need for and interest in the programme topics and methods.[29] Second, boys examined the programme more critically concerning the sessions *Relationship within Family* (part 2=38%), *Body Anatomy* (47%) and *Sexual Abuse* (part 1=33%; part 2=41%).

Three assumptions for these gender differences are possible which are not to be answered satisfactory in this study. Either the used methods or topics were less interesting to the boys because they have received information through other channels while the girls used the sessions as a source of not discussed or unavailable information in their social and cultural surrounding. The boys expressed a greater sensitivity towards the content of the sessions than the girls or the information given in the sessions were more appropriate to the girl's need, for example because of their continued developmental stage, compared to the boys' need of information. Apart from the gender differences, the results gathered also show that the class reached a state of equilibrium over time in terms of their attitude towards the project (not reflected in the graphs).

8.3.2 Comfort with Programme Content and Methods

When it came to the children's level of comfort regarding the programme content and methods applied, the learners were additionally asked to express if they liked or disliked the topic presented in a particular session. The majority of girls (96%) and boys (91%) liked the outlined topics in Intervention I. Girls reported the greatest dislike (≤10%) of three sessions: *Self-Esteem* (12%), *Relationships and Family* (12%), and *HIV/AIDS* (15%) (Figure 8.5). Boys, again, tended to be more critical in their attitude than girls. The dislike category was chosen by boys in all topics, except for the session *Sexual Abuse* (part 1) (Figure 8.6). Boys also reported the greatest dislike (≤10%) of the sessions *Self-Esteem* (18%), *Body Anatomy* (12%), *Health and Hygiene* (20%), *HIV/AIDS* (Part 1=12%), *Sexual Abuse* (Part 2=12%) and *Care and Death* (11%).

---

29 It was relinquished to present the results in figures at this point.

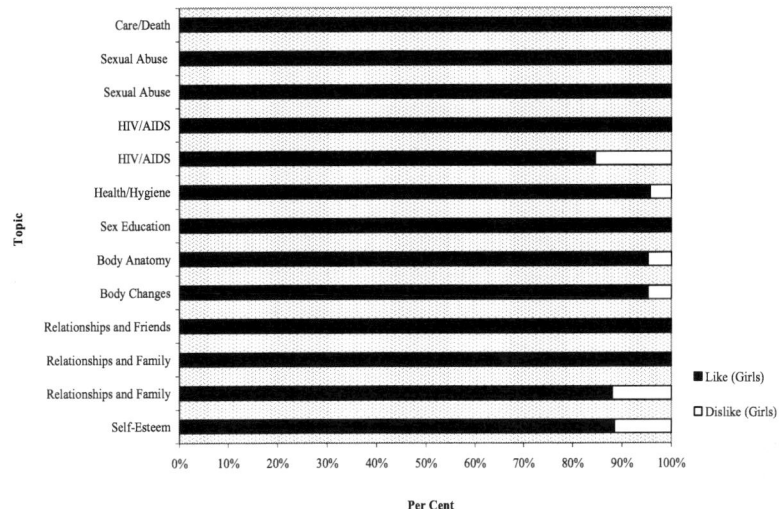

Figure 8.5. Illustration of the Results on the Assessment of Like and Dislike towards Content and used Method by Girls of the Intervention Group.

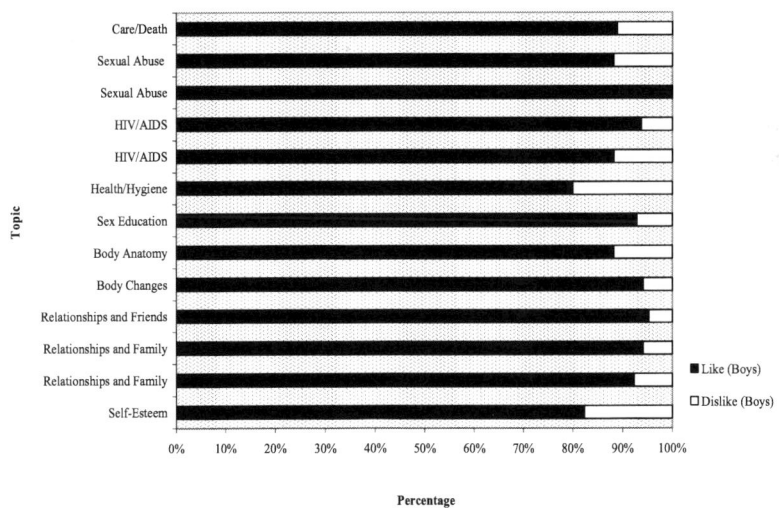

Figure 8.6. Illustration of the Results on the Assessment of Like and Dislike towards Content and used Method by Boys of the Intervention Group.

Boys and girls were also asked to assess the methods applied during the sessions by expressing their like or dislike. The methods were divided into seven categories: (1) games (fun games and sport), (2) art (music, making collages, and drama), (3) group discussion, (4) brainstorming, (5) frontal teaching, (6) food event, and (7) video. The majority of girls and boys enjoyed the methods applied in the sessions. Only a small percentage disliked the used methods. Those boys who expressed their dislike criticised frontal teaching (20%), the video (21%), and group discussion (13%) specifically in mixed gender groups. Girls expressed the greatest dislike of games (15%) and the video (9%).[30]

8.3.3 Relations within the Classroom Setting

The assessment of the quality of relations between learners and HPTs and learners and learners of the same and of the other gender is a defining indicator for prevailing classroom atmosphere or feelings of comfort among attendees. The majority of the girls (99%) and boys (90%) emphasised that they had felt comfortable working with female HPTs. However, looking at specific sessions it becomes obvious that almost 20% of the boys disliked working with female HPTs during the sessions *Body Changes* (18%), *HIV/AIDS* (19%), *Abuse* (18%), and *Care and Death* (18%). One assumption that can be drawn from these results is that boys expressed a dislike of working with female HPTs in sensitive and culturally relevant sessions. Although the HPTs divided the group into homogenous groups and one HPT specifically worked with boys, they still expressed that they felt somewhat uncomfortable to work with the (female) HPT. Without being able to provide data in greater detail, one can assume that a male HPT would possibly increase the feeling of comfort within the participating boys when it came to these intimate issues.

The learners' attitude towards the same and the opposite gender reflect the working relationships between girls and boys during the sessions. In addition, it should be assessed if there were any changes in gender relation during Intervention I. Girls as well as boys express a high percentage of feeling comfortable to work with the same gender. When certain sessions are clustered however, gender differences become evident in the data. While 40% of the girls enjoyed working with boys, only 29% of the boys enjoyed working with girls throughout Intervention I. Only in four of the sessions

---

30 As a side note, the video was shown in English during the sexual abuse session. The learners had great difficulty to follow the story and it had to be repeatedly interrupted to clarify the content with learners.

more boys said that they enjoyed working with girls than girls working with boys, namely the sessions *Body Changes* (41%), *Sex Education* (44%), and *Care and Death* (47%). The most interesting finding is that in the session on body changes and sex education boys and girls were seated separately, which obviously helped to make the boys feel more comfortable – but not the girls. This finding could suggest a local separation of genders especially when dealing with intimate elements.

In summary, although no change in relations was found over time, the work relations between boys and girls and learners and HPTs can predominantly be assessed as supportive for the duration of Intervention I – no negative interactions, events and refusals are known which indicates a positive class atmosphere. Most importantly, these data on the children's' comfort provide important clues towards changing lesson designs and/or implementing methods to increase the participants' comfort.

8.4 Evaluating Social Behaviour of Four Children

A good description of children's behaviour (reaction) within an educational programme such as a life skills programme is a precondition to evaluate whether the outlined intervention is based on the specific needs of the children (Pellegrini et al., 2004) – their developmental stage and tasks considered – and whether it has reached its aim to support the development of social and cognitive competencies among participants. In other words, the participant observations intended to provide information on the expressed social behaviour of the participants who attended the Intervention I and II over a period of six months. The observations also intended to observe the development of the children's verbal and body language, their ability to communicate with other learners, and the expression of their own opinion in interaction with others, especially peers (boys and girls in class) and facilitators (health promotion trainers and participating teacher) during the sessions of Intervention I and II.

Observation Phase I took place during Intervention I for four-and-a-half months from March 2003 until June 2003; Observation Phase II for one-and-a-half month during Intervention II from October 2003 until November 2003. Four children were observed, two boys and two girls within the age range 9 to 12 years. All observations took place during intervention sessions in the specific classroom of the observed children at Ikaya Primary School in Kayamandi. Each participant was observed for 15 minutes every second week during the intervention sessions. Taking into consideration that the results of the interobserver reliability and the interobserver agreement (see chapter 6, par. 3.4) were merely unsatisfactory, the following observation results described were mainly taken from the descriptive part of the instrument.

8.4.1 Participant (A) – Observation Results

Participant A is female and 10 years old. Her position in the classroom changed during Intervention I as she moved from a group with the youngest girls (9 years and younger) in the class to a group with seven girls of her age (10-11 years). She showed a 'willing' attitude towards the sessions in Observation Phase I. In Observation Phase II, she expressed a combination of a willing and an undecided attitude towards the sessions without preference for group or individual work. It can be assumed that the undecided attitude is linked to the activities in the classroom (topic and method), her seating position (she sat with her body turned to the HPTs due to the crowded classroom conditions and table positions) and/or the relation to the HPTs who changed their composition in the second session.

> Participant A expressed predominantly a willing attitude in Observation Phase I and was undecided in Observation Phase II.

Participant A started off with a passive body language at the beginning of Observation Phase I and expressed an active body language at the end of this observation phase, with a shifting combination in Observation Phase II. Active body language was expressed by sitting straight, looking in the direction of the HPTs and concentrating on their explanations. Passive body language was expressed by putting her upper body on the table and playing with something in her hands; an expression of boredom. Most of the positive body language was directed towards other female classmates at the table where she was seated.

> *The participant's body language was mainly positive and open and stabilised during Observation Phase I. An unbalanced character of body language was observed in the two sessions in Observation Phase II.*

In regard to communication level, participant A kept quiet half of the time. Although her use of language decreased from Observation Phase I to II, she maintained a constant language use towards other female learners at her table only, and communicated freely and openly with other girls in the class and the HPTs. Her behaviour towards the trainers was more open in the course of Observation Phase I and she started to freely ask the HPTs questions towards the end of Observation Phase I, again, with an unsteady character in Observation Phase II.

> The participant's communication increased with the formation of a group of four girls in her age from Observation Phase I and II observable.

During Observation Phase I, participant A socialised and physically interacted after being seated at a table with girls of her age. During this phase, she started to express her own opinion mostly during interactions with other female learners among whom she expressed to feel comfortable. In the last two sessions of Observation Phase I, she established a friendship with a girl next to her; the friendship was observed to still exist in Observation Phase II. Other interactions with boys or other girls not sitting at her table could not be observed. However, the use of these data is restricted due to limitations in the observation process in Observation Phase II.

> In Observation Phase I participant A developed her interaction skills with one girl in particular; establishment of same-gender friendship.

> Because of difficulties in the observation process, the observers were not able to evaluate the third category in Observation Phase II due to missing visual contact; the last category isn't therefore part of the analysis.

8.4.2 Participant (B) – Observation Results

Participant B is female and 10 years old. She kept the same position in the classroom, but the composition of learners at the table changed from a table with six girls (Observation Phase I) to a table with four boys and two girls (Observation Phase II). The participant's character was assessed as strongly introverted; her attitude was therefore assessed as varying between willing and undecided. Due to the participant's passive/immobile body language, nonverbal expression and communication, it was often difficult for the observer to judge her attitude towards the programme in Observation Phase I. In the two observation sessions during Observation Phase II, she showed a willing attitude towards the programme sessions.

➤ Participant B expressed an ambivalent attitude towards Observation Phase I and a willing attitude towards Observation Phase II.

Shyness and a cautious body language were observed half of the time due to her introverted character; her body language became less positive when she had to perform in front of the class (as happened once). In both observation phases she limited her body language to moving the upper body in the trainers' direction, expressed lapses in concentration whilst fulfilling the outlined task, and observed processes in class without becoming actively involved. Participant B's body language only became more active during individual work sessions on topics that were mentally and emotionally more demanding (drama play). The participant did not change her body expression over time.

➤ The participant did not show a significant change in body language throughout Observation Phase I and II.

Special communication with other classmates could not be observed in Observation Phase I. She hardly showed any active/direct communication with the group at the table during observation time. When she communicated with others she made no distinction between male and female and it was of a friendly nature. An exception regarding communication was during the session on HIV/AIDS (repetition), where she increased her communication with other female and male learners during group work. A completely opposite behaviour was observed in the following session where individual work was required. Again, she did not communicate at all with classmates at her table.

➤ Participant B's communication skills remained unchanged from Observation Phase I to II.

For the most part of the observation participant B expressed a willingness to participate in the sessions by concentrating on the explanations of the HPTs, or on achieving the task in both observation sessions. Due to her low communication or interaction skills, no change could be observed in her ability to express her own opinion towards others – neither in Observation Phase I nor in Observation Phase II. Only in one group work session on HIV/AIDS a greater frequency of interaction with other learners in the group was observed.

➤ Because changes in interaction skills could not be observed, consequently, no direct expression of her own opinion was visible.

8.4.3 Participant (C) – Observation Results

Participant C is male and 9 years old. His position in the classroom was mainly in a group of boys. In the last sessions, participant C sat in a group with two boys and three girls. Participant C expressed a willing attitude throughout both observation phases. He showed a positive attitude towards trainers/authorities, for example, his general orientation together with his ability to listen and follow advice. He did not make a distinction between group and individual work sessions.

- Participant C showed a positive general attitude towards the intervention in Observation Phase I and II.

He expressed a predominantly positive body language. However, restless body movements were observed in both observation sessions. When he was working on an individual task he displayed a positive body language as a sign of concentration. However, whenever participant C was bored he tended to express a restless and negative body language (e.g. lying on the table, playing with something). In those sessions, he could be easily distracted from work. Also in stressful situations (e.g. volume level in class, sex education session), he reacted with increased physical activity. However, the occurrence of restless behaviour decreased over the course of Observation Phase I and II.

- Participant C increased his open and positive body language in the course of Observation Phase I and II.

Regarding communication participant C used spoken language for half the time in both observation sessions. At the beginning of Observation Phase I, he communicated more often through nonverbal expression (e.g. facial expression). His communication with the boys and girls was balanced and most of the time friendly. During the second observation session, there was an ongoing communication with the girls and one boy at his table.

- At the beginning of Observation Phase I, he had a preference for using nonverbal communication tools. This changed during the course of Observation Phase I to an increased use of verbal communication with others without preference to communicate with girls or boys.

Participant C generally expressed his own opinion well among learners and HPTs, with the result that he attracted the most attention at his table. Participant C functioned well in both mixed and same gender groups. For example, during Observation Phase I, a girl hit him with her hand; he reacted with neither physical nor verbal aggression but used ignorance. He never dominated discussions and was willing to accept girls' and boys' opinions equally. Although he accepted the HPTs' authoritative role he expressed his own opinion when he talked to or answered questions of the HPTs. For example, during the session on abuse (drama play) he was one of the few learners who asked questions with courage and self-esteem. This can be regarded as the ability to express his opinion. He showed a higher potential for participation during group work sessions. Participant C established a friendship with another boy towards the end of Intervention phase II.

> Participant C expressed throughout both observation phases well-developed interaction skills, as well as an ability to express his own opinion.

8.4.4 Participant (D) – Observation Results

Participant D is male and 12 years old. Initially his position in the classroom was in a group of mixed gender. At the end of Observation Phase I, he was seated with his back to the HPTs in a group of four boys. Participant D has an introverted character. He expressed a constant willing attitude throughout the duration of Observation Phases I and II.

> Participant D's general attitude remained stable throughout Observation Phase I and II.

Participant D was predominantly open and active in his body language in both observation phases. Cautious body language that expressed a particular interest could be observed depending on the different topics in the lessons (e.g. HIV/AIDS). Higher levels of passive body language were expressed during communication with others. His body was usually turned to the HPTs during black board teaching, which expressed attentiveness, as opposed to his original seating position where he had to sit with his back to the HPTs.

> The participant's body language remained open and active throughout Observation Phases I and II. Characteristics and movement were clearly linked to the acquisition of information in specific topics during the sessions.

Although participant D increased his communication skills over time, it remained unsteady and on a low level during both observation phases. After the gender composition at his table was changed to include only boys, he expressed an increased ability to communicate. Participant D never communicated actively out of his self and he spoke foremost with the boys at his table. He showed a strong increase in communication frequency in the session on inner organs (Observation Phase I) in which he communicated directly with several boys while being locally separated from girls.

- The participant's language ability increased over the observation periods, although on an inconsistent basis. He clearly expressed a preference to communicate with boys.

His willingness and expression of his own opinion increased from Observation Phase I to II, although he did not often communicate with peers. On the one hand an increase in interaction with others (boys) and an expression of own opinion was observed (e.g. when his neighbour asked him a question or when he did not understand the task he would ask another boy at his table). On the other hand an increase in his ability to express his own opinion was observed (e.g. an increased/improved ability to question the trainers about the presented material/information) at the end of Observation Phase II. However, due to the fact that he was older than the other learners, participant D was easily bored and not challenged enough in tasks; other learners often needed more time. Although he was capable of effective group work, his preference for individual work corresponded with his preference for becoming active without 'wasting time' by talking with others, that is, by avoiding negotiation processes with the group. This was not only due to an increased capability to express his opinion, brought about by the influence of the programme or its developmental stage, but most likely also due to environmental factors – he possibly felt more secure with an increased and established social network in the class (friendships/community of boys).

- The participant expressed a change in interaction and an increased ability to express his own opinion from Observation I to II. This was also shown by an increased/improved ability to lead the group of boys at his table and to ask for more information and presented material in the sessions.

8.4.5 Summary of the Results of Participant Observation

With regard to social learning processes, the following can be deduced regarding the participants from Observation Phase I to II (Table 8.1).[31]

(1) All four participants showed a positive, or at least, an ambivalent attitude towards the sessions, in other words, none of the participants expressed a refusal to participate in the sessions of the programme.
(2) Three of the four participants developed a more open and positive body language from Observation Phase I to Observation Phase II.
(3) Three of the four participants showed an increased use of language and all four improved their interaction skills over time.
(4) All participants interacted well in work relations with the same gender; one female (B) and one male (C) participant did not distinguish between interaction with boys and girls.
(5) None of the participants expressed extreme forms of behaviour, for instance aggressive body language, rude language, or dominant or subordinate behaviour, during Observation Phase I and II (Table 8.3).
(6) The level and stability of changes among variables such as body language, communication and interaction skills were assessed as not constant due to the short duration of the intervention and the children's developmental change from late childhood to early adolescence.

However, the positive results of the participant observations can not only be taken as proof of the positive effects of the model, i.e. the life skills programme on AIDS and sex education. For example, with regard to same gender relations, two of the four participants (A, C) established a friendship, and one participant (D, male) started to build a friendship with one boy. The occurrence of same gender friendships can be linked to the developmental transmission stage of late pre-adolescence to early adolescence, which includes the establishment of stronger peer relations.

---

31 In addition, these results were not found to be prevalent in the analysis of Observation Phase III, which was cancelled as a result of conditions during 'normal' lessons.

Table 8.1.
Observation Results from Observation Phase I and II of the four Participants
– Verification or Falsification of the applied Research Hypothesis.

Hypotheses	A	B	C	D
I. If the participant expressed a more positive general attitude towards the intervention over time, the participant has affected his/her social behaviour.	X/–	X/–	X	X
II. If the participant showed a more open and positive body language in the intervention over time, the intervention has affected the participant's social behaviour.	X	–	X	X
III. If the participant increased his/her ability to use language as a way of communicating with others, the intervention has affected the participant's social behaviour.	X	–	X	X
IV. If the participant increased his/her ability to express his/her opinion towards others within situations of interaction and communication, the participant's social behaviour has increased because of the intervention.	X/–	–	X	X

Note. X = hypothesis is verified, – = hypothesis is falsified, X/– = result not unequivocal

With regard to the question whether the participants reacted differently during group work and individual work, the result was the following: One female participant (B) and the two male participants (C, D) reacted on specific topics, namely drama play, HIV/AIDS repetition, inner organs or AIDS (first session). Group work seems to have encouraged participants to increase their communication skills and demanded more interaction with others. Only participant A did not make a distinction in her attitude towards individual or group work methods. Thus, method preference seems to be linked to participants' character, as expressed by participants B and D who showed a preference for individual work due to their introverted character, while the more extroverted and physically restless participant C preferred both methods as long as he was kept active.

Finally, it must also be emphasised that structural frameworks such as seating position, gender composition at tables, and available physical space affected the feeling of comfort experienced by the participants. The prevailing tight space in the classroom and reversed seating positions most likely discouraged individuals and left them feeling physically uncomfortable; this probably also diverted their attention during sessions – a hindering factor for the acquisition of new information or the practise of new skills. Another important point, and a fundamental basis for the well-being of the participants during the intervention, was ensuring their emotional and physical safety through the implementation of safety measures (e.g. code of conduct). Once, during Observation Phase II, the participating teacher intervened the action by the HPTs with corporal punishment (beating on hands), when participant A and C were observed (Buchinger & Lindner, 2003). How this violent incident affected the social behaviour of the participants can not be judged in the retrospect. However, it can be certainly assumed that it had an effect on the normal behavioural pattern of the individual and therefore influenced the observation results.

8.5 Conclusion

After analysing all data gathered over a period of more than half a year, the following conclusions can be made. The health promotion trainers assessed their own qualifications as generally good and increasing over time (mainly applied to HPT2), although they were originally inexperienced women who were trained specifically for this learning programme. The HPTs regarded the applied methods as generally suitable, even though they had preferences or animosity towards specific methods. This fact becomes more obvious when the two scales, the Self-Confidence and Suitability of Method Scale, are compared with each other. The results of this comparison reflect the trainers' need for further training in more complex teaching methods like frontal teaching and group discussion in order to stabilise their confidence to practice new teaching skills within the classroom setting. Even though teaching can be demanding, both women intimated that they increasingly identified with their work over the course of time and demanded respect by children and parents participate. Although they regarded their relationship with the children as very positive and based on mutual respect, their relationship with the parents of the children in the intervention group was described as ambivalent.

In regard to the gathered data from the learners' reports, the majority of the learners rated the working relationships with the two HPTs as positive ('like'). However, it could have been of great advantage, especially to the boys, if the team consisted of one female and one male HPT. The idea is that the team composition would represent optimistic male and female role models who are experienced in educating pre-adolescent children starting to develop their own sexual orientation, so that they would be able to fulfil their male and female roles in (intimate) relationships and society later.

The implemented methods were generally assessed by learners as appropriate to the content of the sessions. However, there are indications of gender differences in terms of their like and dislike of the topics. In general, boys tended to be more critical while girls tended to be more unanimous in expressing their general attitude towards the programme and in being comfortable with the applied methods. It can be assumed that girls have a greater need for and interest in the programme topics and methods which are difficult to obtain through other sources. Although boys of this age were in general more bored with sessions, they were at the same time more sensitised to specific culturally sensitive topics such as *Body Changes, HIV/AIDS, Abuse,* and *Death and Care.*

The last instrument – participant observation – was intended to clarify the effects of the intervention on the basis of the expressed social behaviour of four children. Two girls and two boys aged 9 to 12 years were observed over six months in two observation phases. It was found that three of the four participants attended the sessions with a positive attitude and increased their communication level towards others or the HPTs. One participant was unbalanced in her attitude, however, never expressed any refusal to participate in the sessions. All four participants improved their interaction skills over time, although on an inconsistent basis. Because three of the four children started to establish friendships, it can be assumed that children entering the phase of early adolescence feel vulnerable and therefore establish friendships with the same gender. It is possible that the intervention provided a platform for these same gender relations; for example, a simple method such as choosing their own seating place and encouraging the participants to interact and communicate with each other freely and openly. Gender differences were evident in the participants' ability to express their own opinions. Only the male participants clearly increased their ability to express their own opinions during interaction. During Intervention I and II no kind of refusal, aggression or extreme subordination was ever observed, which can be identified as a positive result; it means that all four participants felt predominantly comfortable with the programme as it was outlined.

CHAPTER NINE
Results of the Outcome Evaluation

9.1 Introduction

The outcomes of the Intervention (X), the CMP learning programme, are evaluated by means of two main instruments, a questionnaire and an opinion poll, together with a subsidiary instrument, namely the project documentation. The self-administered questionnaire is used containing five psychological and social research variables. This instrument is analysed by means of a quasi-experimental research design applied to the intervention group (IG) and (quasi-)control group (CG)[32], with four test phases. Specific learning outcomes of particular segments of the model were gathered by means of the project documentation. These results are meant to derive additional information on the level of knowledge, attitudes and skills development among children in the intervention group. These paragraphs start with a description of already existing unsafe health intentions, for instance regarding pregnancy, and are followed by an explanation of possible steps that need to be taken to implement sessions on HIV/AIDS and sex education in order to meet parents' educational requirements and to ensure the emotional safety of the children. The preceding is followed by results of active learning tests regarding attitudes towards a fictitious HIV-positive child and the level of knowledge on HIV/AIDS in Intervention (X) II.[33] The last part of the chapter 9 deals with results from the opinion poll (part 1) conveying long-term attitudes among children in the intervention group towards the programme.

---

32 As the control group unexpectedly turned into a quasi-control group after being subjected to the governmental life skills programme on AIDS, most of the presented results cover results from the intervention group participating in the non-governmental programme the Child Mind Project.
33 'X' refers to the non-governmental intervention.

9.2 Effects of the Programme Regarding Individual Protective Variables

In the following section the results of the quantitative instrument, the self-administered questionnaire, are presented in four parts: (1) presentation of socio-demographic variables, (2) outcomes regarding psychological and social competencies variables, (3) investigation of particular outcomes surrounding children's knowledge of HIV/AIDS, and (4) fine adjustment of particular messages conveyed in Intervention I and II.

9.2.1 Comparison between Intervention Group and Control Group Regarding Socio-demographic Variables

In this paragraph socio-demographic variables that were being used in the quantitative instrument, the questionnaire (part A), are presented. The variables are age and gender composition, ethnic heritage and family background. The family composition in particular is presented to provide guidelines to: (1) identify existing family units, and (2) examine possible influences on the mounting psychological and social variables in the socio-demographic background of children in the intervention and control group.

A total number of 80 children, grade 4 level, were asked to participate in the questionnaire (see chapter 6, par. 4.1). Forty-one children were from to the intervention group (Ikaya Primary School) and 39 children from the control group (Nomlinganiselo Primary School). The gender distribution was balanced with 40 girls and 40 boys. The ages of participants ranged from eight to 14 years. More than three quarters of the children (77.5%) were nine to 11 years old; five children (6.3%) eight years old and 11 children (13.8%) 12 years and older. The participating boys and girls were all of African ancestry and lived in disadvantaged settings. The ethnic distribution among learners was predominantly Xhosa; the minority of the samples were Tswana and Sotho.

According to the reports by the *children in the intervention group* (N=41), as illustrated in figure 9.1[34], the most common type of family unit was single-headed family units (44%), with the majority of families headed by women (98%). Thirty-seven percent of the children of the intervention group reported that they lived with both parents and with or without other siblings in so-called nuclear families. In addition, almost 9% of the children reported that they lived with one biological parent and one stepparent with or

---

34 All results were rounded up following mathematical procedures.

without other siblings ('nuclear & stepparent'). Finally, 10% of the children seemed to grow up without their biological parents in family units composed of other siblings, aunts and uncles or other legal guardians ('special'). 'Extended' or 'extended with stepparents' family units were not listed by children in the intervention group.

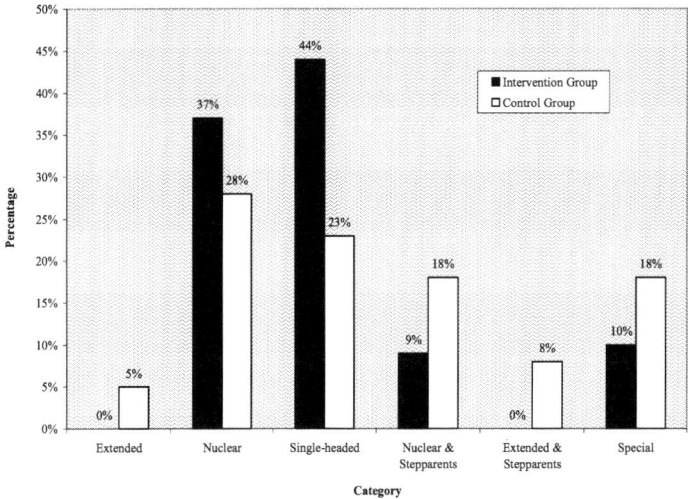

Figure 9.1. Responses on – "Who do you live with at the Moment?" (Eleven Responses clustered in Six Categories) – Existing Family Units in the Intervention Group and Control Group at Pretest in March 2003.

The *children in the control group* ($N=39$) mentioned a greater variety of family units than those in the intervention group. The most common family unit in the control group is the nuclear family unit (28%). The second most common family type is the single-headed family unit (23%), and again the majority of these units are headed by women (98%). Eighteen percent of the children of the control group reported that they lived with one biological parent and one stepparent with or without other siblings (nuclear & stepparents). The same number of children (18%) stated that they lived in family units with siblings and with/without grandparents (special). Half of these special family units were exclusively headed by other children, and can consequently be defined as child-headed households. Almost 8% of the children of the control group reported that they lived in extended family units with stepparents and only 5% of the children stated that they lived in a multigenerational family unit. According to the reports, grandparents were present in half of the extended family units.

According to the statements by the children, the findings illustrate that the children in the intervention group, who live in a semi-urban area and the children in the control group, who live in an urban area, experience different family structures. Although the majority of the children in both groups grow up in nuclear and single female-headed family units, more children in the control group than in the intervention group live with stepparents and grandparents, and in so-called special family units headed by siblings or other relatives due to the absence of biological parents.

Regarding the second objective, to examine possible statistical correlations between the variable 'family' and five dependent psychological (self-esteem, self-efficacy, knowledge) and social (gender communication, social responsibility) variables, no statistically significant interaction was found either among children in the intervention group or among children in the control group.

9.2.2 Changes of the Psychological and Social Research Variables

The results regarding the psychological variables were disappointing in terms of the formulated hypotheses. The results showed that the factorial ANOVA of the four psychological and social variables could not reveal a significant correlation between the variables 'group' and specific 'test phase'. This means, none of the expected changes over the four test phases occurred, neither among the samples who attended the non-governmental Intervention (X), nor among the samples who attended the governmental Intervention (Y), and finally no effects could be detected, not in the non-governmental Intervention (X) I or in the governmental Intervention (Y). For a better understanding figure 9.2 and 9.3 display the means for the intervention and control group of the used psychological and social variables over the four test phases.

For closer examination, means of the dependent variables with regard to the variable gender (male and female) in the intervention and control group are presented over four test phases in appendix G. Only two gender-specific effects in gender communication and social responsibility were detected in the intervention group due to the ceiling effect. In test phases 1 to 3, the boys have significantly higher results regarding inter-gender communication than the girls. With regard to the variable social responsibility girls reach significantly higher results in test phases 2 to 4 (Appendix H).

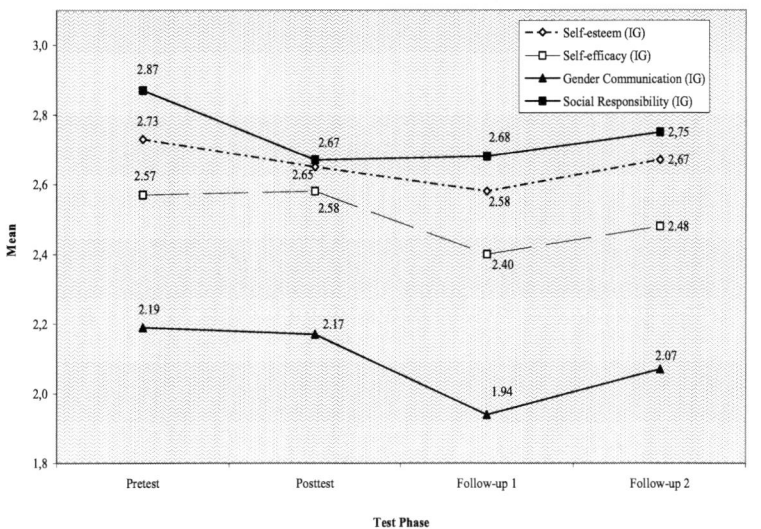

Figure 9.2. Means of the Psychological and Social Variables for the Intervention Group (IG) over four Test Phases.

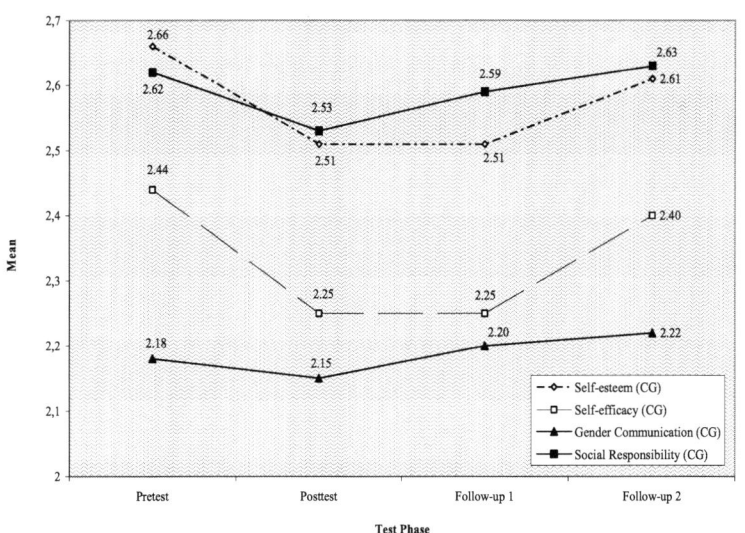

Figure 9.3. Means of the Psychological and Social Variables for the Control Group (CG) over four Test Phases.

Of the four test phases the intervention group reached the highest scores in the scales of self-esteem, gender communication and social responsibility already at pretest level. Between 44.3% and 50% of the learners had already reached the maximum of the scale during the pretest phase regarding the variables of self-esteem and social responsibility, whilst between 87.3% and 97.4% of the learners assessed gender communication and self-efficacy with the highest possible scores.

At this point a detailed description of the scales will be omitted, because these results can be regarded as a sign of the inability of the instrument to detect possible changes within these variables over time. One explanation for this phenomenon is possibly that the 3-point scales applied are not detailed enough to detect more specific changes throughout the intervention. In the preparation phase of this evaluation, debates were held with experts in the field whether it would be possible to use a 4-point or even 5-point scale. The conclusion was to avoid a detailed scale at this stage of the research as, based on their early development phase and inadequate reading and writing skills, the children were unable to understand the envisaged questionnaire format.

9.2.3 Examining the Variable 'Knowledge of HIV/AIDS'

Despite the fact that the changes in the psychological and social research variables were not convincing, the more convincing results were nevertheless derived from knowledge scales 1 and 2, which recorded the samples' level of knowledge of HIV/AIDS. The factorial ANOVA of knowledge scale 1, examining general knowledge of HIV/AIDS, found significant main effects for the variables 'test phase' ($F_{(2.7, 186.4)} = 22.45$; $p<.001$; Partial-$\varepsilon^2=.246$) and a significant 'interaction' ($F_{(2.7, 186.4)} = 14.72$; $p<.001$; Partial-$\varepsilon^2=.176$) (Table 9.1). The 'group' variable is not significant ($p=.121$), which can be ascribed to the descriptively low starting point of the intervention group during the pretest phase. The probability values, as well as the following factorial ANOVA, are measured in accordance with the Greenhouse-Geisser corrected degree of freedom for the assessment of critical coincidence of the F values. Figure 9.4 gives an overview of all means of knowledge scale 1 for the intervention group (IG) and control group (CG) in the four test phases.

Table 9.1.
Results of the Factorial ANOVA of Knowledge Scale 1 with Group Variable (A) and Repeated Measurement Variable (B).

	SS	df		MS	F	p	Partial-ε^2
A	0.17	1		0.17	2.46	.121	0.034
in S	4.90	69		0.07			
B	1.68	3	(2.7)	0.56	22.45	.000 (.000)	0.246
A x B	1.10	3	(2.7)	0.37	14.72	.000 (.000)	0.176
B X N	5.16	207	(186.4)	0.02			

Note. A = group variable, in S = differences between N among both Groups, B = repeated measurement variable, N = number of subjects, A x B = interaction between variables, B x N = interaction between test phase and N, SS = sum of squares, df = degree of freedom, MS = mean square, F = F value, p = probability of F value, Partial-ε^2 = Partial Eta square, values in brackets = Greenhouse-Geisser corrected df and p values.

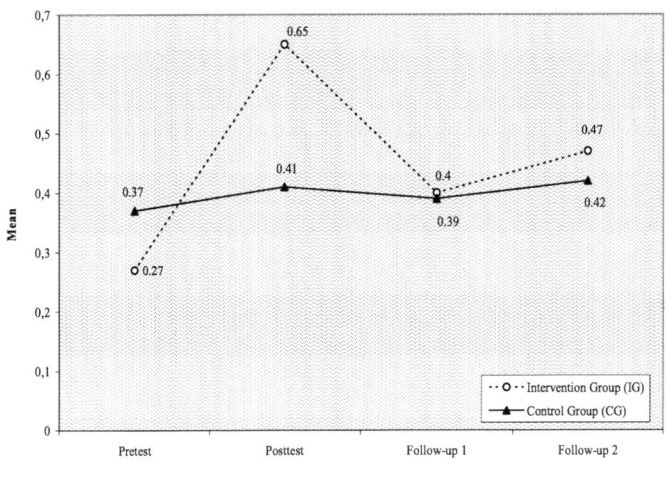

Figure 9.4. Means for Knowledge Scale 1 for Intervention Group (IG) and Control Group (CG) over four Test Phases.

With regard to the research questions, the interpretation of the 'interaction' is of special interest. Therefore a Scheffé-test for the comparison of pairs was measured (measurement by hand in accordance with Bortz, 1999). The evaluation of the variances of error was also done with a Greenhouse-Geisser corrected degree of freedom. Table 9.2 shows the absolute values. The significant differences between the means are marked with ** and * in accordance with the Scheffé-test on a 1% or 5% interval.

The indication of means in table 9.2 is equivalent to the research design with one intervention and one control group (factorial ANOVA) with repeated testing. The six differences in italics on the upper left side of the matrix show the means of the intervention group and the six differences in italics on the lower right side of the matrix show the means of the control group. The differences in bold print illustrate the differences in comparison with all means of the intervention and control group at the four test phases. The result in bold print of -.10 in the middle of the first line in table 9.2 is the difference between $\overline{x}_{11} - \overline{x}_{21}$, that is the difference between the means of both groups at the first test phase.

Table 9.2.
Differences between Means with regard to Knowledge 1 between Intervention Group (IG) and Control Group (CG) over four Test Phases.

	$\overline{x}_{12}$	$\overline{x}_{13}$	$\overline{x}_{14}$	$\overline{x}_{21}$	$\overline{x}_{22}$	$\overline{x}_{23}$	$\overline{x}_{24}$
$\overline{x}_{11}$	-.38**	-.13	-.20**	**-.10**	-.14	-.12	-.16
$\overline{x}_{12}$		.25**	.18*	.28**	**.24****	**.26****	**.23****
$\overline{x}_{13}$			-.07	.03	-.01	**.01**	-.02
$\overline{x}_{14}$				.10	.06	.08	**.04**
$\overline{x}_{21}$					-.04	-.02	-.05
$\overline{x}_{22}$						.02	-.02
$\overline{x}_{23}$							-.04

Note. $\overline{x}_{11}$ = difference of means; first number refers to group (1 = intervention group, 2 = control group), second number refers to test phase (1 = Pretest, 2 = Posttest, 3 = Follow-up test 2, 4 = Follow-up test 2).

At the pretest phase no statistical significant difference between the intervention group and the control group was detected. The two groups only differ regarding their level of knowledge of HIV/AIDS. While the intervention group displays a strong increase in values in knowledge scale 1, the control group does not show a significant change in knowledge scale 1 from pretest to posttest; this means the intervention group has significantly higher values than the control group at the posttest. With regard to the knowledge presented in knowledge scale 1, the Intervention (X) shows an effect. The intervention group shows a significantly higher mean of knowledge scale 1 from pretest to follow-up test 2; however, the sustainability of this increase is less clear. When compared with the posttest results, the means of knowledge scale 1 significantly decrease in the intervention group from test phase three to four. In other words, the means of the intervention group in test phases three and four are not significantly different from the means of the control group at all four test phases.

In summary, the intervention group, in comparison with the control group, starts at a descriptively lower point at the pretest, reaches significantly higher values at posttest, and falls back to the same level as the control group in test phases three and four. A sustainable effect of the Intervention (X) can only be found to a limited extent. However, the governmental Intervention (Y) does not show any significant effect, which means that all paired differences within the control group are insignificant.

The factorial ANOVA on knowledge scale 2, examining HIV transmission and protection, revealed two significant main effects in the variable 'test phase' (variable test phase: $F_{(2.53;\ 172)}=12.44$; $p < .001$; Partial-$\varepsilon^2=.155$/variable group: $F_{(1;\ 68)}=16.62$; $p < .001$; Partial-$\varepsilon^2=.196$) and revealed a significant interaction between both variables ($F_{(2.53;\ 172)}=4.44$; $p < .01$; Partial-$\varepsilon^2=.061$) presented in table 9.3. The underlying means are presented in Figure 9.5.

Table 9.3.
Results of the Factorial ANOVA of Knowledge Scale 2 with Group Variable (A) and Repeated Measurement Variable (B).

	SS	df	MS	F	p	Partial-ε^2
A	2.11	1	2.11	16.62	.000	0.196
in S	8.61	68	0.13			
B	1.24	3 (2.53)	0.41	12.44	.000 (.000)	0.155
A x B	0.44	3 (2.53)	0.15	4.44	.005 (.008)	0.061
B X N	6.80	204 (172)	0.03			

Note. A = group variable, in S = differences between N among both groups, B = repeated measurement variable, N = number of subjects, A x B = interaction between variables, B x N = interaction between test phase and N, SS = sum of squares, df = degree of freedom, MS = mean square, F = F value, p = probability of F value, Partial-ε^2 = Partial Eta square, values in brackets are Greenhouse-Geisser corrected df and p values.

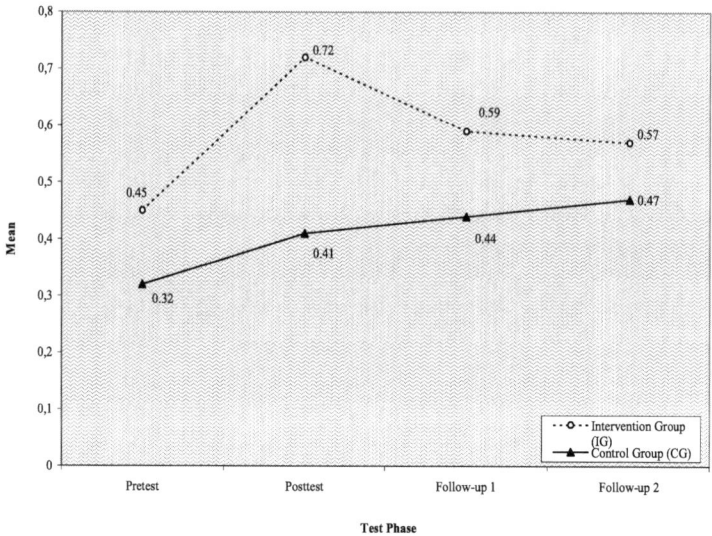

Figure 9.5. Means of Knowledge Scale 2 of the Intervention (IG) and Control Group (CG) over four Test Phases.

Again, at the centre of the interpretative presentation of the results is the interaction effect. Table 9.4 shows the statistically significant differences between means on the 1% to 5% interval. No significant difference exists at the pretest phase between the intervention and control group, although the value of the intervention group is descriptively higher than the value of the control group. Within the intervention group a highly significant increase in the knowledge scale 2 values occurred from pretest to posttest phase, whereas within the control group no significant changes could be detected. Thus, the Intervention (X) shows the predicted effect from pre- to posttest. However, from posttest to follow-up test 2 the means of knowledge scale 2 within the intervention group decreased, though not significantly, and no significant difference to the pretest can be detected. Again, the success of the Intervention (X) is not sustainable

This result is confirmed when the values in both groups are compared. Although the means of the intervention group in the third and fourth test phases are different from the means of the control group at pretest phase, they are similar at posttest and both follow-up tests phases. The sustainability of the effect of the Intervention (X) exceeds the effects of practice and maturation in the control group, which possibly took place between the first two test phases, but in a non-significant manner.

Table 9.4.
Differences between Means in Knowledge Scale 2 between Intervention Group (IG) and Control Group(CG) over four Test Phases.

	$\bar{x}_{12}$	$\bar{x}_{13}$	$\bar{x}_{14}$	$\bar{x}_{21}$	$\bar{x}_{22}$	$\bar{x}_{23}$	$\bar{x}_{24}$
$\bar{x}_{11}$	-.27**	-.14	-.12	.13	.04	.01	-.02
$\bar{x}_{12}$		.13	.14	.40**	.31**	.28**	.25*
$\bar{x}_{13}$			.02	.27**	.18	.15	.12
$\bar{x}_{14}$				.25*	.16	.13	.10
$\bar{x}_{21}$					-.09	-.12	-.15
$\bar{x}_{22}$						-.03	-.06
$\bar{x}_{23}$							-.03

Note. $\bar{x}_{11}$ = difference of means; first number refers to group (1 = intervention group, 2 = control group), second number refers to test phase (1 = Pretest, 2 = Posttest, 3 = Follow-up test 2, 4 = Follow-up test 2).

The assessment of the governmental Intervention (Y) is unproblematic because no two-tailed significant means exist within the control group. In other words, the values in knowledge scale 2 increased within the control group from one test phase to another, but the changes are non-statistically significant. On the whole, the governmental Intervention (Y) did not increase the knowledge on HIV/AIDS among the children in the control group. Thus, the following investigation of results from knowledge scales 1 and 2 will only present results from the variable of knowledge of HIV/AIDS from the intervention group Interventions (X) I and (X) II.

Tables 9.5 and 9.6 show the changes of knowledge of HIV/AIDS in the intervention group in the course of the four test phases. To carry out a full investigation into each item a McNemar-test was done between the values at pretest and the values at the three subsequent test phases. Tables 9.5 and 9.6 show whether the values of the posttest and both follow-up tests are significantly different from the pretest (**p<.01; *p<.05) in knowledge scale 1 and 2. All results in tables 9.5 and 9.6 were rounded up following mathematical procedures. All significant differences display an increase in knowledge.

Table 9.5.
Percentage of Right Answers in Knowledge Scale 1 in the four Test Phases and Significant Changes in the Number of Right Answers compared to Pretest Results of the Intervention Group (IG).

Knowledge Scale 1	Right answer	Pre-test	Post-test	Follow-up test 1	Follow-up test 2
Is AIDS a disease where the immune system of a human being is destroyed and infections make the body weak against other infections?	Yes	28.9	71.1**	78.9**	60.5*
Did the HI-Virus come from the USA?	No	15.8	23.7	21.1	15.8
Is the origin of AIDS unknown?	Yes	28.9	18.4	42.1	31.6
Can the HI-Virus survive outside the body for a few minutes?	Yes	15.8	23.7	21.1	7.9
Can the HI-Virus survive outside the body for some hours?	No	15.8	42.1*	31.6	15.8
Is safer sex a method to prevent pregnancy?	Yes	23.7	42.1	15.8	21.1
Does safer sex mean using a condom during sexual intercourse?	Yes	28.9	68.4**	47.4	50.0
Does safer sex mean practising abstinence from sex?	Yes	21.1	57.9**	52.6*	34.2
Can a policeman get an HIV infection?	Yes	13.2	81.6**	15.8	55.3**
Can a prostitute get an HIV infection?	Yes	52.6	89.5**	63.2	68.4
Can everyone (people) get an HIV infection?	Yes	28.9	84.2**	31.6	57.9*
Can women get an HIV infection?	Yes	23.7	84.2**	31.6	86.8**
Can men get an HIV infection?	Yes	21.1	89.5**	34.2	71.1**
Can you do an HIV-test at an office of public health?	Yes	18.4	86.8**	47.4*	44.7*
Can you do an HIV-test at a doctor?	Yes	63.2	89.5*	65.8	65.8
Can you do an HIV-test at a community clinic?	Yes	26.3	89.5**	39.5	63.2**

Table 9.6.
Percentage of Right Answers in Knowledge Scale 2 in the four Test Phases and Significant Changes in the Number of Right Answers compared to Pretest Results of the Intervention Group (IG).

Knowledge Scale 2	Right answer	Pre-test	Posttest	Follow-up test 1	Follow-up test 2
Can you get the HI-Virus from unprotected sexual intercourse?	Yes	50.0	65.8	57.9	63.2
Does saliva/spittle carry the HI-Virus?[1]	No	34.2	81.6**	44.7	52.6
Does semen carry the HI-Virus?	Yes	42.1	60.5	44.7	34.2
Do tears carry the HI-Virus?	No	47.4	86.8**	73.7*	63.2
Does blood carry the HI-Virus?	Yes	63.2	84.2	78.9	71.1
Does urine carry the HI-Virus?	No	36.8	73.7**	36.8	42.1
Does sweat carry the HI-Virus?	No	44.7	81.6**	73.7*	55.3
Does secretion of the vagina carry the HI-Virus?	Yes	47.4	71.1*	47.4	50.0
Does watching TV with your friend without sleeping with him or her protect you against the HI-Virus?	Yes	44.7	47.4	65.8	55.3
Does using condoms during sexual intercourse protect you against the HI-Virus?	Yes	42.1	65.8	68.4*	86.8**

Note. [1] Due to the young age of children it was well-considered to avoid teaching knowledge that are deeply rooted in medical knowledge, thus, all presented items are to be understood in their dangerous and non-dangerous context. For example, it is medical knowledge that tears carry the HI-Virus (Which liquid of the body includes the HI-Virus? Do tears carry the HI-Virus?), however, not to an extent that can be easily infectious for human beings in everyday situations.

With regard to knowledge scale 1, 12 of the 16 items are significantly different between pretest and posttest. This means 75% of the items contained significantly more right answers at posttest. The corresponding number of significant differences is reduced to three between pretest and follow-up test 1 and increased to seven between pretest and follow-up test 2.

This is surprising, but can most likely be attributed to the developmental stage of the target group, as the intervention group did not receive further intervention in this field of knowledge between follow-up test 1 and follow-up test 2.

The analogue analysis of the 10 items defining the knowledge scale 2 revealed five significant differences from pretest to posttest. Three items significantly changed from pretest to follow-up test 1 and only one changed significantly from pretest to follow-up test 2 (Table 9.6). The analysis of the items from knowledge scale 2 also shows that there exists an insufficient sustainability of the Intervention (X) effect: merely the preventive effect of the condom use is known to more children at the follow-up test 2 than at the pretest.

In summary, at follow-up test 2, compared with the pretest, more children know (1) what AIDS is, (2) who can be infected (police officers, human beings, women, men), (3) where you can go for an HIV-test (Office of Public Health, Community Clinic), and (4) that the use of condoms protects you against HIV infection. Finally, no significant differences between gender regarding knowledge could be detected. Only one age-specific effect regarding knowledge of HIV/AIDS was found in the intervention group. In follow-up test 2 in knowledge scale 2 it was found that older children (13 years) learned more than younger children (10 years) (see also Appendices I and J).

9.3 A Descriptive Analysis of Particular Segments of the Learning Model and Outcomes Regarding HIV/AIDS

Bandura (1986) assumes in his Social Cognitive Theory that every social learning process is based on the individual's need to experience attention, retention, reproduction and motivation in order to demonstrate certain behaviours. The following examples should allow the child to observe, as a result of above listed observational learning processes, and practise personal actions in specific modelled and health-related situations. These examples further describe existing health-related intentions and role allocations among pre-adolescent children, followed by the presentation of particular segments of HIV/AIDS and sex education. These segments illustrate the way to the acquisition of knowledge (level and gaps) regarding HIV/AIDS and attitudes towards an HIV-positive child as a representative of any human. The data are taken from the descriptive project documentation of the sessions on relationships with family and friends, sex education, HIV/AIDS, and the booster session on self-esteem.

9.3.1 Findings of Health-related Intentions

As outlined in chapter 7, a secret box was introduced to encourage learners to ask any question they had on the programme, specific sessions or topics. Several of the questions asked dealt with three fields: sex education, HIV/AIDS and pregnancy. The first field included questions on sex and HIV/AIDS and related issues, for example what happens during or after sexual intercourse, abstinence, and condom use:

(1) If you have sex without a condom what happens?
(2) You can't sleep with a girl when you are not 16. First, he has to be a man.
(3) Why is the vagina wet and the penis erect?
(4) If you sleep with a boy what happens afterwards?

The second field contained questions on HIV/AIDS. Related questions were about the definitions of the term AIDS, the origin of the virus, or whether people can live with the virus. These questions are most probably related to public discussions in the media and immediate surroundings which are obviously picked up by children at this young age. Examples of questions are:

(1) If I have HIV, will I live?
(2) Where does AIDS come from?
(3) Why do you have/get HIV/STIs?
(4) Is AIDS a killer disease?/And when are you going to teach us about it?

The last field of interest was pregnancy and (early) motherhood. Especially the girls expressed great interest in pregnancy-related topics such as the prevention of pregnancy and a few of the girls, aged 10-12 years even expressed that they wished to have a baby. Questions and statements included the following:

(1) If you do not want to have a baby, how can you prevent it?
(2) When can I have a baby?
(3) I want a baby.

In sum, all three listed fields of interest illustrate that children in this pre-adolescent stage express their need for information on topics that target HIV/AIDS and sex education, and their susceptibility to stigmas and messages that surround these 'taboo' topics. Another finding is that the questions and statements on pregnancy in particular most probably reflect a vulnerability to unsafe (sexual) behaviour, especially among girls.

As a second example of health-related intentions among participants, the understanding of the term 'relationships' is described with regard to role allocations of boys (men) and girls (women) in 'intimate' relations. At the beginning of the session children were asked to define role allocations between the father and the mother in a family. They explained that while men work outside of the house (e.g. paid work/occupation) mothers organise the household. According to these statements the composition of a family was defined in a generally traditional way. These understandings of male and female roles seem to be encouraged by socialisation processes children in the intervention group are exposed to in the position they hold in their families.

Underlining this assumption are the following two examples: in one session learners were asked to complete a 'body map' (self-esteem) to list physical activities. Whereas girls tended to list household activities, such as washing clothes or the body, cleaning, cooking, or sensitive physical contacts with other human beings such as hugging or touching, boys recorded mainly activities to their own doings, such as sport activities, eating, washing, and hanging around with friends. After this activity children were asked how they would define the word 'relationship'. They stated that it is merely a traditional unity of a man and a woman, functioning by economical means and glued together by sex and reproduction, parallel to above role allocations of men and women in relationships. They defined non-relationships as, for example friendships and relations within a family (e.g. parents).

This is in itself a concerning finding because the children's conviction was that *all* relationships between the two genders are mainly sexual relations and aimed at reproduction. In the light of this definition manifold relations between same and other gender, whether non- or sexually based, can be recognised as fruitful for their emotional state and social life. Campbell (2003) found in her study with learners at secondary school level that the young people clearly distinguished between friendship and sex and defined them as being mutually exclusive territories. In both these relationships between boys and girls she found communication to be generally low (Campbell, 2003); this reduced the ability between genders to use communication as a health preventive act. In interventions, special attention must be paid to those symbols that define different kinds of relationships to avoid misinterpretation and confusion about the different qualities of emotions to and relations with people, including family or friends, and/or emotions for and activities with each other. In addition, interventions should strive to support the establishment of a social network outside of the family system at the time those children reach adolescence.

9.3.2 HIV/AIDS and Sex Education: Potential Steps and Findings

In the planning phase of the programme it was considered that various steps be taken to sensitise and prepare children to be taught on personally demanding topics such as sex education and HIV/AIDS in order to avoid any emotional overload or negative stimulus. Thus, the topics of sex education and HIV/AIDS prevention were integrated in a cluster of several steps outlined over a period of more than four weeks: (1) internal and external organs, (2) sex education by way of story telling and the introduction of the secret box, (3) a visit to the Community Clinic, (4) a brief preparation session on HIV/AIDS associated with a healthy diet to stabilise the immune system, and finally (5) a session on HIV/AIDS by means of contraceptive modelling.

Special emphasis was placed on the final session on HIV/AIDS where different contraceptives for men and women were presented and a contraceptive kit was used. During the presentation of the condoms, each learner received one condom. Only the trainers illustrated the appropriate use of a condom in front of the class using the wooden model of a penis and a real condom. The children were not allowed to open or keep their condoms. The reason for the strict and serious instruction not to open the condom was, on the one hand, to encourage responsible behaviour towards this preventive method (in other words dealing with condoms is not fun but life protecting), on the other hand, to calm the parents' worries that a condom in their children's hands would be an encouragement to have sex.

Findings that arose from the session on sex education and HIV/AIDS were the following. First, both genders were very interested in seeing how a condom is used. However, while girls showed a greater interest in the various contraceptives for women, the boys were more interested in the use of a condom. Children behaved in a serious manner during this session but it is believed that the protective environment and the clear guidance by HPTs through this sensitive learning process encouraged this 'responsible' behaviour. Second, there were no complaints from parents or any other authority to the HPTs after the session regarding sex education or condom 'distribution' to children at this young age. Parents reported in the parent meetings that they checked all information papers and talked with their children about learned knowledge in the sessions. Third, some of the mothers stated in the mothers' meeting that their children obviously responded to the topics, sometimes in different ways than they had expected. One mother reported that her daughter explained that she could protect her from being infected with HIV, because she knew now how to identify HIV-positive people. Although this statement emphasises the false belief that HIV status is visible, the child expressed that she felt capable to perform a specific protective action towards her mother as part of developing self-efficacy regarding this disease. Finally, the discourse between parents and children encouraged by these sessions put children in the position to be educators for their parents, of whom many were illiterate or have left school at primary school level. One mother explained in the mothers' meeting that she was very surprised when her child came home to explain the inner and reproductive organs to her – she had given birth to many children in her life without being aware of these bodily functions.

9.3.3 Selected Outcomes regarding Attitudes towards and Knowledge of HIV/AIDS

After the first session on HIV/AIDS, the children in the intervention group were asked to represent their knowledge by putting certain descriptions of HIV transmission and protection that they have acquired in the phases of attention and retention into a specific action, namely a 'decision-making process'. The following two examples illustrate results of undertaken tasks during sessions which should have encouraged systematic thinking and activated their problem-solving competency regarding the issue of dealing with problematic situations. These tasks were interpreted as assessments on attitudes and knowledge.

Testing Attitudes towards an HIV-positive Child

Six groups were formed on a voluntary basis; three groups of boys, two groups of girls and one mixed group. In their groups the learners were asked to decide on the following task: "Would you, as a principal of a primary school allow an HIV-positive child to attend your school?" The groups had to make a YES or NO decision and were asked to substantiate their decision.

The groups made the following decisions: The male groups decided against the child's participation at the primary school. The listed reasons were: He/she will infect other children; He/she behaves badly towards others and thinks dirty thoughts; the mothers won't like their children to come and study at this school and no one would like to be part of it; he/she will have sores, broken skin and infect other children with AIDS. The female groups decided in favour of the participation of the child. They did, however, ask for intimate information, for instance, "How did the child get the infection?". They also wanted to take preventive measures for all other non-infected human beings: "How can we avoid transmission in the school?"; or felt responsible to take care of the child: "What must he/she eat now that he/she has HIV + (AIDS)?". The mixed group reacted similarly, tending to consider all possibilities for the child and for the protection of others. However, they felt unable to make a decision: "Yes – she must be educated, must tell what AIDS is, people must look after her. No – can infect others through blood, through sores and cuts." It seems, therefore that male learners tended to refuse the attendance of the HIV-positive child more than the female groups. Female groups tended to consider the general well-being of everyone and showed higher social responsibility to deal with this problem. For the only mixed gender group it turned out to be impossible to come to an agreement on this task.

In conclusion, the decisions of the children illustrate that their knowledge on protection and transmission of HIV/AIDS contained also incorrect facts which consequently influenced the final decision-making process on whether an HIV-positive child should attend the primary school. This part of the session also revealed that even such young learners already expressed specific personal fears, attitudinal constructs and gender tendencies towards a fictitious HIV-positive child (human being). The aspect of human rights, namely that everyone has the right to education, has to be more fully and intensely explained in order to break through the surface of fear and to prevent the development of prejudice patterns within the children of the intervention group.

Testing Knowledge on HIV/AIDS in Booster Session

In the booster session on HIV/AIDS, Intervention (X) II, a mixed gender group task was done where learners had to do self-study with material on HIV/AIDS. The questions which had to be answered were: (1) What protects you against HIV?, (2) How is HIV spread?, (3) What does AIDS mean?, (4) What does HIV mean?, and (5) What does it mean if an HIV-test is 'negative'? Each of the five groups had to answer three questions. This session was meant to prove how much knowledge the participants of the intervention group still had of HIV/AIDS.

With regard to question (1) ('What protects you against HIV?'), the groups listed condoms ("Use a condom if you sleep with your boyfriend."), abstinent behaviour ("You cannot sleep with your boyfriend."/"Don't sleep with other people if you are HIV+."), or hygiene in medical terms ("Don't touch blood of your friends."/"Don't use same condom today and tomorrow.") as protection methods. Some other answers that contained false knowledge were: testing protects ("Go to the clinic to test your blood."), or kissing ("Don't kiss your girlfriend in stretch."; referring to French kissing). Thus, children tended to shift between transmission and protection methods.

Question (2) ('How is HIV spread?') was answered with the following statements: transmission by sexual intercourse ("HIV is spread by sexual intercourse with an infected person."); sexual intercourse without a condom ("By not using any condoms."); mother to child transmission ("From an infected mother to her unborn child."). For the majority of the groups it was clear that sexual intercourse is the main way of becoming infected with the HI-Virus. Although question (3) ('What does AIDS mean?') was complicated, children found the appropriate description in the pamphlets. One group transcribed the complete paragraph from the pamphlet: "A sexually transmitted infection which attacks the immune system destroying the mechanism. Over a period of time the virus enters the blood stream ... symptoms ... an infected person can feel healthy for infection/progress to the disease called AIDS the virus."

Question (4) ('What does HIV mean?') was answered in three ways: Some groups correctly copied the explanation from the pamphlets, other groups decided that HIV was AIDS and another group stated that 'HIV means if you have HIV you must use a condom.' and 'Must tell it to your mother that you have HIV.'. The last question (5) ('What does it mean if an HIV-test is negative?') was answered correctly by three of the six groups who knew that a person does not have the HI-Virus if the test result is negative.

According to the results, knowledge of HIV/AIDS was fragmentary seven months after the first session on this topic. The self-study in group work seems to have had an effect on the level of knowledge in follow-up test 1, which was done three weeks after this booster session, because the answers to questions regarding the definition of AIDS, protection against HIV by condoms and abstinence, or testing have significantly improved. However, false knowledge of the ways of transmission (i.e. blood over open wounds or saliva (kissing)) could not be averted, as quantitative results in the follow-up test 1 show. One must consider the young age of the children – an age which is also a far-reaching phase in terms of intellectual development and constant change and information input. In other words, if a stable basis of knowledge, for example about health issues such as HIV-prevention, is built up at this age it will effect the gathered additional knowledge within other life stages. Consequently, any repeated form of intervention will allow the children to progress and acquire additional knowledge in this learning field and affect their developing health-related behaviour in the long-term.

9.4 Results of the Opinion Poll

The opinion poll taken among learners of the intervention group was not only intended to activate long-term memory in regard to Interventions (X) I and II, but was also meant as a proof of the quality of the introduced learning programme. The poll was done eight months after Intervention (X) II and five months after follow-up test 2. Four questions were asked: (1) Did you like or did you not like the life skills programme?, (2) Do you think other children should receive the same life skills programme?, (3) What made you happy or smile in the life skills programme?, and (4) What made you sad in the life skills programme?.

Most children responded positively to the first two questions. Ninety-five percent of the children said that they liked the programme and that they would recommend the programme for other children. The last two questions, which were answered in groups, revealed that all events, topics and elements of the programme were regarded as positive experiences by the six groups: outdoor trips to Cape Town and the clinic, the drama in the youth centre, the food event, talking about HIV/AIDS, sex and abuse, games such as soccer, learning about life skills and bodily changes as well as about the family and community. Even the video and the implemented rules and confidence sentence were listed as positive experiences. The most frequently listed topics learners liked were HIV/AIDS, which was listed by five of the six groups, abuse, and sex education, listed by four of the six groups. With regard to relations within the class, the HPTs and working in groups were also considered positive.

The groups decided to name four experiences that were demanding to them. First, the bus trip to Cape Town turned out to be difficult because the bus was not roadworthy and had a small accident on the way back to Kayamandi. Second, the sessions on sex and abuse were still strongly remembered by the children even eight months after the end of Intervention (X) II. This could be an indicator that those topics have to be implemented with great sensitivity to the target group's age. Lastly, the death of one of the HPTs was remembered as a very sad event.

9.5 Conclusion

The presented results, gained by means of quantitative (questionnaire) and the combined qualitative-quantitative instruments (opinion poll) evaluated the outcomes of the intervention on the personal and interpersonal domains. Results from the qualitative instrument have to be strictly taken as supportive data in an attempt to close the gaps on knowledge and attitudes regarding HIV/AIDS which were not specifically considered in the questionnaire.

Starting with the results of the quantitative instrument, the analysis of the socio-demographic variable 'family', as the main socialisation column, revealed in the comparison of the intervention and control groups that family units within the control group were more varied than in the intervention group. For example, more children in the intervention group than in the control group live in either single female-headed family units or nuclear family units without an older generation like grandparents. In contrast, many more children in the control group than in the intervention group live in family units with stepparents or in so-called special family units, mainly without their biological parents and under the supervision of older siblings. Although the intervention and control group lived in different structural surroundings, no significant difference between the groups regarding psychological and social variables was detected.

Due to the ceiling effect, the results on the psychological indicators do not say much about whether the project managed, for instance, to encourage self-confidence in the children and/or to improve their self-efficacy. During the pretesting of the instrument with a small number of children from the target group, no high scoring, which is not uncommon during ratings, was noticed (see also Bortz & Döring, 2001). It is probable that this effect is the consequence of inappropriate procedures for pretesting the instrument (see chapter 5, par. 6.2), resulting in uncovered cultural barriers that affected psychological and social variables. For example, it could be proposed that the children gave socially acceptable answers, as the socio-cultural environment demands that children follow the instructions given by an authority. To question or even refuse to follow is considered disrespectful and will be punished. On the whole, the insufficient performance of the psychological variables turned out to be a problem in the evaluation of the CMP project, as the reference to the knowledge acquired during the project cannot be sufficiently evaluated.

In conclusion, only three significant interactions were found within the intervention group over the four test phases: (1) girls expressed a higher social responsibility from posttest to follow-up test 2, (2) boys expressed a greater gender-communication competency from pre- to follow-up test 1, and (3) older children (13-year-old) tended to give more right answers than younger children (10-year-old) in the knowledge scale 2 in follow-up test 2. The results of the evaluation of the knowledge indicators are, of course, of interest for the preparation of individual prevention efforts in the field of

HIV/AIDS. The first and most intensive part of the CMP Intervention (X) I was successful regarding the transfer of knowledge in the field of HIV/AIDS: The intervention group showed the predicted increase in knowledge from pretest to posttest phase, while the control group did not show a similar change. Unfortunately, the success of the CMP intervention was not sustainable in the long run. The success of the programme was mainly that at follow-up test 2 more children knew: (1) what AIDS was, (2) who could become infected, (3) that specific body liquids transmit the virus, (4) where to go for an HIV-test, and (5) that the use of condoms protects them against HIV infection during sexual intercourse. This is to be interpreted as a positive result regarding knowledge of the children in the intervention group. Although the target children had an expected advantage as they lived in a semi-urban area with better access to information, the government intervention programme, which started after the posttest, did not result in any significant increase in knowledge.

A possible strategy to avoid such evaluation difficulties through the use of a quantitative instrument may be to consider long-term training with the target group to teach them how to fill in a 4-point rating scale to effect a learning model on an individual level (e.g. with children or people with reading and writing problems) in further similar studies. Another strategy could be that the designed items implement more specific learning goals which are adjusted to the contents of the learning modules so that the children can make connections between the theoretical instrument (questionnaire) and the practical training sessions.

To prove this aforementioned assumption, further analysis was carried out on specific results of sessions to gain more information on knowledge, attitudes and skills development within the children of the intervention group. The session on family and friendship relations, as well as the booster session on self-esteem revealed that defined relationships between the genders are predominantly related to sexual encounters between men and women with the goal of reproduction. It is not only alarming that, according to the children, those relationships do not require any preventive measures; what is even more concerning is that children exclude the idea of friendship and other fruitful interpersonal relations between the same and the other gender that are important for establishing a strong safety-net in times of crisis. These findings are a possible indication of unsafe health intentions among children in the intervention group and, most probably, favourable for planning preventive initiatives with this target group at an early stage before they become sexually active.

Regarding the decision-making process as to whether an HIV-positive child can attend the school, it was found that while male groups in the intervention group tended to express negative attitudes towards the fictitious child and denied him/her access to the educational facility, the female groups showed positive attitudes but took into account the protection of other people. The assessment of a decision-making process regarding the attendance of a fictitious HIV-positive child at school illustrates the already existing fear of confrontation as well as a gender-based tendency of how the participating girls and boys make decisions regarding a problematic situation. Even if the findings have to be interpreted with care, and are not fully applicable for the target group, findings indicate that this young age group is already exposed to the topic and linked attitudes existing in their social environment. Thus, the recommendation is to implement such constructs on HIV/AIDS in learning programmes to allow for reflection on those constructs of fear and stigmatisation.

In regard to knowledge of HIV/AIDS, in Intervention (X) II a revision session of HIV/AIDS was held and questions were asked on the definition of the disease and the ways of transmission and protection. The results show that knowledge among children in the intervention group is fragmentary and unstable seven months after the first intervention. This result proves that any preventive intervention has to be planned on a long-term basis.

On a positive note, it can be reported that ninety-five percent of the children in the intervention group recommended the programme to other children in the opinion poll. Even eight months after the booster session, the opinion poll revealed that the children still regarded the implemented Child Mind Project (learning model) and the relationship between the HPTs and learners – and between male and female learners – as a predominantly positive experience.

CHAPTER TEN

Developing an Understanding of the Evaluation of the Proximal and Distal Context

10.1 Introduction

The following paragraphs present foremost results from field interviews with nine experts working in governmental and non-governmental institutions in the field of education, health, social and community welfare in Kayamandi. The purpose of these interviews was to identify risks and resources influencing the social life, physical health and mental well-being of children in the case study community. In other words, this data reflects cultural, socio-economic, family, health, and educational conditions which form the fundamental columns for the participating children's development in their growing-up process so that they can enter the adult generation in good physical and mental heath. Thus, the underlying objectives of this chapter are firstly to integrate the gathered data in chapter 10 with data presented in chapter 4, in order to provide an in-depth view of the strengths and challenges facing children in Kayamandi; and secondly to detect influences that had an influence on the intervention and research outcomes presented. The chapter concludes with statements made by the children in the intervention group – gathered by the opinion poll – regarding their attitudes towards, and the challenges facing them in their community.

10.2 Ethnic Diversity and Cultural Heritage

According to the interviewees, Kayamandi is a community diverse in cultures and ethnic groups from South Africa and other African countries:

> There are many different people in Kayamandi with different cultures from other parts of the country: Xhosa (majority), Tswana, Sotho, Coloureds/Afrikaans, Ethiopians, Nigerians, Somalis. (A)

The movement of other South African groups into Kayamandi is recognised as a slow but stable process (E). The majority of residents have their cultural heritage in the Eastern Cape Province and belong to the ethnic group of the Xhosa. Among the different cultures and nationalities, isiXhosa is the interlinking language of all groups in Kayamandi (B).

The cultural background is described as important in the upbringing of children and has a positive and causal effect on children's development.

> They should grow up in their own culture for learning traditions and culture. Indeed there are many ethnical groups, but because the universal language is Xhosa, they seem to develop in a balanced way... Yes, it is much better to grow up in your own culture for being able to communicate and you interact with your own culture. So children can learn their culture and traditions. (B)

One interviewee added that educating children about their blood line and family tree, thereby incorporating the entire extended family, is part of a culture-based educational process (A). According to the statements above, the role of heritage and culture is to encourage a cultural identification process in the socialisation of children at family and community level.

10.3 Physical Environment – Prevailing Risks to Health

The physical environment of Kayamandi is characterised by overcrowding in a geographically limited space (B), considered to have a great impact on children's development. The interviewees considered the informal settlement areas as extremely critical for the mental and physical growth of children (G). These areas were described as overcrowded, with the predominant housing unit, the shack, offering less privacy for occupants (F; B; A; C; H; A).

In addition, overcrowding was also mentioned as causing risky spaces and situations for children, e.g. the danger of fire that spreads quickly in the densely populated areas (A; E) especially during hot dry seasons. The insufficient water supply and waste management, and the "absence of acceptable ablution facilities" (G) for such a large number of people were identified as the causes of an extremely unhygienic living environment (D; H; I; B) that poses health risks to children in informal areas. In addition, the limited physical space within the informal settlement areas presents not only a safety and security problem for children, but also a threat to children's emotional and physical well-being (D; C). Finally, interviewees also mentioned that the whole of Kayamandi (C; D) lacks playgrounds and green spaces for recreational purposes where children can create their own experiences and be safe.

In summary, the interviewees identified limited physical space, shacks as housing units, unhygienic living conditions and the lack of safety as the prevalent physical environmental constrains on the mental and physical development of children in Kayamandi.

10.3.1 Risky Health Conditions and Child Diseases

As already explained in chapter 4, the health service for 28 000 people consists of one day care clinic in Kayamandi. The clinic is visited by a doctor only once a week for two hours (E; C). Apart from the staff shortage, the clinic's general infrastructure was described as being both too small as well as under-equipped for the number of patients to be cared for. Although the interviewees criticised the quantity of the health facilities, they did not mention the quality of the health facilities nor staff qualification as critical in the medical service that is provided.

One interviewee makes recently in-migrated people from former homelands and rural areas responsible for the overcrowding in this health service in Kayamandi (G). Another interviewee working for an administrative facility in Stellenbosch supported this statement and added his criticism that patients from Kayamandi put additional pressure on the health systems in town. When asked for a more detailed explanation, the interviewee quoted three factors that impact upon this situation: (1) the lack of enough health facilities within the community, (2) the high number of health problems within the community itself, and (3) the existing stigma attached to tuberculosis (F) that forces people to use health facilities outside of Kayamandi to prevent public disclosure of their status. After asking how many children actually lived in Kayamandi, the interviewee was unable to answer this question. It can be argued that the absence of an exact census widens the gap between the supply of and the demand for health facilities within a town area that accommodates more than 28 000 residents. A situation like this puts enormous pressure on every working individual dependent on this overstrained health system described by interviewees.

The general health standard of children is described as disquieting and is proved to be an obstacle for the physical and mental growth of children.

The poor health conditions in nutrition and hygiene are hindering factors for the physical and mental growth of children in Kayamandi. (I)

One interviewee from the health sector described the poor health status of children within the Kayamandi community as an interaction between unhygienic conditions, low standards of living and poverty, which results in malnutrition (G). The shack areas in particular, in being densely populated, are identified as pools of poverty where diseases spread easily and malnutrition predominates (H; D). Children that live in these dense areas play in the streets and spaces between shacks where people dispose of waste and waste water, and pick up germs and bacteria (G; H; C; Es). Infections are described as a result of strained unhygienic and poor living and sanitary conditions (I; E). The main diseases of children listed are lower respiratory tract infections, e.g. tuberculosis, bronchitis and pneumonia, and lower body infections, such as diarrhoea (F). Further problems reported are scabies, sores, ring worms on the body and scalp, chicken pocks and malnutrition (G). Malnutrition seems to be a serious problem in the Kayamandi community because several experts stated this health problem in different sequences in the interview sessions as a risk to children resulting in a low immune-resistance (D; I; H; C).

> Their low resistance because of malnutrition puts them at extra risk of smear infections, lower respiratory infection (TB, pneumonia, bronchitis), or diarrhoea. (G)

Another health problem seems to be teenage pregnancy. Experts (D; A; I) testify that teenage pregnancy can already be found at primary school level – sometimes even at the age of nine years (F).

> There is a problem of a high teenage pregnancy rate. It starts in Grade 5 and then after the first child, teenagers often get another child because they want to apply for another child grant. (A)

As an important side note: children in Grade 5, for example, are not older than 12 or 13. Any sexual act with this age group is illegal and professionals are obliged to report child sexual abuse if the pregnant teenager is younger than 16 years. Although some interviewees referred to existing abusive sexual acts by peer pressure or coercion, they did not directly interlink sexual abuse with the high rate of teenage pregnancy within the community. Teenage pregnancy was connected by the interviewees to several societal problems, e.g. applying for child grants in order to avoid unemployment after school, which are perceived by professionals to contribute to early sexual activity of pre-adolescents. Another explanation given by the interviewees was that the risky behaviour of young people appears to be indicative of an absence of fear of infection caused by a difficult social situation that does not offer long-term life perspectives, especially for girls. This lack in perspective in turn supports emotional distress or deprivation (H) among individuals. Other interviewees see early sexual activity as a result of living in one-room shacks (F; G) where the children are likely to observe the sexual activities of their parents.

The problem of teenage pregnancy is not linked to a lack of information provided by health and education facilities or parents, who tend to avoid talking about taboo issues (A), rather, teenagers who fall pregnant are in a certain way made jointly responsible for a behavioural "problem" (A) and for the spread of HIV within the community.

> They are taught about HIV/AIDS and STIs, how to prevent pregnancies (G); and
> The problem with high teenage pregnancy is the spread of HIV. (A)

A further specific health problem was mentioned by one interviewee: Premature Baby Syndrome (H). He commented:

> Premature babies are weak and (poor) families cannot take care of them. What happens to these babies if nobody takes care of them? (H)

Premature birth can be caused by a state of bad health including malnutrition and/or infections, risky health behaviour (including alcoholism) and the youth of pregnant women. Although Premature Baby Syndrome was not quoted by any other interviewee as a health problem within the Kayamandi community, this comment should be taken seriously and investigated in regard to high teenage pregnancy and widely distributed alcohol addiction among individuals within the community.

10.3.2 Lack of Security and Violence against Children

In general, crime is considered a threat to the stability of the community and a safety risk for children.

> Any situation that threatens the stability of a community, high crime, for example, will affect children negatively (G).

The two forms of violence that cause a lack of security for children are: community conflict and forms of child abuse. The interviewees ascribed the major security threats to in-migration, which seems to aggravate an ongoing conflict between recently immigrated and long-term residents, although most residents belong to one ethnic group, namely Xhosa (C). The separation is visible in Kayamandi's structural layout: Recently in-migrated people, expected to have come from areas within the Eastern Cape Province, dominate the informal settlement areas, whilst long-term inhabitants predominantly live in formal areas. The in-migration causes community conflict, as urban/modern-westernised and rural/traditional values and life styles collide.

> The people from the Western Cape Province in Kayamandi look down on the migrants from the Eastern Cape. They often call them 'mongo'. This is a swear word and means stupid person or someone who knows nothing. (B)

Interviewees stated that the two groups do not socialise or communicate with each other due to stigmatising processes and insults, like:

> This is the reason why places like the school and Kayamandi are dirty because of the untidy behaviour of the foreign (add: migrants) people. (B)

Furthermore, it can also be argued that the conflict is not only a conflict between people from poorer and better-off areas (in the community), but rather a power struggle between groups about who rules the community. Although such statements were not made directly in the interview, any struggle within the community give cause for concern since they create additional threats to the youngest members of society, namely children, who are exposed to diverse problems and remain in the middle of the conflict, being heavily dependent on the older generations.

Neglect, violence and sexual abuse were mentioned as prevalent forms of emotional and physical abuse, causing security problems for children in Kayamandi. Alcohol (and drug) addiction was testified as a widespread health risk in Kayamandi – social life in the community seems to centre around alcohol selling places like shebeens and taverns (G; F). Interviewees described alcoholism among adults in families as the reason for the neglect of children. They also stated that alcohol-related problems are predominantly found in informal settlement areas and expressed the concern that risky health behaviour of children is learnt from parents who function as role models (G).

> The drug/substance abuse by parents, e.g. drinking parents (alcohol abuse) is mainly to be found in informal settlements and drug and substance abuse by children will follow. They later show the same behaviour...Neglect, violence – children do not learn the rules from their parents. (H)

Social research (e.g. Berry & Guthrie, 2003) provides additional information showing that alcohol addiction deeply affects family life, as it increases stressors and violence levels and creates a high level of vulnerability in children as they are consequently neglected by their inebriated guardians. Alcoholism in the community should form part of a community-wide health intervention strategy.

Only one interviewee mentioned corporal punishment as a form of physical violence (B) after the interviewer had remarked that this seemed to be a problem at school. During the interview sessions the interviewer had observed several scenes of corporal punishment at school. The interviewee answered that he/she did not understand why teachers were so angry with the children, but was of the opinion that, from personal experience, a heavy beating created a better person (B).

Another form of child abuse mentioned is the sexual abuse of children. This form of violence was affirmed by several interviewees at different times in the interview sessions. Sexual abuse was described as widespread and starting at a very early age (H; A; F; B). One interviewee counted 15 incidences of sexual abuse at the primary school in the year 2001 (A). Official statistics (presented in chapter 4) do not support this statement. The interviewees did not mention emotional threats the children are exposed to as being a form of abuse.

10.4 Insights into Family Structures and Realities

The interviewees identified the following systems as the predominant family types in Kayamandi: the single-headed, urban-extended, legal guardian or child-headed system. Nuclear and rural-extended family systems were less frequently listed.

Single-headed families are described as the predominant family system in Kayamandi, and the result of high divorce rates, new partners or long-term separation of partners prevalent in informal settlements (B). The majority of single-headed families are ruled by women (F; C; H; E). The female- and single-headed families are associated with poverty and malnutrition (B); one interviewee expressed his concern that the predominance of single-headed households and the lack of extended families cause an absence of support systems and safety for children (H).

The second most common listed family system is the urban form of the extended family. The existence of a rural-extended family system which accommodates different generations over a longer period of time and is ruled by older generations was denied in interviews (H). The urban form of an extended family is described as a system of different family members who stay together for a short period of time. Two findings on the existence of an urban-extended family lead to this conclusion: First, the interviewees only described the existence of "big family members" (C), and second, the absence of grandparents who live mainly in the Eastern Cape Province (E) leads to a combination of people or blood relatives staying together without being ruled or regulated by the oldest authorities of the family as is the case in rural-extended family systems. Despite the fact that the traditional form of an extended family cannot be established within the urban community because of the absence of older generations, some interviewees still expressed the belief in traditional rural-extended family systems.

> Extended families still exist, hopefully lending support to children, motivating them and hopefully older ones setting example by way of their lifestyles, shaking up of young unmarried is bad example. (G)

Other types of family units that accommodate children in the absence of parents are either legal guardians (e.g. aunt, uncle) or child-headed families where children of secondary school age take care of younger siblings (B; C). These systems are established to safeguard young children when father and mother have passed away (D; H). The consequence for the older siblings is a shortened childhood; in addition, they are prone to terminate school attendance prematurely.

> First-born in poor families or oldest children bear early and high responsibility for other children. If the parents are away, they take over the parents' role and sometimes they do not go to school. (I)

Some interviewees mentioned that migration processes cause families in Kayamandi to be overburdened by unstable family systems; poverty with its related financial and psychological strains; and difficult and overcrowded living conditions within their physical environment. According to the interviewees, such an environment causes extremely unstable psychological and social situations for children and hinders them to have emotionally stable relationships with family members or peers. In the interviewees' opinion, this instability causes an emotional disturbance that prevents the development of 'normal behaviour', thereby putting children at risk of abuse or of becoming sexually active through peer pressure (F).

Several interviewees criticised the fact that many families cannot meet their children's basic need for food and shelter (C; I). Poverty and a high rate of unemployment (E; F; D; C; H) were noted as predominantly negative social conditions at the root of malnutrition and the generally low health status of children in Kayamandi (D; I).

One interviewee described two kinds of parents, those that are "dead tired" when they come home from long working hours, and those that "drink themselves to dead" as they are unemployed and spend most of the time at home (B). Both examples show that working conditions for the low paid strata of the society are difficult, with high social instability due to high unemployment levels. Other interviewees stated that there is a lack of parental responsibility, because parents are not there for their families (D) and, consequently, their absence causes a lack of control and protection of their children (B). Despite these criticisms, the families are recognised as playing a tremendous role in the mental and physical development of children.

> The role of families is to teach children in the ways of life and how to be independent. This includes points like supporting self-esteem, motivation, love, and care. (A)

10.5 The Existing Educational System

The role of education is to empower children because knowledge is power (F). All interviewees agreed that the education of children plays an important role in their mental development and their future perspectives.

> Schools, library, crèche can offer a ray of hope, if only children are motivated to study hard and want to change their lives and have a desire for better life. (G)

The existing school system in Kayamandi lacks material, financial and structural shortages, among other. The system is considered overcrowded due to too many children and too few schools. The only primary school accommodates 1 700 pupils in a community of 28 000 residents. Schools are described as overburdened with a shortage of teachers, materials (e.g. books), and classrooms that are too small (E; F).

> There are currently too few teachers, too small classrooms, poor access to educational support structures, toys, books (E); and to some extent they prepare children for their future. Schools are overloaded (classes are overcrowded, great lacks/gaps, teachers come too late). There is much to do (F).

One interviewee from the educational sector comments that, in his/her opinion, Ikaya Primary School is an 'abnormal' school with too many learners (some classes with up to 73 children): "As teacher you cannot work with all" (A). The interviewee explained that teachers work with 55 children in Grade 1. In total, seven Grade 1 classes exist at Ikaya Primary School.

The educational facilities are also influenced by the social conflict within the community which also escalates during the school day as learners and/or teachers have to socialise with each other. This is described as "cultural clashes" by one interviewee (F) who attributes the problem of violence in the school setting foremost to children from rural areas.

> They grew up in the Eastern Cape, were brought here for schooling. That change causes confusions in their minds resulting in a very unruly behaviour. The children come from the Eastern Cape Province to the Western Cape Province. They experience a transmission and confusion phase from extremely rural living conditions and behavioural rules to a semi-urban setting like Kayamandi. Conflicts develop because of confusion, e.g. the language difference. They have difficulties to socialise and conflicts are expressed in violence – stabbing with knives and stealing – and a lack of social responsibility. (B)

Vandalism, e.g. breaking of windows and doors, and burglaries are described as further forms of crime at Ikaya Primary School. An alarm system exists in the reception area, but even if the alarm goes off, it is ineffective because security services from Stellenbosch do not come to the school in Kayamandi. Even though the school has an alarm system it is thus not insured against burglaries. One consequence is that if something gets damaged or is stolen, the school lacks the finances to make the necessary replacements (e.g. broken windows or doors) (B). Another problem which seems to be caused by neighbouring residents is the regular destruction of the fence around the school terrain. People destroy the fence to create a short cut between two areas of the community. The behaviour is commented on:

> We seem to have a community that does not care about school. (B)

There also appears to be a problem with the payment of school fees. The strained financial situation of families is consequently linked with material shortage, which ultimately affects the children's education (D). In addition, another interviewee referred to the human rights of parents. The interviewee asked parents to learn more about their parental rights and duties as part of their responsibility to support their children in the educational process and to co-operate with teachers.

> In educational structures there is lack of cooperation with parents. Parents do not know what to do; they do not know their human rights. (C)

The above interviewees' statements do not consider the fact that it is most probably the parents' illiteracy and the socially marginalised position of the parents intellectually and emotionally which hinders them from exercising their rights and assuming their responsibilities at school.

10.6 Conditions in Kayamandi – Strengths and Challenges

One interviewee expressed his conviction that the Kayamandi people are trying their best in this difficult situation (A). Another interviewee said that there was still hope to solve any difficulty if the existing resources were well-managed and life for the inhabitants in Kayamandi was improved.

> There is hope for the better. They can improve their lives in Kayamandi through the present resources they can use and if people who use now resources just stop mismanaging the resources. (H)

Some experts are hopeful that resources and strengthening protective factors will influence children in their mental and physical growth. The following paragraphs define such health-enhancing factors within the environmental, family, and educational situation in this community.

10.6.1 Demands for Structural Changes

Interviewees agreed that the difficult and disadvantaged living conditions in the area impact greatly on the emotional state (or mental health) of children from an early age on. Children were described as growing up in "emotionally distressed and/or deprived and degrading circumstances" (G; H), which have a great impact on their "emotional welfare" (H). Interviewees therefore demand a complete change of the present geographical structure of Kayamandi that includes physical expansion, better access to water and toilets (E), and proper housing (H). The living environment has to be changed in such a way that children can enjoy entertainment and recreational activities on safe playgrounds and sports fields (E; A).

> There must be a sports field and playground or park and after school activities and more school. (A); and sport facilities are needed. Sport would allow for a more structured focus. (B).

A new concept of planning and networking would therefore not only create more options for children to develop their physical and emotional competencies but would also protect them.

> It is dangerous for children to play in the streets because cars have to pass playing children. (A)

Those places of activity and relaxation constitute places of safety where children are kept busy after school and receive care regarding rape and abuse (A). Listed risk factors for children are manifold and the insecurity within homes and the community, caused by crime such as burglaries, stealing of cars, clothes, or cell-phones, and rape, is heavily criticised by the interviewees. The present crime prevention strategies, e.g. the neighbourhood watch or police, do not specifically accommodate children. In addition, the police are not perceived as present in the Kayamandi community (A).

Another specifically mentioned problem is the fact that Kayamandi has a very young age structure. A sustainable development plan of the area ought to include that many young people will set up their own living places and will therefore need private space that is unavailable at present (H). According to a non-governmental interviewee, maps of and statistics about Kayamandi are preconditions for an exact planning and measuring of the strengths and challenges demanded (H). In conclusion, the uncontrolled population increase in Kayamandi will worsen the emotional, health and social conditions for all residents in the near future if no action is taken by the Municipality of Stellenbosch.

10.6.2 Strengthening the Support of Families

The absence of stable family systems and the growth of new family types create new demands for the community and the society on the whole. Many single parents or children who grow up in newly formed family systems, e.g. legal guardian or child-headed family units live in Kayamandi. Some interviewees criticise the absence of long-established family systems in the community where a positive family life is based on biological kinship.

> Loving and taking care of children would mean that biological parents take care and love their children so that they can grow up to be better human beings. Otherwise there is less chance of growing up healthy. (H)

However, other interviewees discern the difference between the functions of biological kinship in a family system and the new potential family units, and suggest that families have to provide stability (F) and a fostering home that teaches good family values which stimulate the child's mind and discipline (I). One interviewee strongly emphasises the preconditions for a functioning and positive family life, namely parents who are not only role models, but also offer "a loving and caring home" for their children (G).

As family life in Kayamandi is often characterised by extreme poverty, health hazards and exposure to violence, families need to be supported by the professionals within the community. All interviewees agreed that the "cycle of hopelessness" (F) can only be broken if a strong health promotion service for parents is offered within the community (G). Mothers in particular, as main care-takers, should receive training in social skills and family values so that they can educate and take proper care of their children regarding "nutrition", "hygiene", and "respect" (I). These services, however, have to be connected with the provision of basic requirement for the home, e.g. good nutrition (I) to make them sustainable.

The establishment of cooperative relationships between people in public institutions and non-governmental organizations and adults or parents in the community is equally important. According to one interviewee, the Community Clinic, for example, offers health promotion courses, but parents do not attend these courses (G). An interviewee from the educational sector tried to explain this perceived irresponsibility of the parents in taking care of their children with a feeling of incompetence on the part of adults. Workshops on child development for parents are a suggested solution (A). On the one hand, this statement supports the idea of increased health promotion intervention within families and on the other hand displays an acceptance of and comprehension for different attitudes between professionals and parents.

10.6.3 Demands for the Improvement of the Educational System

The educational system is seen as playing a vital role in developing the mental capacity of the child. One of the interviewees stated that he/she was convinced that all children – whether from urban or rural areas – had the same skills and abilities, but that differing access to educational institutions created dissimilarity between the children (I). Thus, the mental capacity of a child should be developed from an early age on in crèches and pre-primary schools. Although there are crèches in Kayamandi; they are often regarded as being inappropriate in terms of facilities offered or they have insufficient funds (I).

Ikaya Primary School could serve as an example of the strain on the educational system in the community. One interviewee is convinced that 800 of the 1 700 learners at the primary school would either need social, psychological, learning or financial support. In the interviewee's opinion the employment of a social worker at the school might be a step towards addressing the children's problems (A). Another interviewee mentioned that he/she hoped that the new system would take care of especially the "black" families, together with the mental and physical growth of the children (H). He/she thought that education would play a vital role in the early identification of psychological and/or physical problems preventing difficult living conditions for children.

> The educational system was supposed to have a multi-disciplinary diagnostic system where a child who suffers from emotional/behavioural condition and malnutrition can be detected early in the school system. (H)

Indeed, the change to Outcome Based Education (OBE) by the National Department of Education and the introduction of Curriculum 2005 is as confusing for children as for teachers (B). The demands on teachers to fulfil all expectations of the department and society are high.

> The school has an overloaded schedule that pushes teachers hard to write tests, reports, teach, and care about the social needs of the learners. (B)

Another interviewee feels the educational sector favours only the very few children with talent and intelligence. He/she is hopeful that the new OBE system can change this situation in time.

> The educational system brings a change to a few individuals. Many do ...leave school without finishing. The reasons are: apartheid, parental situation, changes from the old to the new system. It needs time to create more 'successful' individuals. (B)

Some interviewees feel that additional programmes that offer new forms of entertainment (e.g. soccer) should be introduced and guided by professionals to support children's playing skills (I). The concept that sport development (e.g. soccer) might increase children's chances to reach higher education through sports scholarships, and possibly enable children to experience success in a field other than education was expressed by another interviewee.

> It is good to focus on sport because some children are not good in reading or mathematics and sport can give them a chance to apply for scholarships for universities so that they can be someone. Also, children find positive role models on the sports field and they can have happy feelings apart from failure at school. (A)

One expert sees the building of a new primary and secondary school as the solution (B). He/she stated in one interview that the Stellenbosch Municipality had bought a plot to build a new school and is waiting for the National Department of Education to provide funds for the construction (B). Apart from the demanded increase in educational facilities, the lack of activity both by teachers and parents was also criticised. Teachers were criticised for being late for work or for showing a lack of responsibility (F). Another interviewee raised the point that teachers did not solve problems at school (H) while another one added that the schooling of teachers needed to be improved and adapted to international standards (A). However, it was also mentioned that there are teachers who show a high commitment to working with children, e.g. training teams in netball and soccer or support families that apply for grants, often without the support of the parents. Parents' lack of responsibility is expressed by their absence during parent meetings or refusal to check their children's books or attend school performances. The interviewees expressed their helplessness when parents do not cooperate when teachers need information on the background of the child, e.g. living conditions, family conditions, or traumatic experiences that would help them to support children in the educational process (A).

The above mentioned interviewee expressed the wish that he/she would like to see well-educated children in his/her community; that he/she would like to teach children in such a way that one day they would understand there is something that they can gain from "their" school and that they can be proud of their educational heritage.

> If they come back they can say: 'Thank you!' (A)

Finally, when asked what impact an additional learning programme, such as the undertaken life skills intervention, could have, the interviewees agreed that it could positively affect the teaching of skills for present and future life demands (I). In addition, it could enable participants to support their parents (C) in sharing learned knowledge with them (F). One interviewee believed that such health promotion initiatives could change children's perceptions in life (G).

> It will enlighten them. It will teach them that there is more to life than partying, sex, and alcohol. It will make them think about life, that they have life to live, that there is much for them to do. They will meet interesting people and places and enjoy life. (G)

However, interviewees were also aware that to ensure the quality of such an educational intervention, structural frameworks (I) will have to be put in place, for instance, the implementation must be planned for longer than one year (D; A) and the quality of training for trainers must have special importance (E). Finally, one interviewee felt that a health promoting initiative has to be undertaken with young children; to him, childhood seems to be a good time to undertake a "transfer of the mind" because children are still "fresh" and for them is it therefore "easy to learn to change" (B).

10.7 Children's Analysis of their Demands

In August 2004, an opinion poll was held with 47 children from the intervention group. The short questionnaire session included three questions about the children's observation of positive and negative elements in their physical and living environment. The opinion poll does not claim to be representative of all children living in Kayamandi. However, it gives a small group of children a voice to express their views.

The first question was: "What do you think, what is Kayamandi like?" Possible answers were "ugly", "beautiful", "ugly and beautiful" or "I do not know", which were pinned on posters to the black board. Children could answer this question by standing next to the appropriate poster. The second question was: "What do you think? – What is beautiful in Kayamandi?" and the third question: "What do you think? – What is ugly in Kayamandi?" The results were gathered during a brainstorming session in which the children were asked to give two ideas for each question.

The following results were revealed: More than half of the children (52.7%) felt incapable of answering the question on "What is Kayamandi like?", 28% of the children found Kayamandi beautiful and ugly and only 17% assessed their living environment as beautiful. These results reveal that more than half of the children have an ambivalent or no relation at all to their community.

When it came to the children's opinion on their physical environment, the majority of children decided that the school ($N=15$), newly built flats ($N=12$) and houses ($N=3$) were beautiful. A small number of children regarded the hospital ($N=1$), home ($N=1$), people ($N=1$) and the township ($N=1$) itself as pretty. Some found the town Stellenbosch ($N=4$) and the houses in the town ($N=1$) beautiful, although these answers articulated dreams and wishes and the ability to make comparisons with living standards in town.

The children saw a need for change in their place of residence. The majority of the children suggested that prevalent housing types, such as hostels ($N=20$), shacks ($N=13$), and halls ($N=1$), were ugly. Five noted prevailing hygienic conditions (dirt ($N=4$)), stalls that sell meat) as revolting. Three expressed the demand for a clean environment with proper accommodation "Shacks where all the papers are everywhere so they make Kayamandi dirty".

In summary, the results signify the children's demand for a change of the township structure. The children mainly criticised housing types and hygienic conditions in informal settlements. These densely populated areas are filled with noise, odour, dirt and waste and do not offer children the retreat and safety they require.

10.8 Conclusion

In regard to the physical and mental health, as well as the social well-being and development of children in the community of Kayamandi, the following factors were identified: cultural, socio-demographic and socio-economic conditions, and health/security and educational infrastructures (see also Richter et al., 2004).

Despite the importance of cultural and tribal heritage as element of socialisation for children, Kayamandi was overwhelmingly regarded as a multi-problem community that negatively affects child development and reduces quality of health even before birth.

All odds are against the growth of children in Kayamandi area. (I)

Based on existing socio-economic and socio-demographic conditions, poverty was described as an intrinsic factor in creating extensive risks for the physical and mental well-being of children. The living area of children is characterised by overcrowding and an extremely overburdened infrastructure regarding housing, sanitation and public services. The entire area lacks public places, e.g. markets or parks/green areas which might function as peace zones or recreation places for the purpose of physical and mental well-being.

More than two thirds of the settlement area consists of informal housing. The dense, chaotic and disorganised nature of these areas compresses the poorest strata within it, namely single female-headed households with children and recently migrated people. These people are the most vulnerable to social and economic inequity in Kayamandi; children that grow up in these households are consequently most susceptible to the shortages in basic needs and often suffer from malnutrition and lack of security, and are exposed to abuse, depression or demoralisation. In addition, interviewees also agreed that the combination of population density, inappropriate sanitation facilities, and widespread malnutrition not only favour diseases like tuberculosis and diarrhoea, but optionally reduce the immune-resistance of children and finally threaten quality of health in the long run for them.

The absence of a hierarchical structural layout prevents not only a safe but also a supportive community life, thereby increasing the existing atmosphere of conflict in the community. The existing long-standing conflict between residents living in formal and residents living in informal areas within the borders of Kayamandi is mentioned as a major security risk for children, apart from other prevalent forms of violence like neglect and child (sexual) abuse. On the one hand, the conflict can be interpreted as a collision of westernised urban lifestyles and traditional rural value systems within a densely populated and overcrowded area. On the other hand, it can be seen as a power struggle between the ruling strata living in formal areas and the poorest strata living in informal areas with sparse resources, which threatens the wellbeing and even survival of all inhabitants of this area.

The correlation between poverty and migration was identified as a further problem with regard to family life and protective measures for children. The large-scale migration of people from rural to urban areas or between urban areas in their search for work has a tremendous effect on children's socialisation. This relates to the fact that parents and other adult caretakers were described as influential in the development of the child's personality and behaviour, and that their influence might be beneficial or detrimental to success in adulthood.

For example, families that migrate from a rural to an urban living often experience the destruction of traditionally based family systems and a growth in single-headed family units. Parents or adults, who are by themselves in a process of value transition, can often not provide their children with the orientation and stability they require, or transfer the responsibility to other institutions such as schools. The assumption that can be drawn is that any disturbance in the interaction of the child with his/her parents or a lack of adequate attention, care, love and support from the family (or even from the community's side) leads to psychological stressors that hinder the development of health-related psychosocial competencies, e.g. self-esteem, mastery or resilience. It can be argued that the absence of protective or stable social systems that provide social support in a situation of deprivation, isolation and inhumane living conditions does also bear health risks, such as early sexual performance, for example, as substitute for emotional satisfaction and absent social support (see also Campbell, 2003).

The educational system, another pillar of socialisation, is described as a reflection of societal problems. Several interviewees expressed their concern that the change to OBE leaves teachers to deal with both the expectations of the National Department of Education and an impoverished community where individuals have little long-term perspective. Furthermore, the problematic interaction between parents and teachers creates a barrier for the mutual support of children and is a great disadvantage for the intellectual development and social skills of children.

The named risk factors influencing child development in Kayamandi can be assumed to weaken their health status, and most worryingly, make them vulnerable to developing risk-taking health behaviour during their process from childhood to adulthood. Experts in the field agree with and strongly demand structural changes (that match suggestions made from the results of the opinion poll among children), list strategies for strengthening the family systems, and emphasise the improvement of the educational system. However, they also clearly state that they as experts often feel helpless when confronted with the magnitude of problems, and that working in an extremely underdeveloped infrastructure requires support from a broader platform of society. The final future prognosis on the great responsibility of every person involved, according to one interviewee:

> The goal should be a changing society – a society with values. (I)

CHAPTER ELEVEN
Discussion of Research Findings

11.1 Introduction

Life skills programmes, in general, set high standards in their aim to be holistic and multileveled models, ultimately enabling human beings to develop a sound and positive mental health (see also Elias & Weissberg, 2000 in WHO, 2005). Contents of teaching are diverse and fundamental skills and competencies (e.g. social and emotional skills such as problem-solving, creative and critical thinking, self-awareness, communication, interpersonal relations, empathy, and emotional self-control) that influence not only the individual health but also the way of living and acting together with other human beings.

The presented life skills programme in this book, the *Child Mind Project*, evaluated the effects of a school-based life skills programme on HIV/AIDS and sex education, which was specifically designed for pre-adolescent children (10-11 years of age). Because children have an ability for psychosocial adaptation and a great enthusiasm for new learning input; it was therefore assumed that by early developmental and positive empowerment, protective factors for health behaviour could be encouraged and risk factors endangering their mental health be stemmed. In other words, the project aimed at developing social and psychological competencies required to cope with prevalent life tasks and to enhance the development of health behaviour, thereby reducing the risk of HIV infection among pre-adolescent children, i.e. before they become sexually active.

According to Mukoma and Flisher (2004), the challenge for the evaluation of school-based health promotion initiatives lies in achieving a balance between scientific rigour and consideration of practical possibilities and needs. In other words, social and living conditions have not only a tremendous effect on the individual level but also on the project and research level. For this reason, another goal of the study was to identify risk and protective factors influencing the mental and physical development of children in their social and physical sphere and to identify specific hindering and/or supporting factors, which influenced the ventured intervention itself. Thus, those data also enabled the researcher to modulate the learning programme on the actual needs and demands of the targeted group and guaranteed the building of a link between social/scientific sphere and individual need.

In summary, the points of discussion in the chapter 11 summarize specific research results in accordance with the gathered data in relation to the evaluation of needs, process and outcome. Thus, the final frame of the evaluation study will be built between theory, actual challenges, and research findings presenting one initiative for pre-adolescent children in the field of health promotion.

11.2 The Applicability of the Coordination Structure

In South Africa, public schools face specific problems when located in extreme socially-disadvantaged areas. In their day-to-day life, these schools deal with children whose life is indelibly marked by a multitude of social problems, e.g. unhygienic living conditions, extreme poverty, malnutrition, and instable family systems often shaped by work migration. The expansion of children's cognitive capacity and their ability to deal with social demands can easily emphasise the children's problematic background and the schools own difficult and underequipped structural, personnel and financial situations. The existing strains and stressor influence learner-teachers, as well as learner-learner relations, and learning situations can often lead to an administration of interpersonal behaviour practised by authoritarian pedagogical ideologies (e.g. corporal punishment).

A comparable situation was found to exist in the case study school, the Ikaya Primary School, in Kayamandi (Stellenbosch). The exhaustion of teachers working with children, who are often hungry when they come to school, their feeling of overstrain and isolation in facing a magnitude of social problems certainly provide some explanations why the governmental life skills programme on AIDS was not implemented in the schedule of the case study school as an additional learning area. Another important factor why the governmental life skills programme was not applied for the children were the difficult and often strongly socially stigmatised topics on AIDS, sex, death or disease. Teaching about taboos affords the improvement of own value and behavioural systems and the opening as a role model. For many teachers talking in front of a class about intimate information is an understandable hurdle and, moreover, talking about taboo issues within a closely interweaved social network system in the community can also be risky for anybody who dares to speak out the most feared issues.

Although, teachers from the Ikaya Primary School participated in workshops on the governmental life skills programme on AIDS, the school was unable to implement the programme as an additional educational offer due to its own staff provision. Outside support for this process was urgently needed for the school to achieve the curriculum in the field of life skills on AIDS and sex education set by the South African National Department of Education.

A solution for this shortage of structural capacity was seen in an educational cooperation with an outside partner, who was able to organize and permute a life skills programme on AIDS and sex education for pre-adolescent children at this particular primary school. From 2002 until 2004, the following coordination structure for the life skills programme on AIDS and sex education was characterised by two columns – cooperation partners and stakeholder/community network.

11.2.1 Strengths and Challenges of the Cooperation Structure

The cooperation partners for the programme were the Ikaya Primary School, the Ikamva Lethu Center (former SAA unit) and the Joy for Life Organization. The outcomes of this *cooperation model* can be identified as very positive and valuable during the pilot study; which gave the programme design extreme diversity. The three institutions combined their staff and material resources and professional expertise to make the programme function properly and appropriate for the target group. This was done, for instance, by emphasising the schooling and qualification of the HPTs. Further valuable input included free teaching material, the organization of the support by specific segments within the community (e.g. religious) and the protection of staff/project, maintaining public relations with the school governing board, and the application of workshops for HPTs and female legal guardians of the participating children. Finally, with this support system, the CMP gained a large amount of material resources and personal support to keep the intervention functioning on a low cost basis throughout all of its phases.

However, right from the beginning of the pilot study, a difficult situation for the project was caused by *structural changes within the organization structure*. During the planning phase of the study, the unit of the SAA carrying out health promotion interventions with youth in Kayamandi became an independent Section 21 Company, called the Ikamva Lethu Centre. These structural and financial transformations led to a change in the local partners' character. Thus, already at the outset, the first and community-based cooperation partner lost its strong anchor position for the pilot project and was consequently unable to make any integral and/or long-term plans to sustain the evaluated programme.

The *fragmentary cooperation* model, caused by a low capacity building and a magnitude of instabilities and uncertainties between the partners, can be seen as a main hurdle to finally sustain the project into a stable educational offer for pre-adolescent children in Kayamandi. The necessity to establish a strong project partner system and a clear system of responsibilities right from the beginning would have been a precondition of the *Child Mind Project* to reach sustainability.

11.2.2 Strengths and Challenges of the Community Network

As stated by Guba and Lincoln (1989), the involvement of various stakeholders means responding to local needs within an acceptable cultural framework. This consequently means that if research is to be regarded as an integral part in the increased effect of the intervention, it then also encourages *constant monitoring* and provides a practical way to cross boundaries between theory and practice (Guba & Lincoln, 1989). For this reason, several efforts were made to develop a network with specific governmental and non-governmental institutions in the community in order to strengthen this pilot project in its larger physical environment.

The negotiations involved a network of various institutions and local experts who were encouraged to support the CMP, namely: a civic group, a religious-based organization, the Kayamandi Community Clinic, the Social Welfare Organization (to a certain extent), the youth centre and the primary school as partners, and local artists. This network turned out to be extremely important for staying in touch with institutions and ensuring the direct involvement of stakeholders and experts in the case study community (e.g. the community clinic, youth centre and drama group). Thus, the pilot project could be implemented in its physical environment, and the effect of several sessions could be expanded (e.g. the drama on abuse, or medical support) during the time of the intervention.

The main column of the negotiation process was the accomplished action research approach. That is to say, the researcher assumed a 'dual position' in project and research management as this was most likely to affect the relationship with the community and especially the case study school. Here it became obvious, that the case study school increasingly associated the project with the researcher's persona, thus providing a gateway between field work (practice) and research (theory). The action research approach finally effectuated that various local organizations played an advisory role in the evaluation of the intervention in terms of cultural, environmental and political determinants, with the result that their expertise had an effect on the research and project level of this study. Holding regular meetings ensured a constant discussion on research findings and proved the steady loss of objectivity by the local experts and the evaluator.

Furthermore, it was vital for the evaluator, as a cultural outsider coming from western European background, to understand (South) African cultural patterns, social convictions and/or prevalent value systems in order to reduce research bias due to contrary value systems. In reverse, *negotiation procedures* were especially important in building an understanding among local experts for the need of this health initiative that targeted sensitive topics such as HIV/AIDS and sex education, particularly as these issues are normally rejected and stigmatised. Further, the negotiating procedures also served to establish a net of safety measures to protect the health promoting initiative as well as the HPTs living in the community.

Although negotiation processes within the Kayamandi community were effective in that they *safeguarded the pilot study*, they were ineffective in gaining community support to introduce the project as a new community-based approach for children. This was due to (1) the project partner organizations being identified as the responsible institutions, (2) the fragmentary and overburdened infrastructure within the community, which led several organizations to feel incapable to join the project as partners, and (3) the project lacking the complete support of people in powerful positions, such as in the town council or local political parties. Especially the last point, support of people in powerful political and/or financial positions, is detrimental to obtain further funds for any pilot project(s). Finally, the non-allocation of financial funds and the unresolved question of ownership of the project resulted in the termination of the *Child Mind Project* in 2004.

11.3 The Main Columns – Incorporation of Parents, Class Teacher and Health Promotion Trainers

Without any doubt, the two main socialisation columns with the most influence on child development in pre-adolescent stage are parents (or families) and teachers (schools). To give parents and the class teacher a reasonable role and say, the *Child Mind Project* incorporated specific initiatives and activities to involve parents and teachers in the pilot study.

11.3.1 Parents on Board – A Both-Sided Support System

Several attempts were made to involve parents more closely in the project in their function as the most important emotional role models and legal guardians of their children. During the pilot project, more than four *parent meetings* were held to inform parents about the content of the sessions, their children's learning achievements and to ask their feedback on the positive or negative effects of the intervention regarding their children's behaviour.

Some of the outcomes of these meetings were that, after the considerable mistrust towards the project was partly overcome, parents were relieved that 'someone' took over this sensitive field of education. The use of educated 'outsiders', the health promotion trainers, did not appear to be a point of critique; however, it was clear that parents controlled taught knowledge and checked information papers. According to statements given by parents, the intervention positively affected the communication between parents and their children.

In addition, as the parents' own level of education is sometimes so low that they often feel incapable of fulfilling a supportive educational role for their children, *further initiatives, e.g. health-promoting workshops* or other informal platforms for interaction were found to be a very effective way of passing on knowledge to the parents. It was found that an awareness workshop on HIV/AIDS – whereby the children's female caretakers participated in the intervention group – was an effective method to offer a platform for discussion. Despite the fact that only five mothers joined the workshop, it unexpectedly changed into a meeting where mothers discussed problems relating to child care as well as personal problems affecting their own emotional state, for example feelings of overstrain and helplessness in a situation of extreme poverty.[35]

However, experience has shown that a once-off workshop is not recommended. To be effective, these kinds of interventions have to be organized on a regular and continuous basis. Parents need to be supported to enable them to function as emotional and physical 'bodyguards' and social role models for their children; especially children growing up in impoverished settings. Furthermore, parents and educators involved in these programmes need to be prepared and supported to find a balance between different educational approaches towards providing health-enhancing knowledge and skills for their children, as life skills programmes often

---

[35] As a side note, a further unexpected outcome of this meeting was that women, who had never talked about HIV/AIDS, walked home with five boxes of condoms that they wanted to distribute at shebeens in Kayamandi.

convey strongly westernised messages, which stand in contrast to observed and adapted attitudinal constructs with regard to their setting, convictions and behaviour. It is thus recommended that workshops for parents be planned parallel to the undertaken life skills programmes to (1) allow parents to keep up with their children's development in the programme, (2) reduce the pedagogical attempts of the parents and the approach of the life skills programme to a common denominator, and (3) put parents in a position to be role models for their children, which most likely could contribute to normalising child-parent relations and reducing stressor within families.

11.3.2 The Class Teacher – Inputs on Project and School Level

The roles of the class teacher in this educational cooperation model encompassed three areas of input: (1) to form a bond between the school (e.g. management, other grade 4 teachers, case work) and the CMP, (2) to support the preparation for parent meetings (e.g. name lists, room arrangements), and (3) to give expert pedagogical input to the health promotion trainers. From this experience it is recommended that *support teachers* be involved at the start of such an educational cooperation model because they are familiar with daily schedules and procedures at school. This means, with the support of the teacher it was much easier to manage the project from within the school setting, including the organization of outdoor trips and parent meetings.

Despite the fact that the support teachers were often not able to attend the full duration of the sessions due to an administrative workload, their involvement in classroom activities were also found to be effective in supporting the project team in case work and in the preparation and adjustment of lessons.

Another positive outcome for the support teacher personally, is the fact that the programme allowed her to gain more knowledge on the taught topics. As an example, while many evaluations of school-based life skills programmes report that teachers often feel overburdened or ashamed to convey key preventive messages such as condom use, the teacher at the case study school used the opportunity to gain more information on HIV/AIDS and preventive barriers. In the session on HIV/AIDS, for example, she came to the front of the class and expressed her interest in the use of female condoms. The teacher's increased and open interest in the topics taught might be an indication of her feelings of relief and comfort in the presence of other educators which then created a more relaxed position for her in the class without having the full responsibility of an individually-working educator.

The most negative finding of the cooperation model was that old *behavioural codes* between the teacher and children could not be fully broken. In the last session of the booster unit, the class teacher hit latecoming learners with a stick on their hands.[36] Although, it was only an exceptional incidence throughout the time of the intervention, two problems arise from this type of behaviour with regard to the programme and its outcomes. First, it can be considered a risk-taking enterprise to involve a teacher at the case study school where rigid conflict-solving methods are used which contradict approaches to create a healthy learning environment in the classroom. Second, the same example can also be used to illustrate a life skills approach whereby children are taught non-violent conflict management and given the opportunity to express his/her own opinion with confidence. In other words, the encouragement of more self-confidence and open behaviour in children may often be seen as disrespectful acts towards an authority and results in problematic interpersonal relations at the school between learners and teachers. Further research is clearly needed to examine whether children are exposed to confusion or further threats when they act in two different social interaction systems, and to detect what these threats are, in order to implement safety measures among life skills programmes.

11.3.3 The Health Promotion Trainers – A Challenged Opportunity for Educational Support

Besides the fact that those findings have an alarming nature, they can also provide a fertile ground for new ways and challenges. An hypothesis can be: if an educational system remains in deep contrast to health enhancing values and behavioural rules then the involvement of outside educational partners, who provide new constructs of behavioural interactions for the existing school system can be a supportive instrument in conveying new strategies and competencies for interpersonal relations within the school setting.

For the accomplishment of the *Child Mind Project* it was decided to integrate an educational and cultural bridge: health promotion trainers. The implementation of a cooperative teaching model was to support the school in personnel infrastructural strains and to moderate as objective outsiders between teachers and parents of the participating children; symbolizing an alternative educational methodology.

The involved health promotion trainers, two unemployed women from the Kayamandi community, were already involved in volunteer work in the

---

36 The health promotion trainers did not intervene in the teacher's action. The most likely cause of this inactivity was not having clearly defined responsibilities among HPT's and class teacher in the sub-unit, as well as a general lack of conflict-solving skills on how to deal with the stressor situation.

field of child welfare and medical support for HIV and STI counselling at the office of public health in Kayamandi. Before the start of the intervention both women received substantial training over three months based on the manual of the life skills programme.

Although, the HPTs' reports revealed that they assessed their own self-confidence more positively in combination with an increased experience in teaching and the use of learning methods over the course of Intervention I and that the applied teaching methods were generally well-managed in the classroom, there were, nevertheless, certain identified problem areas. These were particularly time management and the application of complicated methods such as frontal teaching, group discussion and conflict-solving management in the classroom. *Continuous training* is recommended to assure the accuracy of taught specialised knowledge as a precondition for increasing the precision of modelled situations and stabilising and manifesting individual teaching competencies and skills over a prolonged period among the health promotion trainers.

The HPTs reports also show that the management of group work sessions or class management was supported by their teamwork. Working in a team obviously helped these two women to put them at ease in the classroom setting and to decrease stressor in teaching situations. In time, this also served to increase their self-confidence to manage new demands and challenges. Therefore, in the opinion of the HPTs the lack of skills and competencies could be well-balanced by their teamwork.

Another area of further training can be recommended for *case work*. During the intervention phase, children reported cases of (sexual) abuse to the HPTs. Handling such cases independently outside of the classroom requires specific professional competencies to be able to react sufficiently and provide further support for the children. If this cannot be provided, the helper easily finds him/herself in a situation of helplessness – in other words, the HPT experiences a feeling of excessive pressure as a result of the support. Based on this experience, the incorporation of socio-psychological support and on-going workshops for teaching staff is recommended so that they will be able to cope with such additional stressor. Furthermore, another recommendation is the employment of a social worker who concentrates on case work in the programme, so that HPTs can concentrate on teaching. This should be considered in the run-up of the planning phase in every health-promoting initiative in a comparable social setting.

11.4 Applied Methods for Creating Emotional and Intellectual Safety

The subjective nature of assessing positive social relations is determined by the quality of psychosocial learning processes, which in turn affects the individual's ability of self-motivation and his/her behaviour. Positive social relations create an atmosphere of equity and fairness; good relations between all involved persons were assumed to be a precondition for *transferring social competencies* regarding positive norm constructs.

11.4.1 Implementing Safety Measures

A precondition to create an environment leading to positive relations between human beings is the formation of a setting characterised by clear regulations and safety. With regard to the unstable, and often rigorous, school atmosphere at the case study school, it was of special importance to create an atmosphere of tolerance, respect and solidarity within the classroom to motivate and empower learners to enlarge their cognitive, emotional and social competencies. The implemented framework, rituals and code of conduct were finally found to be effective methods to ensure reliable and accountable relations between all participants and to provide children and educational personnel with a healthy learning environment.

The specific *safety measures*, for example, the code of conduct, turned out to be vital in an environment where physical punishment is commonly applied as a disciplinary measure. In retrospect, had it not been for the creation of an emotionally safe framework, where children could act and speak freely and openly, the most important precondition for the implementation of a life skills programme on HIV/AIDS and sex education would have been imperilled right from the beginning. Regulations and codes of conduct that apply equally to learners and educators in the classroom setting are strongly recommended. These will then provide a constant structure of the programme and form a basis for orientation and clear preferences in interpersonal contacts (HPTs, learners, and supporting teacher).

11.4.2 Interpersonal Working and Learning Relations

Because one of the main goals of the programme was to develop social competencies among participants, it was necessary to *enhance encouraging interpersonal working and learning relations* between girls and boys, as well as between the children and the HPTs.[37]

Although, the vast majority of the boys and girls expressed a positive attitude towards the HPTs, more boys expressed a dislike of working with HPTs on culturally and individually sensitive topics such as body changes, HIV/AIDS and abuse. During the phase of team establishment, several consulted experts working for organizations in the case study community were divided on whether to insist on a male HPT in the project. Some argued that the involvement of a man would bear the danger of abuse for female learners, due to the high prevalence of rape in South African schools; others made it clear that it would increase the risk of power struggles within the team that could ultimately undermine the project. Despite the above mentioned considerations in the planning phase of the intervention, in retrospect it became evident that employing both male and female HPTs would have been of great advantage for male and female participants to experience 'models' of both genders in the classroom. It can be assumed that a heterogeneous gender of the HPTs would have especially strengthened the feeling of comfort for boys and their interest to learn more about the topics taught in the programme, and with it, supported a growing relation to a male role model who stimulates an identification process of boys for their later male role in family and society.

With regard to same-gender relations: in general both sexes liked working and learning with children of the same gender. Intergender relations were assessed more positively by girls than by boys in Intervention I. Only in three sessions (*Body Changes*, *Sex Education*, and *Care and Death*) more boys than girls preferred working with the other sex. This is most interesting because in sessions on body changes and sex education gender-specific group work was used. It can therefore be deducted that both genders agreed to be separated in sessions on sensitive topics; furthermore, while boys enjoyed being separated from girls in one room, girls expressed more clearly that the local separation in those sessions in the same location was insufficient for them.

While no changes in intergender relations were revealed over the duration of Intervention I, the participant observation of four children disclosed that, firstly, the programme provided an environment in which boys and girls learned and acted with each other without any refusal or dispute and, secondly, three of the four children established friendships with the same gender from Intervention I to Intervention II. These findings most likely correlate with the developmental stage of the children: during the transition

---

37 The children's relation with the involved teacher could not evaluated due to her absence from many sessions.

phase from late childhood into adolescence children tend to enlarge their social networks and establish more stable same gender relations – a pre-step before turning into intimate gender relations. Besides the fact that such a health-promoting initiative like the *Child Mind Project* offers an environment that enhances positive interpersonal relations important for emotional comfort and the practice of social competencies, it can also accompany children in their developmental process to adolescents outside of school and family sphere. This fact asks for a greater emphasis on the establishment of friendship systems in the programme, as well as the enhancement of children's safety and social networks both in and outside the classroom.

11.4.3 The Efficacy of Applied Topics and Methods

The *Child Mind Project*, as a life skills programme focusing on AIDS awareness and sex education, is a multimodal intervention which uses specific topics that are related to the HIV/AIDS pandemic. Due to the socially-disadvantaged setting of the pilot study, several sessions and methods were also assessed and re-modulated during the evaluation process in order to make them more appropriate to the culture and the living standards of the children and to closely interweave them with specific demands and needs.

Specific *re-modulations* were made in the sessions on healthy nutrition (e.g. food), sexual abuse (e.g. drama play), the planning of outdoor trips (e.g. community clinic or youth centre) to make existing infrastructures more accessible to the children, HIV/AIDS (condom promotion), and sex education (sexual intercourse, contraception). Further information for re-modulations were gathered from the secret box, field trips, and literature review. Especially the secret box was found to be a valuable instrument to detect fields of interest directly from children.

As an example, one field of interest of the children was the issues of HIV/AIDS or sex. In regard to the high number of teenage pregnancies at primary and secondary school level in the case study community, supported by the results of the literature review, the topics were incorporated in the intervention in Grade 4. The incorporation of those topics were against the planning of the governmental programme which introduced the most important health messages on the prevention of unplanned pregnancy and HIV-transmission in grade 6.

The learners' reports and opinion poll revealed that with regard to gender differences, boys expressed a greater feeling of boredom (when also defining a stable group of boys in the intervention group) during the sessions than girls, who almost unanimously stated that they found the sessions to be fun.

The gender differences were mainly found in the analysis of attitudes towards specific topics and applied methods. While girls expressed a great interest in most of the topics and enjoyed applied methods, boys were more critical and expressed the greatest dislike in topics on hygiene, body anatomy, HIV/AIDS and sexual abuse.

These findings could lead to the assumption, namely, that boys had obtained knowledge on those topics through other channels. However, this can not be verified by a gender difference in terms of quantitative outcomes when it comes to knowledge of HIV/AIDS. Two other and more convincing explanations for the gender differences in the general attitude towards the programme could be the following. First, the absence of a positive male role model might have avoided the development of interest for the topics especially among boys. Second, the topics taught were more relevant to the developmental stage of the girls than that of the boys and therefore resulted in more interest among girls than boys. Despite the right or wrong of the formulated assumptions, there should be paid more attention to the gender specific re-modulation of topics and methods in comparable health-promoting initiatives for pre-adolescents.

An additional, and not to be underestimated, understanding was that the young age of the children required a great *sense of empathy* when applying sensitive and emotionally demanding topics. The social-cognitive (thought and consciousness) processes between models and individuals (e.g. observation) play a paramount role in Bandura's *Social Cognitive Theory* (1986). However, when working with children, emotions are vital for encouraging interest and motivation. The cognitive and emotional dimensions and their interplay are decisively dependent on the function of the social dimension, which means that, if the model (or its lesson sessions) is not acceptable regarding content and emotions, the learning processes will be distorted (Illeris, 2002). This assumption can be supported by the results of the opinion poll. In the children's long-term memory all of the applied topics (including HIV/AIDS and abuse) were positively assessed; however, some children still regarded emotionally demanding topics such as HIV/AIDS or abuse as demanding even eight months after Intervention II.

In general, when working with a young age group all applied methods should be lively and enjoyable aimed at increasing an interest in the discussion topics and geared at *motivating children* to perform and adopt health behaviour later in life. It is therefore recommended that a stronger emphasis should be put on examining emotional competencies (e.g. empathy) and should subsequently be included in the research model.

11.5 Research Gaps – Considerations Regarding Learning Outcomes on the Individual Level

The outcome evaluation of psychological and social variables on the individual level, can be defined as being extremely limited due to the inability to analyse the cognitive and social variables other than those relating to a knowledge on HIV/AIDS. The only references which could be made to the sustainability of the effect of the programme showed significant changes in the knowledge of HIV/AIDS from pretest to posttest in conveying the four main messages. It was found that significantly more children at the posttest were able to define AIDS as a disease that destroys the immune system. More children were convinced that everyone, gender or social position regardless, can get infected. Many more children knew that the community clinic or the office of public health were medical institutions where they could go for an HIV-test, whilst significantly more children knew that the use of condoms protects you against an HIV-infection.[38]

11.5.1 Causes of Knowledge Instability among the Participating Children

However, as the quantitative results on knowledge also show, the acquisition of knowledge was not sustainable among participants; furthermore, knowledge increased significantly in several items at follow-up test 2 without any intervention taking place. Thus, a train of thought is given to formulate assumptions for this phenomenon at this point.

Pre-adolescent children are still in the *process of absorbing*, acquiring and organizing knowledge in their minds, thus, knowledge is generally far-reaching and not immediately relevant and parts of it is therefore lost over time. In other words, children can simply forget what they have learned, or rather that the correspondence to reality is lower; children at this age are not yet sexually active and the acquired knowledge might be of no practical relevance to them. The increase in knowledge after Intervention II can also be a *'delayed processing'* of knowledge regarding HIV/AIDS. This means, children build new knowledge on the volume of information and symbols (meaning of words) they gathered during the intervention. Another factor that can be supported by a delayed processing can be that this new knowledge is confirmed and improved by *observations* in their environment, for example

---

38 No significant differences in knowledge levels between genders were found.

peer groups or families, and other stimuli, for example media. Similarly to this process, they carefully weigh up what is of importance to them and finally *reformulate information* so that it makes sense to them. Again, the precondition for this process is an increased sensitivity, which might be foregrounded by the intervention.

Bandura's *Social Cognitive Theory* (1986) emphasises that health behaviour is mainly shaped by conscious decisions of rational individuals and by rationalising a complex situation with a multitude of influencing factors on the individual level (Campbell, 2003). According to his theory, it can be assumed that individual and interpersonal factors which encourage certain behavioural strategies are very much determined by the extent to which community and societal contexts enable and support the performance of such behaviour outside the intervention. Thus, the instability of knowledge of HIV/AIDS could also be ascribed to an insufficient belief in the accuracy or relevance of the knowledge in the children's physical or social environment.

As an illustration: children grow up in a very ambiguous environment where they interact with people who either believe in scientific information, pass on a limited understanding of the disease to their children, simply do not talk about such issues or do not believe in scientific arguments at all. For example, in the presence of two different medical approaches – African and western – these different medical/scientific systems also present two different methods of prevention of the HI-Virus or cure for AIDS. While the former explains everything from a very holistic point of view including the belief in ancestors; the latter presents knowledge from a purely scientific understanding taught in the *Child Mind Project*. The real danger of the existence of two different health-promoting systems is that children, who are heavily dependent on the transfer of knowledge from authorities and older age groups, obtain incomplete or false knowledge in spite of what they have learned in a modelled situation from people such as (female) health promotion trainers. From this perspective it seems possible that the lack of sustainability of the results is not only due to the children simply forgetting what they have learned, but also to their not believing in what they were taught during the *Child Mind Project*.

Although children in this pre-adolescent phase have not yet developed health behaviour, the information, skills and competencies can only manifest in an individual's mind if the social and community contexts actually create the basis for the absorption and performance of learned health behaviour. Such *causal opportunities* can be resources, social support, integration in social networks and/or rational systemic structures and cultural convictions. Thus, these two different belief and value systems described above need to be included in health promoting initiatives, in order for individuals to weigh up their personal (behavioural) strategies to ensure health. With this course of action the individual can form his/her opinion, e.g. on AIDS, by proving the different belief systems and, given time, interweave such knowledge with his/her personal belief system under the guidance of experts.

11.5.2 Social Factors Shaping Individual Outcomes and Projects Possibilities

Factors which lie outside of the behavioural constructs of the individual, but greatly influence the strategies for protection and the realization of a health lifestyle, can most likely be traced to the living conditions of human beings. Most of the children in the study experience a *shortage of basic needs*, such as food, shelter, or security. Many of the issues raised concerning HIV/AIDS are assumed not to be particularly relevant to the individual's daily life. For example, many children in the intervention group were often hungry during the sessions; this whilst taking part in a programme proclaiming high values such as well-being, a healthy lifestyle and/or protective methods for the future. The lasting success of a programme that targets well-being, self-fulfilment and appreciation can only be measured if the satisfaction of such tremendously important basic rights is fully ensured (Maslow, 2002). In order to reinforce the personal conviction that there is a real life threat, interventions not only need to be more relevant to the individual's daily health demands but also provide real opportunities for the increase of physical health and well-being. Funding proposals must incorporate a section on the provision of food to children living in extreme poverty, so that they can concentrate on higher values such as creative and critical thinking, self-awareness, and self-control aimed by life skills programmes.

Regarding the investigated cognitive variables, it is recommended that further research has to be done in order to examine the acquisition of knowledge and skills that bear a relation to the everyday life of children. In this way, the focus shifts towards the children's lifestyle, instead of only concentrating on the development of a certain protective health behaviour. The shift of research paradigm must be accompanied by a long-term approach on life skills to fill possible gaps and stabilise knowledge and are able to influence the establishment towards creating protective, non-risky behavioural constructs for the socialisation process from pre-adolescents to adulthood.

11.6 Conclusion

The perspectives for future generations of South African children are considered to be more problematic as the consequences of poverty in combination with the AIDS epidemic will fall foremost on their shoulders. One of the most effective currently existing health promoting instruments to prepare children for life and future demands and to inform about HIV infection are life skills programmes. These programmes provide a wide spectrum of positive individual experiences, a broad general knowledge, and comfort, at the same time practicing health-related skills and competencies in an enabling environment.

However, from the experiences of the *Child Mind Project* it is concluded that if such life skills programmes are to be more effective, the entire school setting (and, at best, the whole community) should be targeted as a health promoting institution that provides emotional, educational and administrative structures for all individuals to practise health-related behaviour. If this goal is not met, however, the effects of health promoting initiatives, like the evaluated one, will be unsteady and the outcomes fuzzy, especially within a very impoverished and/or socially-disadvantaged community, such as case study community "Kayamandi".

The highest priority for health promoting initiatives, and the key goal for the prevention of the further transmission of HIV among the younger segments of society, is to reduce growing risk factors in the socio-interpersonal and socio-economic sphere. Due to the conviction that health is determined by the physical, mental and social well-being of an individual, important data were gathered on *risk and protective factors* that affect child development in the case study community Kayamandi. Socio-demographic and socio-economic conditions, and health/security and educational infrastructures were identified as relevant areas to incorporate specific risks and protective factors. However, most of the factors identified make children vulnerable to unsafe mental and physical health, like insecurity due to instable family units and exposure to poverty, risks of violence, exposure to ill physical health by malnutrition and unhygienic living conditions, a rapid social change by large-scale migration processes, and hopelessness due to low standards of education and reduced future prospects (see also WHO, 2005, p. XIIX). These sets of vulnerabilities to health risks during childhood are expected to increase with maturation unless preventive health promoting initiatives are not undertaken to equip these vulnerable children with competencies that would enable them to cope with prevailing developmental and life demands.

The greatest precondition to turn the tide is an open public and society-wide discussion, as well as clear actions from the part of the South African government to target health and social problems that increase exposure e.g. to HIV for individuals would provide both a real as well as an acknowledged platform for health initiatives to enhance the health of many human beings.

In the knowledge that politically, economically and socially developing countries are hit especially hard by the AIDS pandemic, the fact must also be emphasised that the dimensions of this pandemic are beyond the experience of everyone involved, as it demands overcoming psychological barriers and creates personal stress for every human being involved. There is great concern that another generation will bear the burden of the AIDS pandemic should there continue to be a lack of appropriate protection and preparation of children for such an enormous and often incomprehensible pandemic with all its short-term and long-term effects.

To be able to bring together meaningful research results on the individual and programme level the link to the social environment and its participation urges for effectiveness and efficiency of such pilot studies as described in this book. As this study and its outcomes also reflect, a change from behavioural prevention to structural prevention is urgently needed. Because social determinants are so overwhelming for research and programme implementation, first and foremost research needs to focus on local needs and those needs should be described and shaped by local people, guided by experts, and met with a framework of stable cooperation and financial constructs. Such a participative approach is even possible in a very socially-disadvantaged setting as the involved citizens of the community of Kayamandi have verified in the *Child Mind Project*.

EPILOGUE

At the time the majority of children who participated in this study are 18 years old, the epidemic will have reached its highest level (approximately around 2010); they will be young adults just starting their independent lives and establishing families. The biggest question now is: Will they, as the new South African generation, be equipped to cope with the demands of life in an epidemic situation under the most difficult living constraints?

After all my experiences in the field of health promotion and AIDS prevention, I am still undecided on the right answer of the question raised above. For this reason, I would like to give voice to a South African woman, who, I think, is the real expert to make a statement on ways of protecting the next generation in avoiding a continuance of an HIV/AIDS pandemic.

S. G. Gedze, a South African woman belonging to the ethnicity of Xhosa survived apartheid, an abusive marriage and impoverished living conditions in which she, as a single mother, successfully raised her four children. She is now in her mid-fifties and faces another problem she never expected to be exposed to. Within four years she lost two of her four children – her youngest daughter and one son, as well as, one of her grandchildren to AIDS. Despite her great emotional suffering and devastation, which is evident in her physical change, her mind is still strong and courageous. She is one of the few people who have started to speak openly with the young people about taboo issues such as HIV, sex and condom use and against ignorance and fear in her community. In our last meeting she asked me to write the following message in this book "for the people in my country and anywhere else in the world".

> "Protect your children and speak with them, otherwise you will have to bury your children – as we do here – before you as a parent leave this world." (S.G.G.)

This statement emphasises how the onus is on us as adults (e.g. parents, teachers or members of society and government), to guarantee each and every child in an endangered situation the right to live a healthy and protected life.
To fulfil our role, we have to overcome our own personal barriers.
To do justice to this duty we have to allow child participation.
To prepare the children for the world we live in today, and leave them a better world for tomorrow, means their personal involvement at their level of understanding.
A Child's Mind Required!

REFERENCES

Aaro, I. E., Flisher, A. J., Kaaya, S., Onya, H., Fuglesang, M., Klepp, K.-I., & Schaalma, H. (2005). Promoting sexual and reproductive health in early adolescence in South Africa and Tanzania: Development of a theory- and evidence-based intervention programme. *Scandinavian Journal of Public Health*, Preview article, 1-9.

Abraham, C., Sheeran, P. & Johnston, M. (1998). From health beliefs to self-regulation: The advances in the psychology of action control. *Psychology and Health, 13*, 569-591.

Adler, G. & Qulo, O. (1999). HIV/AIDS and STDs. In: N. Crisp & A. Ntuli (Eds.), *South African Health Review*. Durban: Health System Trust.

Alem, A. & Kebede, D. (2003). Conducting psychiatric research in the developing world: Challenges and rewards. *British Journal of Psychiatry, 182*, 185-187.

Angless, T. & Schefer, T. (1997). Children living with violence in the family. In: C. De la Rey, N. Duncan, T. Shefer & A. Van Niekerk (Eds.), *Contemporary issues in human development: A South African focus*. Johannesburg: International Thomson Publishing Southern Africa.

Applegate, M. (1998). AIDS education for adolescents: A review of the literature. *Journal of HIV/AIDS Prevention & Education, 2*(1), 5-29.

Armitage, C. J. & Conner, M. (2000). Social cognition models and health behaviour: A structured review. *Psychology and Health, 15*, 173-189.

Azjen, I. (1985). From intention to actions: A theory of planned behaviour. In: J. Kuhl & J. Beckman (Eds.), *Action-control: From cognition to behaviour* (pp.). Berlin: Springer.

Azjen, I. & Fishbein, M. (1970). The prediction of behaviour from attitudinal and normative beliefs. *Journal of Personality and Social Psychology, 6*, 466-487.

Badcock-Walters, P. (2002). Education. In: J. Gow & C. Desmond (Eds.), *Impacts and interventions: The HIV/AIDS epidemic and the children of South Africa*. (pp. 95-109). Pietermaritzburg: University of Natal Press.

Baldwin, S. A. & Hoffmann, J. P. (2002). The dynamics of self-esteem: A growth-curve analysis. *Journal of Youth and Adolescence, 31*(2), 101-113.

Bandura, A. (1977). *Social learning theory*. Englewood Cliffs, NJ: Prentice Hall.

Bandura, A. (1986). *Social foundation of thought and action: A Social Cognitive Theory*. Englewood Cliffs, NJ: Prentice Hall.

Bandura, A. (1991). A social cognitive approach to the exercise of control over AIDS infection. In: R. DiClemente (Ed.), *Adolescents and AIDS: A generation in jeopardy* (pp. 1-20). Beverly Hills: Sage.

Bandura, A. (1997). *Self-efficacy: The exercise of control*. New York: Freeman.

Bandura, A. (1998). Health promotion from the perspective of Social Cognitive Theory. *Psychology and Health, 13*, 623-649.

Barbarin, O. A. & Richter, L. (2001). *Mandela's children: Growing up in post-Apartheid South Africa*. New York: Routledge.

Barnes, J. M. (2002a, January). *Pollution, sanitation and community education campaigns in Kayamandi: A dense settlement in South Africa* (Interim report and final report). Tygerberg: University of Stellenbosch, Department of Community Health and Medical Faculty.
Barnes, J. M. (2002b, March 13). *Report on water quality analysis of the Plankenbrug River.* Tygerberg: University of Stellenbosch.
Barnett, E., de Koning, K. & Francis, B. (1995). *Health and HIV/AIDS education in primary and secondary schools in Africa and Asia* (Overseas Development Administration, Education Resource Group, Serial No. 14), Liverpool, England.
Becker, M. H. (1974). The health belief model and personal health behaviour. *Health Education Monographs, 2*, 324-508.
Bednar, R., Wells, M. & Peterson, S. (1989). *Self-esteem: Paradoxes and innovations in clinical theory and practice.* Washington, DC: American Psychological Association.
Bekker, S. B. (Comp.). (2002). *Migration study in the Western Cape (2001). Main Report.* Compiled for the Provincial Government of the Western Cape. Cape Town: Provincial Government of the Western Cape.
Berger, I. (2002, October 22). HIV/AIDS education falling on deaf ears. Schools offer very little support for children affected by HIV/AIDS. *PlusNews.*
Bergmann, K. E. & Bergmann, R. L. (2004). Prävention und Gesundheitsförderung im Kindesalter. In: K. Hurrelmann, T. Klotz & J. Haisch (Eds.), *Lehrbuch Prävention und Gesundheitsförderung* (pp. 55-62). Bern: Huber.
Berman, S. (1997). *Social consciousness and the development of social responsibility.* New York: State University of New York Press.
Berman, S. & La Farge, P. (1993). *Promising practices in teaching social responsibility.* New York: State University of New York Press.
Berry, L. & Guthrie, T. (Eds.). (2003). *Rapid assessment: The situation of children in South Africa.* Cape Town: Children's Institute.
Bhana, A., Brooks, H., Makiwane, M. & Naidoo, K. (2005, January). *Evaluation of the impact of the life orientation programme on HIV/AIDS in Gauteng schools: Pilot study.* Johannesburg: Gauteng Department of Education.
Bicher, A. K. (2005). *Insights from Kayamandi.* Berlin.
Blecher, M. S., Steinberg, M., Pick, W., Hennick, M. & Durcan, N. (1995). AIDS-knowledge, attitudes and practices among STD clinic attenders in the Cape Peninsula. *South African Medical Journal, 18*, 1281-1286.
Bolognini, M., Plancherel, B., Bettschart, W. & Halfon, O. (1996). Self-esteem and mental health in early adolescence: Development and gender differences. *Journal of Adolescence, 19*, 233-245.
Bortz, J. (1999). *Statistik für Sozialwissenschaftler.* Berlin: Springer.
Bortz, J. & Döring, N. (2001). *Forschungsmethoden und Evaluation.* Berlin: Springer.
Boshoff, P., Pretorius, G. & Ungerer, E. (1993). *Education modules for primary students. Puberty: Time for facts. Presenter's manual with work sheet masters for the classroom.* South Africa: Educational Technology.
Boult, B. E. & Cunningham, P. W. (1991). Black teenage pregnancy in Port Elizabeth. *Early Child Development and Care, 75*, 1-70.

Bower, C. (2003a). RAPCAN. Personal communication. Data from South African Police Services. In: L. Berry & T. Guthrie (Eds.), *Rapid assessment: The situation of children in South Africa*. Cape Town: Children's Institute.
Bower, C. (2003b). RAPCAN. Personal communication. In: L. Berry & T. Guthrie (Eds.), *Rapid assessment: The situation of children in South Africa*. Cape Town: Children's Institute.
Bower, C. (2005). Global study on violence against children. *Article 19, 1*(1).
Bowley, D. M. & Pitcher, G. J. (2002). Child rape in South Africa: An open letter to the Minister of Health. *SAMJ, 92*(10), 744.
Brack, C., Orr, D. & Ingersoll, G. (1988). Pubertal maturation and adolescent self-esteem. *Journal of Adolescent Health Care, 9*, 280-285.
Bray, R. (2002). *Missing links? An examination of contributions made by social surveys to our understanding of child well-being in South Africa*. (CSSR Working Paper No. 23). Cape Town: University of Cape Town, Centre for Social Science Research, Social Surveys Unit.
Bray, R. (2003, April-May). Child work and well-being. *Children First, 48*, 12.
Brooks, H, Shisana, O. & Richter, L. (2004). *National household survey HIV prevalence and risk survey of South African children*. Cape Town: Human Sciences Research Council.
Brown, K. M., McMahon, R. P., Biro, F. M., Crawford, P., Schreiber, G. B. & Similo, S. L. (1998). Changes in self-esteem in black and white girls between the ages of 9 and 14 years. *Journal of Adolescent Health Care, 23*, 7-19.
Buchinger, C. & Lindner, M. (2003). *Observation report. Observation phase 2.* Unpublished report.
Buga, G. A., Amoko, D. H. & Ncayiyana, D. J. (1996). Adolescent sexual behaviour, knowledge and attitudes to sexuality among schoolgirls in Transkei, South Africa. *East African Medical Journal, 73*, 95-100.
Bühringer, G. & Bühler, A. (2004). Prävention von Depression und Sucht. In: K. Hurrelmann, T. Klotz & J. Haisch (Eds.), *Lehrbuch Prävention und Gesundheitsförderung* (pp. 179-189). Bern: Huber.
Burlington (2005). *Dictionary*. Retrieved March 28th, 2005, from www.burlington.ca/Planning/Official%20Plan/Part_VII/.
Business Intelligence Menu. (2004). *Detail reporting: Case summary per offence. Statistics of the South African Police*. Retrieved April 13, 2004, from http://.../DEREPCKOFFENCE.run?comp_cd=1853&geolvl=Station&date_from =2002-09-01&dat2004/08/13.
Cairns, E., McWhirter, L., Duffy, U. & Barry, R. (1990). The stability of self-concept in late adolescence: Gender and situational effects. *Pers. India Differ, 11*, 937-944.
Campbell, C. (2003). *Letting them die: Why HIV/AIDS prevention programmes fail*. (The International African Institute). Cape Town: Double Storey.
Cassimijee, N. (1998). *The role of gender in black adolescent sexuality: An eco-systematic approach*. Unpublished master's thesis,. University of Pretoria, Pretoria, South Africa.
Chiam, H. (1987). Change in self-concept during adolescence. *Adolescence, 22*, 69-76.

Child Welfare South Africa. (2005). Retrieved March 28th, 2005, from //welcome.php_childwelfare_principles.htm.
Christofides, N. J., Jewkes, R. K., Webster, N., Penn-Kekana, L., Abrahams, N. & Martin, L. J. (2005). Other patients are really in need of medical attention: The quality of health survivors in South Africa. *Bulletin of the World Health Organization, 83*(7), 495-502.
Chubb, N. H., Fertman, C. L & Ross, J. L. (1997). Adolescent self-esteem and locus of control: A longitudinal study of gender and age differences. *Adolescence, 32*, 113-129.
Commission on Health Research for Development (1990). *Health research: Essential link to equity in development*. Oxford: Oxford University Press.
Compas, B., Hindon, B. & Gerhardt, C. (1995). Adolescent development: Pathways and processes of risk and resilience. *Annual Reviews in Psychology, 46*, 265-292.
Coughlan, F. J., Coughlan, N. S. & Jameson, C. P. (1996). Where knowledge and attitude separate: Adolescent HIV/AIDS knowledge survey as information for social work training. *Social Work, 32*, 255-261.
Crime Information Analysis Centre. (2004, August 19). *Information regarding crime in Kayamandi: Overview of crime in Kayamandi for the period 2003*. Stellenbosch: Stellenbosch Police.
Dalrymple, L. & DuToit, M. K. (1993). The evaluation of a drama approach to AIDS education. *Educational Psychology, 13*(2), 147-154.
Davis, S. F., Palladino, J. J. (2000). *Psychology* (3rd ed.). Upper Saddle River, NJ: Prentice Hall.
Dawes, A. (2002). Sexual offences against children in South Africa: Considerations for primary prevention. In: L. Berry & T. Guthrie (Eds.), *Rapid assessment: The situation of children in South Africa*. Cape Town: Children's Institute.
Dawes, A., Kropiwnicki, Z. (d.S.), Kafaar, Z. & Richter, L. (2005). *Corporal punishment of children: A South African national survey*. Sweden: Save the Children Fund.
De Jesus Mari, J., Lozano, J. M. & Duley, L. (1997). Erasing the global divide in health research: Collaboration provides answers relevant to developing and developed countries. *BMJ, 314*, 390.
De Jong, T., Ganie, L., Naidoo, T. & Prinsloo, E. (1994). Towards a model for school guidance and counselling in South Africa. In: T. De Jong, L. Ganie, S. Lazarus, T. Naidoo, L. Naude & E. Prinsloo (Eds.), *Education support services in South Africa: Policy proposals*. Belville: University of the Western Cape.
De la Rey, C., Duncan, N., Shefer, T. & Van Niekerk, A. (Eds.). *Contemporary issues in human development: A South African focus*. Johannesburg: International Thomson Publishing Southern Africa.
Demo, D. H. & Savin-Williams, R. C. (1983). Early adolescent self-esteem as a function of social class: Rosenberg and Pearl revisited. *American Journal of Sociology, 88*, 763-774.
Dennerlein, J. & Adami, K. (2004). *Sustainable district development in Kayamandi*. Frankfurt: University of Applied Sciences Frankfurt Main.

De Onis, M. & Blössner, M. (2003). The World Health Organization global database on child growth and malnutrition: Methodology and applications. *International Journal of Epidemiology, 32*, 518-526.

Development Action Group. (2002, May 14). *Kayamandi zone F informal settlement socio-economic survey*. Retrieved May 2004, from www.africalife.de/site/dyn/1537.htm.

Dohnke, B. (2003). Emotionale und motivationale Effekte von Erwartungen und erwartungsbezogenen Erfahrungen im Rehabilitationsprozess: Eine Untersuchung von Effekten erwartungsgemäßer und erwartungsdiskrepanter Behandlungsergebnisse. Unpublished doctoral dissertation, Humboldt-Universität zu Berlin, Philosophische Fakultät, IV Institut für Rehabilitationswissenschaften.

Donaldson, S. (1990). *Kayamandi: Eksterne skakeling van 'n swart stedelike woonbuurt*. Unpublished paper.

Dorrington, R., Bradshaw, D., Johnson, L. & Budlender, D. (2004). *The demographic impact of HIV/AIDS in South Africa: National indicators for 2004*. Cape Town: Center for Actuarial Research, South African Medical Research Council and Actuarial Society of South Africa.

Dryfoos, J. G. (1991). Adolescents at risk: A summation of work in the field – programs and policies. *Journal of Adolescent Health, 12*, 630-637.

Du Bois, D., Felner, R. D., Brand, S., Phillips, R. S. C. & Lease, A. M. (1996). Early adolescent self-esteem: A developmental-ecological framework and assessment strategy. *Journal of Research on Adolescence, 6*, 543-579.

Duncan, N. & Rock, B. (1997). Inquiry into the effects of public violence on children. In: L. Berry & T. Guthrie (Eds.), *Rapid assessment: The situation of children in South Africa*. Cape Town: Children's Institute.

Eaton, L. & Flisher, A. J. (2000). HIV/AIDS knowledge among South African youth. *Southern African Journal of Child and Adolescent Mental Health, 12*, 97-124.

Eaton, L., Flisher, A. J. & Aaro, L. E. (2003). Unsafe sexual behaviour in South African youth. *Social Science & Medicine, 56*, 149-165.

Eccles, J. S., Midgley, C., Wigfield, A., Buchanan, C. M., Reuman, D., Flanagan, C. & Maclver, D. (1993). Development in adolescence: The impact of stage-environment fit on young adolescents' experiences in schools and in families. *American Psychologist, 48*(2), 90-101.

Education Atlas. (2002). *Children's Budget Unit: Budgeting for child socio-economic rights. Government obligations and the child's right to social security and education. The popular version*. Cape Town: Budget information service, IDASA.

Education Labour Relations Council. (2005, March 31). *Results of a comprehensive survey of factors determining educator supply and demand in South African public schools* [Media Statement].

Educational Support Services Trust. (2003) *The court is my friend. Information paper*. Department of Justice and Constitutional Development.

Elias, M. & Weissberg, R. (2000). Primary prevention: Educational approaches to enhance social and emotional learning. *Journal of School Health, 70*, 186-190.

Elkins, D., Maticka, T., Kuyyakanond, T. & Miller, P. (1997). Towards reducing the spread of HIV in northeastern Thai villages: Evaluation of a village-based intervention. *AIDS Education and Prevention, 9*(1), 49-69.

Elkonin, D. S. (1993). *Acquired immune deficiency syndrome: Knowledge, attitudes, and sexual activity among university students.* Unpublished master's thesis, University of Port Elizabeth, Port Elizabeth, South Africa.

Erhard, A. (2000). Informelle Wirtschaft und Informelle Siedlung: Globale Phänomene und das Beispiel Südafrika, GW-Unterricht 79/2000.

Everatt, D. & Orkin, M. (1993). *Growing up tough: A national survey of South African youth for the Joint Enrichment Project.* Johannesburg: Community Agency for Social Enquiry.

Everett, K. (1995). *Get wise about AIDS: Lessons for a safer lifestyle. National AIDS research programme..* Swaziland: Macmillan Boleswa, Medical Research Council.

Farquhar, C. & Kanabus, A. (1998). AIDS and children: What's it got to do with them? Sussex: AIDS Education and Research Trust, AVERT.

Fawole, I., Asuzu, M., Oduntan, S. & Bieger, W. (1999). A school-based AIDS education programme for secondary school students in Nigeria: A review of effectiveness. *Health Education Research, 14*(5), 675-683.

Finger, B., Lapetina, M. & Pribila, M. (2002). *Intervention strategies that work for youth: Summary of the Focus on Young Adults End of Program Report.* Virginia: Family Health International.

Fitzgerald, A. M., Stanton, B. F., Terreri, N., Shipena, H., Li, X. & Kahihuata, J. (1999). Use of western-based HIV risk reduction interventions targeting adolescents in an African setting. *Journal of Adolescent Health, 25*(1), 52-61.

Flexner, S. B. (1980). *The Random House Dictionary.* NJ: Random House.

Flisher A. J., Cloete, K., Johnson, B., Wigton, A., Adams, R. & Joshua, P. (2000). Health promoting schools: Lessons from Avondale Primary School. In: D. Donald, A. Dawes & J. Louw (Eds.), *Addressing childhood adversity: Psychosocial interventions in South Africa* (pp. 113-130). Cape Town: David Phillip.

Flisher, A. J., Ziervogel, C. F., Chalton, D. O., Leger, P. H. & Robertson, B. A. (1993). Risk-taking behaviour of Cape Peninsula high school students, Part 7: Sexual behaviour. *South African Medical Journal, 83*, 495-497.

Foon, D., Gebhard, F., Mastai, J., Torpe, B. & Van Riesen, V. (Producers). (1984). *Feeling YES and feeling NO.* [Motion picture]. Canada: National Film Board of Canada.

Friedland, R. H., Jankelowitz, S. K., De Beer, M., De Klerk, C., Khoury, V. & Csizmadia, T. (1991). Perceptions and knowledge about the acquired immunodeficiency syndrome among students in university residences. *South African Medical Journal, 79*, 149-154.

Gallant, M. & Maticka-Tyndale, E. (2004). School-based HIV prevention programmes for African youth. *Social Science & Medicine, 58*, 1337-1351.

Gibney, L., DiClemente, R. J. & Vermund, S. H. (Eds.). (1999). *Preventing HIV in developing countries: Biomedical and behavioural approaches.* New York: Plenum.

Goliath, C. G. (1995). *Secondary school pupils' perceptions of AIDS and AIDS education.* Unpublished doctoral dissertation, University of Port Elizabeth, Port Elizabeth, South Africa.

Gow, J. & Desmond, C. (2002). *Impacts and interventions: The HIV/AIDS epidemic and the children in South Africa.* Pietermaritzburg: University of Natal Press.

Groenewald, C. (1992). *The social problems faced by the Stellenbosch community.* Unpublished paper.

Grunsheit, A. (1997). Impact of HIV and sexual health education on the sexual behaviour of young people: A review update. Geneva: UNAIDS.

Guba, E. G. & Lincoln, Y. S. (1989). *Fourth generation evaluation.* Sage: Newbury Park, CA.

Hamber, B. & Lewis, S. (1997). *An overview of the consequences of violence and trauma in South Africa.* South Africa: Centre for the Study of Violence and Reconciliation.

Harter, S. (1990a). Causes, correlates, and the functional role of global self-worth: A lifespan perspective. In: R. J. Sternberg & J. Kolligan (Eds.), *Competence considered* (pp. 67-97). New Haven, CT: Yale University Press.

Harter, S. (1990b). Self and identity development. In: S. S. Feldman & G. R. Elliott (Eds.), *At the threshold: The developing adolescent* (pp. 352-387). Cambridge, MA: Harvard University Press.

Harvey, B., Stuart, J. & Swan, T. (2000). Evaluation of a Drama-in-Education programme to increase AIDS awareness in South African high schools: A randomized community intervention trial. *International Journal of STD & AIDS, 11*, 105-111.

Havighurst, R. J. (1972). *Developmental tasks and education.* New York: Longman.

Heunis, C. (1994). AIDS-related knowledge, attitudes, beliefs and behaviour among students: Survey results. *Acta Academica, 26*, 134-153.

Hill, J. P. & Lynch, M. E. (1983). The intensification of gender-related role expectations during early adolescence. In: J. Brooks-Gunn & A. C. Petersen (Eds.), *Girls at Puberty* (pp. 201-228). New York: Plenum.

H. J. Kaiser Foundation. (1999, January 27-29). *National adolescent sexual health initiative.* Johannesburg: H. J. Kaiser Foundation.

Hosman, C. & Llopis, E. (2005). The evidence of effective interventions for mental health promotion. In: World Health Organization, *Promoting mental health: concepts, emerging evidence, practice.* Geneva: World Health Organization, Department of Mental Health and Substance Abuse in collaboration with the Victorian Health Promotion Foundation and the University of Melbourne.

Hudson, W. W. (1992). *The WALMYR Assessment Scales Scoring Manual: Index of Peer Relations (IPR).* Temp, AZ: WALMYR.

Human Rights Watch. (2001). *Scared at school: Sexual violence against girls in South African schools.* New York: Human Rights Watch.

Human Rights Watch. (2003). *World report 2003. South Africa.* Retrieved January 1st, 2004, from www.hrw.org.

Human Rights Watch. (2004a, January 1). *Human rights overview. South Africa.* Retrieved January 1st, 2004, from www.hrw.org.

Human Rights Watch. (2004b, January 1). *South Africa.* Retrieved January 1st, 2004, from www.hrw.org.
Human Rights Watch. (2004c, January 1). *Human rights overview.* South Africa: Human Rigths Watch.
Human Sciences Research Council (HSRC). (2002). *Nelson Mandela/HSRC study of HIV/AIDS: South African national HIV prevalence, behavioural risk and mass media.* (Household Survey). Cape Town: ComPress.
Human Sciences Research Council (HSRC), Centre for AIDS development Research and Evaluation (CADRE), and Medical Research Council (MRC) (Comps.). (2005). *South African national HIV prevalence: HIV incidence, behaviour and communication survey.* Cape Town: Nelson Mandela Children Fund.
Hurrelmann, K. (1998). *Lebensphase Jugend.* Weinheim: Juventa.
Hurrelmann, K., Klotz, T. & Haisch, J. (Eds.). (2004). *Lehrbuch Prävention und Gesundheitsförderung.* Bern: Huber.
Illeris, K. (2002). *Three dimensions of learning: Contemporary learning theory in the tension field between the cognitive, the emotional and the social* (2nd ed.). Denmark: Roskilde University Press.
Institute of Psychiatry. (2004). *International mental health: Research theme child & adolescent.* London: King's College, Institute of Psychiatry.
Jacobs, M., Shung-King, M. & Smith, C. (Eds.). (2005). *South African Child Gauge 2005.* Cape Town: University of Stellenbosch.
James, W. (1983). *The principles of psychology.* Cambridge, MA: Harvard University.
Janoff-Bulman, R. (1985). The aftermath of victimisation: Rebuilding shattered assumptions. In: C. R. Figley (Ed.), *Trauma and its wake.* New York: Brunner Mazel.
Janz, N. K. & Becker, M. H. (1984). The health belief model: A decade later. *Health Education Quarterly, 11*, 1-47.
Jerusalem, M. (2002a). Gesundheitsförderung in Schule und Elternhaus. In: R. Schwarzer, M. Jerusalem & H. Weber (Eds.), *Gesundheitspsychologie von A bis Z. Ein Handbuch* (pp. 171-174). Göttingen: Hogrefe Verlag.
Jerusalem, M. (2002b). Gesundheitliche Präventionsprogramme. In: R. Schwarzer, M. Jerusalem & H. Weber (Eds.), *Gesundheitspsychologie von A bis Z: Ein Handbuch* (pp. 400-403). Göttingen: Hogrefe Verlag.
Jewkes, R., & Abrahams, N. (2002). The epidemiology of rape and sexual coercion in South Africa: An overview. *Social Science & Medicine, 55*, 1231-1244.
Jewkes, R. & Levin, J. (2002). Rape of girls in South Africa. *The LANCET, 359*, 319-20.
Joint United Nations AIDS Programme (UNAIDS) & World Health Organization. (WHO). (2001). *AIDS epidemic update.* Geneva.
Joint United Nations AIDS Programme (UNAIDS) & World Health Organization (WHO). (2005a, December). *AIDS epidemic update.* Geneva.
Joint United Nations AIDS Programme (UNAIDS) & World Health Organization. (WHO). (2005b). *Violence against women. HIV/AIDS: Critical intersections. Intimate partner violence and HIV/AIDS.* (UNAIDS/WHO Information Bulletin Series No.1).

Joint United Nations AIDS Programme (UNAIDS), World Health Organization (WHO) & United Nations Children's Fund (UNICEF). (2002). *Young people and HIV/AIDS opportunity crisis*. Geneva.
Joy for Life. (2003). *Finding our voices, talking with our children about sexuality and AIDS*. Cape Town: Albion Press.
Kaaya, S. F., Flischer, A. J., Mbwambo, J. K., Schaalma, H., Aaro, L. E. & Klepp. K.-I. (2002a). A review of studies of sexual behaviour of school students in sub-Saharan Africa. *Scandinavian Journal of Public Health, 30*, 148-160.
Kaaya, S. G., Mukoma, W., Flisher, A. J. & Klepp, K.-I. (2002b). School-based sexual health initiatives in sub-Saharan Africa: A review. *Social Dynamics, 28*, 64-88.
Kalichman, S. & Nachimson, D. (1999). Self-efficacy and disclosure of HIV positive sero-status to sex partners. *Health Psychology, 18*(3), 281-287.
Kaplan, M. E. & Van den Worm, Y. (1993). Adolescents' perceptions of AIDS: A preliminary investigation. *Unisa Psychologia, 20*, 9-13.
Kau, M. (1991). Sexual behaviour and knowledge of adolescent males in the Mpolo region of Bophuthatswana. *Curationis, 14*, 37-40.
Keller, H. (1998). *Lehrbuch Entwicklungspsychologie*. Bern: Huber.
Kelly, K. (2000). *Communicating for action: A contextual evaluation of youth responses to HIV/AIDS*. Pretoria: National Department of Health.
Kelly, K. (2001). Bambasinani: Community orientation to HIV/AIDS prevention, care and support (The EQUITY Project/USAID).
Kelly, K., Ntlablati, P., Oyosi, S., Van der Riet, M. & Parker, W. (2002). Making HIV/AIDS our problem: Young people and the development challenge in South Africa South Africa: Save The Children.
Kelly, K. & Parker, W. (2000). *Communities of practice: Contextual mediators of youth response to HIV/AIDS*. Pretoria: National Department of Health, Beyond Awareness Campaign.
Kenyon, C., Heywood, M. & Conway, S. (2000). *Mainstreaming HIV/AIDS, progress and challenges in South Africa's HIV/AIDS campaign*. Health Systems Trust, AIDS Law Project and International Association of Physicians in AIDS Care.
Kinsman, J., Nakiyingi, J., Kamali, A., Carpenter, L., Quigley, M., Pool, R. & Whitworth, J. (2001). Evaluation of a comprehensive school-based AIDS education programme in rural Masaka, Uganda. *Health Education Research. 16*, 85-100.
Klepp, K.-I., Flisher A. J., & Kaaya, S. (Eds.). (in press). *Promoting Adolescent Sexual and Reproductive Health in Eastern and Southern Africa*. Uppsala, Sweden: Nordic Africa Institute.
Klepp, K.-I., Ndeki, S., Leshabari, M. T., Hannan, P. J. & Lyimo, B. A. (1997). AIDS education in Tanzania: Promoting risk reduction among primary school children. *American Journal of Public Health, 87*(12), 1931-1936.
Klepp, K.-I., Ndeki, S. S. & Seha, A. M. (1994). AIDS education for primary school children in Tanzania: An evaluation study. *AIDS, 8*(8), 1157-1162.
Knäuper, B. (2002). Gesundheitsverhalten über die Lebensspanne. In: R. Schwarzer, M. Jerusalem & H. Weber (Eds.), *Gesundheitspsychologie von A bis Z. Ein Handbuch* (pp. 216-219). Göttingen: Hogrefe Verlag.

Knoll, N., Scholz, U. & Rieckmann, N. (2005). *Einführung in die Gesundheitspsychologie.* München: Ernst Reinhardt Verlag.
Kruger, J. M. & Richter, L. M. (1996). South African street children: At risk for AIDS? *Africa Insight, 26,* 237-243.
Kuhn, L., Steinberg, M. & Mathews, C. (1994). Participation of the school community in AIDS education: An evaluation of a high school programme in South Africa. *AIDS Care, 6*(2), 161-171.
Labadarios, D. (Ed.). (2000). *The national food consumption survey (NFCS): Children aged 1-9 years in South Africa, 1999.* Pretoria: National Department of Health.
Lehohla, P. (2000). *Statistician-General: Statistics South Africa 2000* (Discussion Paper 1: Comparative Labour Statistics, Labour Force Survey: First Round Pilot (September 2000)). Retrieved September 2000, from http://www.statssa.gov.za/Publications/DiscussLFS/DiscussLFSSeptember2000.pdf.
Leibbrandt, M., Woolard, L. & Bhorat, H. (2000). Understanding contemporary household inequality in South Africa.
Leviton, L. (1989). Theoretical foundations of AIDS-prevention programs. In: R. Valdiserri (Ed.), *Preventing AIDS: The design of effective programs.* New Brunswick: Rutgers University Press.
Lindner, M. & Otto, C. (2004). *Observation report. Observation Phase 3.* Unpublished report.
Lloyd, C. (2005). *Growing up global: The transitions to adulthood in developing countries.* Washington, DC: National Academise Press.
Lourens, B. (2004, January-February). Creating classrooms where 'I can': Places of emotional safety. *Children First, 53.*
MacLachlan, M., Chimombo, M. & Mpemba, N. (1997). AIDS education for youth through active learning: A school-based approach from Malawi. *International Journal Educational Development, 17*(1), 41-50
Magome, K., Louw, N., Motlhoioa, B. & Jack, S. (1997-98). *Life skills and HIV/AIDS education programme, project.* Pretoria: Department of Education and the National Department of Health.
Magwaza, A. (1997). Children living with violence in the family. In: C. De la Rey, N. Duncan, T. Shefer & A. Van Niekerk (Eds.), *Contemporary issues in human development: A South African focus.* Johannesburg: International Thomson Publishing Southern Africa.
Maslow, A. H. (2002). *Motivation und Persönlichkeit.* Reinbek: Rowohlt.
Mathee, A. (2004, June). *Towards healthy environments for South African children.* Paper presented at the HECA Side Event at the Fourth Ministerial Meeting on Environment and Health, Budapest.
Maticka-Tyndale, E., Wildish, J. & Gichuru, M. (2004). *HIV/AIDS and education: Experience in change in behaviour, a Kenyan example.* Commonwealth Education Partnerships.
Markefka, M. & Nauck, B. (1993). *Handbuch der Kindheitsforschung.* Neuwied: Luchterhand.

McCarthy, J. & Hoge, D. (1982). Analysis of age effects in longitudinal studies of adolescent self-esteem. *Developmental Psychology, 18*, 372-379.
McPhail, C. & Campbell, C. (2000). 'I think condoms are good, but AAI, I hate those things': Condom use among adolescents and young people in a Southern African township. *Social Science and Medicine, 52*, 1613-1627.
Meyer, A. J. (1989). *An exploratory study to establish the effectiveness of a sex education programme which was undertaken in Soshanguve.* Pretoria: Human Sciences Research Council.
Meyer-Weitz, A., Reddy, P., Weijtz, W., Van den Borne, B. & Kok, G. (1998). The socio-cultural contexts of sexually transmitted diseases in South Africa: Implications for health education programmes. *AIDS Care, 10*(Suppl. 1), 39-55.
Mitchell, G. V. (1994). An evaluation of the impact of a ten hour HIV/AIDS prevention programme on male adolescents' HIV/AIDS-related knowledge, attitudes and beliefs. Unpublished doctoral dissertation, University of Cape Town, Cape Town, South Africa.
Morrell, R. (2001). Corporal punishment in South African schools: A neglected explanation for its persistence. *South African Journal of Education, 21*(4).
Morrell, R. (2004). Silence, sexuality, and HIV/AIDS in South African schools. *Sexuality in Africa Magazine, 1*(4), page numbers.
Mukoma, W. & Flisher, A. J. (2004). Evaluations of health promoting schools: A review of nine studies. *Health Promotion International*, 19 (3), 357-368.
Mukoma, W. & Flisher, A. J. (in press). A systematic review of school-based AIDS prevention programmes in South Africa. In: K.-I. Klepp, A. J. Flisher, & S. Kaaya (Eds.), *Promoting Adolescent Sexual and Reproductive Health in Eastern and Southern Africa.* Uppsala, Sweden: Nordic Africa Institute.
Munodawafa, D., Marty, P. J., & Gwede, C. (1995). Effectiveness of health instruction provided by student nurses in rural secondary schools of Zimbabwe: A feasibility study. *International Journal of Nursing Studies, 32*(1), 27-38.
Mvulane, Z. (2003, February-March). The right to food. *Children First, 47*(5).
Mvulane, Z. & Proudlock, P. (2002). Access to basic nutrition and sufficient food in South Africa: What are the obstacles? Draft access document for internal discussion.
Nair, Y. (2005, March-April). Engaging young people, promoting sexual health. *Children First, 60.* .
National Advisory Mental Health Council (NAMHC). (1996). Basic behavioural science research for mental health: Vulnerability and resilience. *American Psychologist, 51*, 22-28.
National Crime Prevention Strategy. (1996). In: L. Berry & T. Guthrie (Eds.), *Rapid assessment: The situation of children in South Africa.* Cape Town: Children's Institute.
National Department of Education. (1996). *Rights and responsibilities of parents: A guide to publicschool policy.* Pretoria: Education Human Resources.
National Department of Education. (1997, June). A resume of instructional programmes in public schools. (Report No. 550). In: K. Magome, N. Louw, B. Motlhoioa & S. Jack (1997-98). *Life skills and HIV/AIDS education programme,*

project. Pretoria: Department of Education and the National Department of Health.

National Department of Education. (2000) (Eds.). *The HIV/AIDS emergency: Guidelines for educators.* Pretoria: Department of Education.

National Department of Health. (2000). *Ubungani: A Parent guide for life skills, sexuality and HIV/AIDS education. Part of the primary school Pilot Project.* Pretoria: National Department of Health.

National Department of Health. (2001). *National Integrated Plan.* Pretoria: Department of Health.

National Department of Health. (2004a). *National HIV and syphilis antenatal seroprevalence survey in South Africa.* Pretoria.

National Department of Health. (2004b, June). Research update National Department of Health: Health systems research. *Research Co-ordination and Epidemiology, 6 (1).*

National Department of Health. (2004c, June). Systems research: Research co-ordination and epidemiology. *Research Update, 6*(1).

National Progressive Primary Health Care Network (NPPHCN). (1996). *Youth speak out for a healthy future: A study of youth sexuality.* Johannesburg.

Natrass, N. (2003). *Unemployment and AIDS: The social-demographic challenge for South Africa.* Cape Town: University of Cape Town, School of Economics, Development Policy Research Unit.

Nottelmann, E. D. (1987). Competence and self-esteem during the transition from childhood to adolescence. *Developmental Psychology, 23,* 441-450.

Oerter, R. (1995a). Kindheit. In: R. Oerter & L. Montda (Eds.), *Entwicklungspsychologie.* Weinheim: Beltz.

Oerter, R. (1995b). *Entwicklungspsychologie* (3rd ed.).Weinheim: Beltz.

Office on the Right of the Child. (2001). The Presidency. In: L. Berry & T. Guthrie (Eds.), *Rapid assessment: The situation of children in South Africa.* Cape Town: Children's Institute.

O'Malley, P. M. & Bachman, J. G. (1983). Self-esteem: Change and stability between ages 13 and 23. *Developmental Psychology, 19,* 257-268.

Padayachee, S. (2004). *Lawyers for human rights.* Child Rights Project.

Page, N. P. (1990). Effectiveness of a sex education programme in changing sexual knowledge, attitudes and behaviour of black adolescents. Unpublished doctoral dissertation, University of the Witwatersrand, Johannesburg, South Africa.

PAWC & KTC. (1989). *A macro plan for Kayamandi.* Stellenbosch.

Peires, J. (2005). *Nazism and Apartheid: Similarities and differences.* Cape Town: Cape Town Holocaust Centre.

Pellegrini, A. D., Symons, F. J. & Hoch, J. (2004). *Observing children in their natural worlds: A methodological primer* (2nd ed.). Lawrence Erlbaum Assoc.

Peltzer, K. (1999). Factors affecting condom use in an urban adult community of the Northern Province, South Africa. *Journal of Psychology in Africa, 9,* 66-77.

Peltzer, K. (2002a). Factors affecting behaviours that address HIV risk among a sample of junior secondary school students in the Northern Province. *Health SA Gesondheid, 7*(3).

Peltzer, K. (2002b). AIDS und HIV als globales Problem. In: R. Schwarzer, M. Jerusalem & H. Weber (Eds.), *Gesundheitspsychologie von A bis Z: Ein Handbuch* (pp. 1-4). Göttingen: Hogrefe Verlag.

Peltzer, K. & Promtussananon, S. (2005). HIV/AIDS knowledge and sexual behaviour among junior secondary school students in South Africa. *Journal of Social Sciences, 1*, 1-8.

Perkel, A. K. (1991). *Psychosocial variables in the transmission of AIDS.* Unpublished doctoral dissertation, University of Western Cape, Cape Town, South Africa.

Perkel, A. K., Strebel, A. & Joubert, G. (1991). The psychology of AIDS transmission: Issues for intervention. *South African Journal of Psychology, 21*, 148-152.

Peruga, A. & Celentano, D. D. (1993). Correlates of AIDS knowledge in samples of the general population. *Social Science and Medicine, 36*, 509-524.

Phurutse, M. C. (2005). Factors affecting teaching and learning in South African public schools: Factors determining educator supply and demand in South African public schools. Cape Town: Human Sciences Research Council and Medical Research Council of South Africa.

Pilots Project in Southern Africa. (PTT) (2004, May). *Kayamandi township.* Retrieved May, 2004, from www.africalife.de/site/dyn/1537.htm.

Pinquart, M. & Silbereisen, R. K. (2004). Prävention und Gesundheitsförderung im Jugendalter. In: K. Hurrelmann, T. Klotz & J. Haisch (Eds.), *Lehrbuch Prävention und Gesundheitsförderung* (pp. 63-72). Bern: Huber.

Planned Parenthood Association of South Africa (PPASA) (1997). *Life Skills and HIV/AIDS education: A manual and resource guide for intermediate phase school teachers.* Compiled by Norton, J. & Dawson, C.. Sandton: Heinemann.

Polce-Lynch, M., Kliewer, W. & Myers, B. J. (1994). *Gender differences in early adolescent self-esteem: The mediating role of body image.* Unpublished manuscript, Virginia Commonwealth University, Virginia.

Polce-Lynch, M., Myers, B. J., Kliewer, W. & Kilmartin, C. (2001). Adolescent self-esteem and gender: Exploring relations to sexual harassment, body image, media influence, and emotional expression. *Journal of Youth and Adolescence, 30*(2), 225-244.

Polk, R. K. (2002). *Social responsibility: Evaluating the national outcomes, program outcomes for youth.* Retrieved May 15, 2005 from http:\\ag.arizona.edu/fcr/fs/nowg/sc_soial.html.

Quaker Peace Centre. (1999). *The South African handbook of education for peace.* Cape Town: Quaker Peace Centre.

Quaker Peace Centre. (2002, July 1-3). Peace education programme: St. Theresa Primary School. *Reflection Journal.* Cape Town: Quaker Peace Centre.

Quatman, J. & Watson, C. M. (2001). Gender differences in adolescent: Self-esteem an exploration of domains. *The Journal of Genetic Psychology, 162*(1), 93-117.

Rape Crisis. (2005). *Rape statistics South Africa.* Retrieved September, 2005, from http: //www.rapecrisis.co.za.

Ratsaka, M. & Hirschowitz, R. (1995). Knowledge, attitude and beliefs amongst inhabitants of high density informal settlements with regard to sexuality and AIDS in Alexandra township. *Curationis, 18*, 41-44.

Reddy, P. & Meyer-Weitz, A. (1997). *Sacred or secret: Psychosocial and contextual determinants of STD-related behaviour.* South African Research Council.

Reddy, P., Meyer-Weitz, A., Van den Borne, B. & Kok, G. (2000). Determinants of condom-use behaviour among STD clinic attenders in South Africa. *International Journal of STD & AIDS, 11*, 521-530.

Resources Aimed at the Prevention of Child Abuse and Neglect (RAPCAN). (2001). *Annual Report 2001.* Cape Town: RAPCAN.

Richter, L. M. (1996). *A survey of reproductive health issues among urban black youth in South Africa* (Final Grant report). Pretoria: Centre for Epidemiological Research in South Africa.

Richter, L., Dawes, A. & Higson Smith, C. (Eds.). (2004). *Sexual abuse of young children in Southern Africa.* Cape Town: Human Sciences Research Council.

Rosenberg, M. (1979). *Conceiving the self.* New York: Basic Books.

Rosenberg, M. (1986). Self-concept from middle childhood through adolescence. In: J. Suls & A. J. Greenwald (Eds.), *Psychological perspective on the self* (pp. 182-205). Hillsdale, NJ: Erlbaum.

Rosenberg, M. & Rosenstock, I. M. (1966). Why people use health services. *Millbank Memorial Fund Quarterly, 44*, 94-124.

Rosenberg, F., Schoenbach, C. & Schooler, C. (1995). Global self-esteem and specific self-esteem: Different concept, different outcomes. *American Sociological Review, 60*, 141-156.

Rosenstock, I. M. (1966). Why people use health services. *Millbank Memorial Fund Quarterly, 44*, 94-124.

Rotter, J. (1954). *Social learning and clinical psychology.* New York: Prentice-Hall.

Sanderson, C. (1999). Role of relationship contact in influencing college students' responsiveness to HIV prevention videos. *Health Psychology, 18(3)*, 295-300.

Savin-Williams, R. C. & Demo, D. H. (1984). Developmental change and stability in adolescent self-concept. *Developmental Psychology, 20*, 1100-1110.

Saxena, S. & Porter, D. (2004, March 10). Mental health research in developing countries. *Mental Health News.*

Schinke, S., Botvin, G., Orlandi, M. & Schilling, R. (1990). African-American and Hispanic-American adolescents, HIV infection, and preventive intervention. *AIDS Education and Prevention, 2(4)*, 305-312.

Schnabel, P.-E. (2004). Gesundheitsförderung in Familien und Schulen. In: K. Hurrelmann, T. Klotz & J. Haisch (Eds.), *Lehrbuch Prävention und Gesundheitsförderung* (pp. 281-291). Bern: Huber.

Schwarzer, R. (Ed.). (1992). *Self-efficacy: Thought control of action.* Washington, DC: Hemisphere.

Schwarzer, R. (1996). *Psychologie des Gesundheitsverhaltens* (2nd edition). Göttingen: Hogrefe.

Schwarzer, R. (1996). *The general self-efficacy scale (GSE).* Berlin: Free University of Berlin.

Schwarzer, R. (2001). Social-cognitive factors in changing health-related behaviour. *Current Directions in Psychological Science, 10*, 47-51.
Schwarzer, R. (2002). Selbstwirksamkeitserwartung. In: R. Schwarzer, M. Jerusalem & H. Weber (Eds.), *Gesundheitspsychologie von A bis Z: Ein Handbuch* (pp. 521-523). Göttingen: Hogrefe Verlag.
Schwarzer, R. & Fuchs, R. (1996). Self-efficacy and health behaviours. In: M. Conner & P. Norman (Eds.), *Predicting health behaviour* (pp. 163-196). Buckingham: The Open University.
Schwarzer, R., Jerusalem, M. & Weber, H. (Eds.). (2002). *Gesundheitspsychologie von A bis Z: Ein Handbuch*. Göttingen: Hogrefe Verlag.
Shuey, D. A., Babishangire, B. B., Omiat, S. & Bagarukayo, H. (1999). Increased sexual abstinence among in-school adolescents as a result of school health education in Soroti district, Uganda. *Health Education Research, 14*(3), 411-419.
Simmons, R. G. & Blyth, D. A. (1987). *Moving into adolescence: The impact of pubertal change and school context*. New York: Aldine de Gruyter.
Simmons, R. G. & Rosenberg, D. A. (1975). Sex, sex roles, and self-image. *Journal of Youth and Adolescence, 4*, 229-258.
Skinner, D. (2000). *A practical application of psychological theory: Use of the theories of reasoned action and planned behaviour to gain a better understanding of HIV related behaviour among youth in the communities of Kayamandi and Mbekweni*. Unpublished doctoral's thesis, University of Cape Town, Cape Town, South Africa.
Smart, R. (2002). Preventing transmission of HIV. In: J. Gow & C. Desmond (Eds.), *Impacts and interventions: The HIV/AIDS epidemic and the children of South Africa* (pp.189-206). Pietermaritzburg: University of Natal Press.
Smith, C. A. (2002). Motivation, attributions, and self-efficacy in children. *Journal of Physical Education, Recreation and Dance, 73*(3), 10-13.
Soet, J., Dudley, W. & Dilario, C. (1999). The effects of ethnicity and perceived power on women's sexual behaviour. *Psychology of Women Quarterly, 23*(4), 707-723.
South African Police Services (SAPS). (2000). Semester report 1 of 2000.
Soul City. (n.d.). *Living positively with HIV and AIDS*. Jacana.
Soul City. (n.d.). *Talking about sexuality and sexually transmitted infections*. Jacana.
Soul City. (n.d.). *Women, children, and HIV and AIDS: Workbook 2*. Kensington: ViVa Books.
Stanton, B. F., Li, X., Kahihuata, J., Fitzgerald, A. M., Neumbo, S. & Kanduuombe, G. (1998). Increased protected sex and abstinence among Namibian youth following a HIV risk-reduction intervention: A randomized, longitudinal study. *AIDS, 12*, 2473-2480.
Statistics South Africa. (2001). *Census 2001 database.*. Retrieved September, 2005, from http://www.statssa.gov.za/census01/Census/Database/Census%202001/Census%202001.asp.
Statistics South Africa. (2005a). *Mortality and causes of death in South Africa: 1997-2003*. Pretoria.
Stellenbosch Police. (2004). *Police zones in Kayamandi*. Stellenbosch.

Stellenbosch School Clinics. (2002, August 6). *Attendance register.* Unpublished report.
Steyn, N. & Labadarios, D. (2002, September). *Nutrition policy implementation: Integrated nutrition programme for South Africa.* National Department of Health.
Stover, J., Walker, N., Garnett, G. P., Salomon, J. A., Stanecki, A. & Ghys, P. D. (2002). Can we reverse the HIV/AIDS pandemic with an expanded response? *The Lancet, 360,* 73-77.
Streak J. (2002). Child Poverty Monitor (IDASA No.1). In: L. Berry & T. Guthrie. *Rapid assessment: The situation of children in South Africa.* Cape Town: Children's Institute.
Strebel, A. & Perkel, A. (1991). *'Not our Problem'. AIDS knowledge, attitudes, practices and psychosocial factors at UWC.* (Psychology Resource Centre Occasional Paper Series No. 4). Cape Town: University of the Western Cape.
Swart-Kruger, J. (2001). In: L. Berry & T. Guthrie (Eds.), *Rapid assessment: The situation of children in South Africa.* Cape Town: Children's Institute.
Thom, A. (2002). *Where the river flows: An impoverished community and a determined Stellenbosch epidemiologist are on a collision course with local authorities about a river so polluted it's potentially life threatening.* Retrieved August 28, 2002, from http://www.healthe.org.za/news/easy_print.php?uid=200 20817.
Turcotte, K. (2003). *The nutritional status of children aged 1-7 years in Kayamandi (Western Cape, South Africa) as determined by 24-hour recall and anthropometric measurements.* Montreal: McGill University.
United Nations. (1989). *Convention on the rights of the child.* Adopted by the General Assembly of the United Nations on 20 November 1989.
United Nations. (1995). *Primary School Kit on the United Nations.* Geneva: UN Publications.
United Nations Children's Fund (UNICEF). (2001). *The state of the world's children 2001.* NewYork: Oxford University Press.
United Nations Children's Fund (UNICEF). (2004, December). *The state of the world's children 2005: Childhood under threat.* London.
University of Stellenbosch. (2001). *Socio-economic survey that was conducted in the Kayamandi residential area of the Stellenbosch municipal area during April to May 2001.* Stellenbosch: University of Stellenbosch, Department of Sociology.
Valois, R. F. & Kammermann, S. (1984). *Your sexuality: A personal inventory.* New York: Random House.
Van Wijk, B. (1994). *The dynamics of HIV transmission amongst a group of school-going adolescents in South Africa.* Unpublished honours thesis, University of Cape Town, Cape Town, South Africa.
Varga, C. & Makubalo, L. (1996). Sexual non-negotiation. *Agenda, 28,* 31-38.
Vergnani, T., Flisher, A. J., Lazarus, S., Reddy, P. & James, S. (1998). Health promoting schools in South Africa: Needs and prospects. *Southern African Journal of Child and Adolescent Mental Health, 10*(1), 44-58.
Visser, M. J. (1996). Evaluation of the First AIDS Kit, the AIDS and Lifestyle education programme for teenagers. *South African Journal of Psychology, 26*(2), 103-113.

Visser, M. J., Roos, J. L. & Korf, L. (1995). AIDS-prevention on the campus. *South African Journal of Higher Education, 9*, 165-173.
Walker, L., Verins, I., Moodie, R., & Webster, K. (2005): Responding to the Social and Economic Determinants of Mental Health: A Conceptual Framework for Action. In: World Health Organization (WHO). (2005). *Promoting mental health: Concepts, emerging evidence, practice.* (pp. 89-106). Geneva: World Health Organization, Department of Mental Health and Substance Abuse in collaboration with the Victorian Health Promotion Foundation and the University of Melbourne.
Western Cape Department of Education. (2002a). *Life skills and HIV/AIDS education: Resource guide.* Cape Town.
Western Cape Department of Education. (2002b). *Life skills and HIV/AIDS education: Activity book. Grade 4.* Cape Town.
Western Cape Department of Education. (2002c). *Life skills and HIV/AIDS education: Teacher's guide. Grade 4.* Cape Town.
Western Cape Stellenbosch Municipality. (2003, January-December). [Sub-Dis WC Stellenbosch Municipality. Facility WC Kayamandi Clinic]. Unpublished raw data.
Western Cape Stellenbosch Municipality Kayamandi Clinic. (2004, August 10). *Tuberculosis programme, Health Facility Report* (WC Kayamandi Clinic Report Nos. Q3 2003 to Q2 2004). Stellenbosch.
Whitefield, V. J. (1999). *A descriptive study of abusive dating relationships amongst adolescents.* Unpublished master's thesis, University of Cape Town, Cape Town, South Africa.
Wigfield, A. & Eccles, J. S. (1994). Children's competence beliefs, achievement values, and general self-esteem: Change across elementary and middle school. *Journal of Early Adolescence, 14*(2), 107-138.
Wild, L. G., Flisher, A. L., Bhana, A. & Lombard, C. (2002). *Psychometric properties of the Self-esteem Questionnaire for South African adolescents.* Cape Town: University of Cape Town.
Wood, C. & Foster, D. (1995). 'Being type of lover...': Gender-differentiated reasons for non-use of condoms by sexually active heterosexual students. *Psychology in Society, 20*, 13-35.
Wood, K., Maepa, J. & Jewkes, R. (1997). *Adolescent sex and contraceptive experiences: Perspectives of teenagers and clinic nurses in the Northern Province.* Pretoria: Centre for Epidemiological Research in South Africa (Women's Health).
World Bank. (1993). *World development report 1993: Investing in health.* New York: Oxford University Press.
World Bank. (2002). *Education and HIV/AIDS: A window of hope.* Washington, DC.
World Bank (2002, March 3). *World development indicators database.* Retrieved March 3rd, 2002, from http://www.worldbank.org/data/databytopic/ILIT.pdf.
World Health Organization. (WHO) (1986). *Ottawa Charta.* Retrieved July 13, 2004 from http://www.who.int/hpr/achive/docs/ottawa.html. *Meeting of senior officials and Ministers of health.* (WHO/HDE/HID/02.8). Johannesburg: WHO.

World Health Organization. (WHO) (1992a). *Study of the sexual experience of young people in eleven African countries: The narrative research method.* Geneva: WHO.
World Health Organization. (WHO) (1992b). *Comprehensive school health education: Suggested guidelines for action.* Geneva: WHO.
World Health Organization. (WHO) (1996). WHO global consultation on violence and health. Violence: A public health priority (WHO/EHA/SPI.POA.2). In: World Health Organization, *Promoting mental health: Concepts, emerging evidence, practice* (World Health Organization report). Geneva: Department of Mental Health and Substance Abuse in collaboration with the Victorian Health Promotion Foundation and the University of Melbourne.
World Health Organization. (WHO) (1999a). *Partners in life skills education: Conclusions from a United Nations Inter-Agency meeting.* (Department of Mental Health WHO/MNH/MHP/99.2). Geneva: WHO.
World Health Organization (WHO) (1999b). *A critical link: Interventions for physical growth and child development.* Geneva: WHO.
World Health Organization. (WHO) (2000, October). *Violence against women and HIV/AIDS: Setting the research agenda.* (Meeting report: Gender and women's health). Geneva: WHO.
World Health Organization. (WHO) (2002). *Child abuse and neglect.* Retrieved 2002, from http://www.who.int/violence_injury_prevention. World Health Organization. (WHO) (2001). *Basic documents* (43rd ed.). Geneva: WHO.
World Health Organization. (WHO) (2005). *Promoting mental health: Concepts, emerging evidence, practice.* Geneva: World Health Organization, Department of Mental Health and Substance Abuse in collaboration with the Victorian Health Promotion Foundation and the University of Melbourne.
World Health Organization (WHO), National Department of Health of the Republic of South Africa & Southern African Development Community. (2002, January 19-22). *Johannesburg declaration on health and sustainable development.*
Wylie, R. (1979). *The self-concept: Theory and research on selected topics* (Vol. 2). Lincoln, NE: University of Nebraska Press.
Yeld, J. (2004, October 25). Dangerous germs found in Cape rivers. *Cape Argus.*
Yoro Badat, N.-J. (2004, July 3). Is your teenager having sex? Many factors determine attitudes towards sexuality. *Weekend Argus.*
Youniss, J., McLellan, J. A. & Yates, M. (1997). What we know about engendering civic identity. *American Behavioural Scientist, 40*(5), 620-631.
Youniss, J. & Yates, M. (1997). *Community service and social responsibility.* Chicago: University of Chicago Press.
Zanobini, M. & Carmen, M. (2002). USAI Domain-specific self-concept and achievement: Motivation in the transition from primary to low middle school. *Educational Psychology, 22*(2).
Zere, E. & McIntyre, D. (2003). Inequities in under-five child malnutrition in South Africa. *International Journal for Equity in Health, 2,* 7.

APPENDICES

Appendix A
Checklist for Casual Observation

Date: _____
Place: _____

Results

1. **Graphic Information:**

   | Grade: |
   | Class teacher: |
   | Number of learners: |
   | Number of girls: |
   | Number of boys: |
   | Ages: |
   | Verification of marks: |

2. **Impressions:**

   | Subject: |
   | Used methods: |
   | Style of teaching: |
   | Atmosphere: |
   | Learners' behaviour: |

3. **Interest of the class teacher to work in the programme:**

Appendix B

Questionnaire for Field Interview

Name: _____
Place, Date: _____

1. Which factors influence children in their mental and physical growing process from childhood to adolescence in Kayamandi?

1.1 Environmental (living) conditions:
_____
_____
_____

1.2 Social factors:
_____
_____
_____

1.3 Health conditions:
_____
_____
_____

1.4 Ethnographic conditions:
_____
_____
_____

1.5 Family structures:
_____
_____
_____

2. What kind of positive factors support children in developing a strong mental and healthy physical growth in Kayamandi?

3. What kind of negative factors hinder children in developing a strong mental and healthy physical growth in Kayamandi?

4. What role do the educational systems play in the mental growth of children in Kayamandi?

5. What role do families play in the mental and physical growth of children in Kayamandi?

6. How can a one-year life skills programme influence children in their mental and (physical) growth?

Date, Place: _____
Signature: _____

Appendix C

Health Promotion Trainers' Report

Name of reporter: _____
Date: _____
Topic of lesson: _____

Mark your opinion with an "X". Mark from "excellent" (1) to "bad" (5).

Description of Method	Suitability of Method					(Self-) Confidence (trainer)					Comments
1.	1	2	3	4	5	1	2	3	4	5	
	○	○	○	○	○	○	○	○	○	○	
2.	1	2	3	4	5	1	2	3	4	5	
	○	○	○	○	○	○	○	○	○	○	
3.	1	2	3	4	5	1	2	3	4	5	
	○	○	○	○	○	○	○	○	○	○	
4.	1	2	3	4	5	1	2	3	4	5	
	○	○	○	○	○	○	○	○	○	○	
5.	1	2	3	4	5	1	2	3	4	5	
	○	○	○	○	○	○	○	○	○	○	
6.	1	2	3	4	5	1	2	3	4	5	
	○	○	○	○	○	○	○	○	○	○	

Appendix D

Checklist for Participant Observation[39]

Date: _____	Place: _____
Name of observer: _____	Signature: _____
Time commenced: _____	Time completed: _____
Topic of lesson: _____	
Short description of activity: _____	
Seat place/description: _____	
Name of girl/boy: _____ Age: _____	

Behaviour	Checklist						
Initiation of role activity	Willing ☐		Undecided ☐		Negative ☐		
Body language	1	2	3	4	5	6	Comments
Open/ free/ active	☐	☐	☐	☐	☐	☐	
Shy/ cautious/ passive	☐	☐	☐	☐	☐	☐	
Use of positive nonverbal language	☐	☐	☐	☐	☐	☐	
Use of negative nonverbal language	☐	☐	☐	☐	☐	☐	
Aggressive	☐	☐	☐	☐	☐	☐	
Use of language	1	2	3	4	5	6	Comments
Friendly	☐	☐	☐	☐	☐	☐	
Unfriendly	☐	☐	☐	☐	☐	☐	
Quiet	☐	☐	☐	☐	☐	☐	
Rude	☐	☐	☐	☐	☐	☐	
Characteristics of behaviour to other gender	1	2	3	4	5	6	Comments
Has the courage to state own opinion	☐	☐	☐	☐	☐	☐	
Does not hold an own opinion	☐	☐	☐	☐	☐	☐	
Willing to accept other opinion	☐	☐	☐	☐	☐	☐	
Unwilling to accept other opinion	☐	☐	☐	☐	☐	☐	
Dominant in argumentation	☐	☐	☐	☐	☐	☐	
Subordinate in argumentation	☐	☐	☐	☐	☐	☐	
Special Comments							

---

[39] The presented formula is reduced in size.

Explanation of the Used Terms for Participant Observation

Behaviour	
Attitude:	General behaviour of participant during observation.
Willing	Participant decides to be a part of the lesson.
Undecided	Participant is not sure whether to agree or disagree to participating in the lesson.
Negative	Participant refuses to be a part of the lesson.
Body language:	Signs, actions and reactions with facial expressions and gestures (including arms, hands, legs, body posture etc.).
Open/ free/ active	Participant shows body language that expresses initiative and motivation.
Shy/cautious/passive	Participant shows minimal initiative or motivation. He/she observes the situation and takes over a passive part.
Use of positive nonverbal language	Participant's body posture shows motivation and willingness to participate (friendly gestures, body posture expresses self-esteem).
Use of negative nonverbal language	Participant's body posture does not show motivation or willingness to participate (no movement, unfriendly gestures, body posture expresses refusal)
Aggressive	Participant's body posture shows readiness to express physical and verbal violence.
Use of language (communication):	Expression with words (comments, sentences, single words etc.); observer pays attention to sound of words.
Friendly	Participant uses positive voice and interacts politely with other learners.
Unfriendly	Participant uses negative voice and interacts impolitely with other learners.
Silent/ Keeps quiet	Participant uses few words, speaks in a low voice and does not communicate much with other learners.
Rude	Participant uses very impolite voice and communicates loudly and incoherently.
Characteristics of behaviour towards other learners (interaction):	Ways of interaction and communication with other learners.
Courage to express his/her own opinion	Participant's body language is open. The form of expression makes clear statements about the personal opinion and opens his/her mind in the presence of other learners.
No expression of own opinion	Participant's body language is defensive. The used language does not represent or express an own opinion or a strong minded attitude towards the reactions or argumentation of the other learners.
Willing to accept a different opinion	Participant's body language is friendly. The communication with other learners expresses the will to find a solution for the problem and he/she accepts the opinion of others.
Unwilling to accept a different opinion	Participant's body language is defensive and reluctant. The communication with the partner does not express the willingness to find a solution or to accept the opinion of the other.
Dominating in discussions	Participant's body language and communication shows superiority to the other learners. He/she does not allow the other learner to finish his/her sentence or argumentation. The participant believes in finding a solution alone without the other learners or is unable to listen to others.
Subordinate in discussions	Participant takes a subordinate role towards the other learners. He/she allows the partner to make decisions and find a solution for a problem.
Special Comments:	The observer can write down any comment about the observation or the action of the participant in interaction with others.

Appendix E
Revised Questionnaire

BOY

TITLE

Imigaqo:
Kulamacandelo alandelayo uzakufumana amahlu amabini akubuza ngezinto ezahlukeneyo. Funda umbuzo ngamnye ngenyameko kwayeuphendule impendulo ngokunyanisekileyonangokukuko. Ungathathi ixesha elide kumbuzo omnye. Akukho mpendulo ilungileyo okanye engalunganga kumbuzo ngamnye. Into efunekayo kukuba unike impendulo ethi ingqamane ngqo nendlela oyiyo. Impendulo zakho ziya kugcinwa ziyimfihlelo.
Ukuba kukho into engacaci ngokupheleleyo xa ugcwalisa kolu luhlu lwemibuzo ungoyiki ukubuza kutitshala okanye lo uqeqeshelwe ukwenza oku.

Siyabulela kakhulu ngempendulo zakho ezinyanisekileyo!

Directions:
In the following two sections you will find items that ask you different things. Read each item carefully and answer honestly and genuinely. Do not take long on each item. There are no RIGHT or WRONG answers for each item. What is correct is to give your answer that typically represents your behaviour. Your answer will be kept confidential.
If there is anything unclear while you are filling in the questionnaire, feel free to ask the teacher or trainer.

Thank you very much for taking part in this interview!

ICANDELO I: Bhala iimpendulo zakho kumabala abonisiweyo okanye ngokuthi ufake u 'X' kwibhokisana kulemibuzo ilandelayo. (PART I: Write your answers on the blank spaces or put an "X" in the boxes for the following items.)

1. Ubuni (Gender):

Ndiyintombazana ☐
(I am a girl)

Ndiyinkwenkwe ☐
(I am a boy)

2. Uzelwe nini (Age):

Ndineminyaka _____
(I was born in)

3. Ibanga (Grade): _____

4. Uhlala nabani ngoku?
(With whom are you living now?)

Nabazali bobabini (Parents)	☐
Nomama (kuphela) (Mother (only))	☐
Nomama kunye notatomncinci (Mother with stepfather)	☐
Nosisi (Sister)	☐
Notatomncinci kunye nomamoncinci (Stepparents)	☐
Notata kuphela (Father (only))	☐
Notata kunye nomamoncinci (Father with stepmother)	☐
Nobhuti (Brother)	☐
Nomakhulu notatomkhulu (Grandparents)	☐
Nomalume/nomalumekazi (Uncle/aunt)	☐

Nabanye abantu (nceda ucacise) (Others, please specify):

_____

ICANDELO II: Kumbuzo ngamnye, khetha ibhokisi esecaleni kwengcaciso ezidwelileyo uze ubeke u "X". (PART II: The next set of questions ask how you feel about yourself. For each question, tick the box next to the statement that best describes how you feel about yourself.)

1.
Ndiyayithanda indlela endenza ngayo izinto ezininzi. (I love the way I can do most things.)
Andivumelani ☐ (disagree)/Ndiyavumelana ☐ (agree)/Andiqinisekanga ☐ (not sure)
2.
Ndiyayithanda indlela endiyiyo.[40] (I love the way I am.)
Andivumelani ☐ (disagree)/Ndiyavumelana ☐ (agree)/Andiqinisekanga ☐ (not sure)
3.
Ndingulomntu kanye ndifuna ukuba nguye. (I am the kind of person I want to be.)
Andivumelani ☐ (disagree)/Ndiyavumelana ☐ (agree)/Andiqinisekanga ☐ (not sure)
4.
Ndizithanda kanye ngohlobo endililo.[41] (I like being just the way I am.)
Andivumelani ☐ (disagree)/Ndiyavumelana ☐ (agree)/Andiqinisekanga ☐ (not sure)
5.
Ndingumntu olungileyo kanye ngohlobo endifuna ukubalulo. (I am as good a person as I want to be.)
Andivumelani ☐ (disagree)/Ndiyavumelana ☐ (agree)/Andiqinisekanga ☐ (not sure)
6.
Ndinganakho ukusombulula iingxaki ezinzima ukuba ndingazama ngaphezulu kokuba ndisenza. (I can always manage to solve difficult problems if I try hard enough.)
Andivumelani ☐ (disagree)/Ndiyavumelana ☐ (agree)/Andiqinisekanga ☐ (not sure)
7.
Ukuba kukho ondiphikisayo (or ochasayo), ndiyakwazi ukufuna eny' indlela yimbi ukuze ndifumane oko ndikufunayo (b). (If someone is against me, I can find the means and ways to get what I want.)
Andivumelani ☐ (disagree)/Ndiyavumelana ☐ (agree)/Andiqinisekanga ☐ (not sure)
8.
Kulula kum ukubambelela kwinjongo zam de iminqweno yam iphumelele. (It is easy for me to stick to my aims and accomplish my goals.)
Andivumelani ☐ (disagree)/Ndiyavumelana ☐ (agree)/Andiqinisekanga ☐ (not sure)

---

40 The word 'love' in Xhosa is preferred, because the words like and love are the same word in Xhosa.
41 In Xhosa, more everyday language, but has the same meaning.

9.
Ndizithembile ukuba ndinganendlela elula yokuphumelela nakwintoni na enokwenzeka kum. (I am confident that I could deal efficiently with unexpected events.)
Andivumelani ☐ (disagree)/Ndiyavumelana ☐ (agree)/Andiqinisekanga ☐ (not sure)

10.
Ndinakho ukusombulula iingxaki ezininzi ukuba nje ndingazama ngokwaneleyo. (I can solve most problems if I invest the necessary effort.[42])
Andivumelani ☐ (disagree)/Ndiyavumelana ☐ (agree)/Andiqinisekanga ☐ (not sure)

11.
Xa ndisengxakini ndingakwazi ukufumana izisombululo zibeliqela. (When I am in trouble, I can usually find several solutions.)
Andivumelani ☐ (disagree)/Ndiyavumelana ☐ (agree)/Andiqinisekanga ☐ (not sure)

12.
Ukuba ndisoloko ndisengxakini ndinakho ukucinga ngesisombululo. (If I am in trouble, I can usually think of a solution.)
Andivumelani ☐ (disagree)/Ndiyavumelana ☐ (agree)/Andiqinisekanga ☐ (not sure)

13.
Ndinakho ukujongana nayo nayiphi na into endivelelayo. (I can usually handle whatever comes my way.)
Andivumelani ☐ (disagree)/Ndiyavumelana ☐ (agree)/Andiqinisekanga ☐ (not sure)

14.
Ndisebenzisana nje ngokulula namantombazana (amantombazana) akwibanga lam.[43] (I get along very well with boys (girls) in my class.)
Andivumelani ☐ (disagree)/Ndiyavumelana ☐ (agree)/Andiqinisekanga ☐ (not sure)

15.
Amakhwenkwe (amantombazana) abonakalisa ukundihlonipha. (Boys (girls) really seem to respect me.)
Andivumelani ☐ (disagree)/Ndiyavumelana ☐ (agree)/Andiqinisekanga ☐ (not sure)

16. Ndiwathanda ngokwenene amakhwenkwe (amantombazana) kwibanga endikulo. (I really like the boys (girls) in my class.)
Andivumelani ☐ (disagree)/Ndiyavumelana ☐ (agree)/Andiqinisekanga ☐ (not sure)

17.
Amakhwenkwe (amantombazana) akwibanga endikulo alunge kakhulu kum. (The boys (girls) in my class are very nice to me.)
Andivumelani ☐ (disagree)/Ndiyavumelana ☐ (agree)/Andiqinisekanga ☐ (not sure)

18.
Amakhwenkwe (amantombazana) akwibanga lam andijongela phezulu. (The boys (girls) in my class seem to look up to me.)
Andivumelani ☐ (disagree)/Ndiyavumelana ☐ (agree)/Andiqinisekanga ☐ (not sure)

---

42 Another possible translation: I can solve most problems if I try hard enough.
43 Note the double meaning of 'Quba': drive and getting along.

19.
Amakhwenkwe (amantombazana) akwibanga lam ayawamkela amacebo am. (The boys (girls) in my class regard my ideas and opinions very highly.)
Andivumelani ☐ (disagree)/Ndiyavumelana ☐ (agree)/Andiqinisekanga ☐ (not sure)
20.
Ndinqwenela kakhulu ukukhathalela abanye abantu kwindawo endihlala kuyo. (I am very much willing to take care of other people in my community.)
Andivumelani ☐ (disagree)/Ndiyavumelana ☐ (agree)/Andiqinisekanga ☐ (not sure)
21.
Ndingathanda ukuthabatha inkxaxheba ekuncedeni abantu abanesifo uGawulayo (AIDS) kwakunye nezinye iingxaki. (I would like to participate in helping people with AIDS or other problems.)
Andivumelani ☐ (disagree)/Ndiyavumelana ☐ (agree)/Andiqinisekanga ☐ (not sure)
22.
Ndenza izinto ekhaya ngalendlela kulindelwe ngayo. (I do things at home as expected.)
Andivumelani ☐ (disagree)/Ndiyavumelana ☐ (agree)/Andiqinisekanga ☐ (not sure)
23.
Ndenza izinto esikolweni ngalendlela kulindelwe ngayo. (I do things in schools as expected.)
Andivumelani ☐ (disagree)/Ndiyavumelana ☐ (agree)/Andiqinisekanga ☐ (not sure)
24.
Ndiya thanda ukunceda abanye. (I am very much interested in helping other people.)
Andivumelani ☐ (disagree)/Ndiyavumelana ☐ (agree)/Andiqinisekanga ☐ (not sure)

ICANDELO III: Uluhlu lwemibuzo elandelayo ibuza malunga nolwazi lwakho ngentsholongwane kaGawulayo (HIV) okanye uGawulayo (AIDS). Kumbuzo ngamnye khetha ibhokisi enempendulo ocinga ukuba yiyo okanye ngendlela owazi ngayo uze ubeke u "X". (PART III: The next set of questions asks you something about your knowledge of HIV/AIDS. For each question, tick the box next to the statement that best describes how you feel about yourself.)

25a)
Lithetha ntoni eligama iHIV? Ingaba HIV sisigulo apho amajoni omzimba womntu athi abulawe lulwesuleleko nesithi senze umzimba ube (bu)wiki ungakwazi ukulwa nezinye izifo? (What does AIDS mean? Is AIDS a disease where the immune system of a human being is destroyed and infections make the body weak against other infections?)
Ewe ☐ (yes)   Hayi ☐ (no)   Andiqinisekanga ☐ (not sure)

26a)
Ivelaphi lentsholongwana iHIV? Ingaba HIV isuka phesheya Kwezilwandle? (Where did the HI-Virus come from? Did the HI-Virus come from the USA?)
Ewe ☐ (yes)   Hayi ☐ (no)   Andiqinisekanga ☐ (not sure)

26b)
Ivelaphi lentsholongwana iHIV? Okanye HIV ayaziwa imvelaphi yakhe? (Where did the HI-Virus come from? Or is the origin of AIDS unknown?)
Ewe ☐ (yes)   Hayi ☐ (no)   Andiqinisekanga ☐ (not sure)

27a)
Unokuyifumana njani umntu lentsholongwane iHIV (f)? Ungayifumana ngokulalana ngokungakhuselekanga? (How can you get the HI-Virus? Can you get the HI-Virus from unprotected sex?)
Ewe ☐ (yes)   Hayi ☐ (no)   Andiqinisekanga ☐ (not sure)

28a)
Yeyiphi incindi yomzimba enokuba nayo lentsholongwane iHIV? Ingaba amathe anayo lentsholongwane iHIV? (Which liquid of the body carries the HI-Virus? Does saliva/spittle carry the HI-Virus?)
Ewe ☐ (yes)   Hayi ☐ (no)   Andiqinisekanga ☐ (not sure)

28b)
Yeyiphi incindi yomzimba enokuba nayo lentsholongwane iHIV? Ingaba incindi yobudoda inayo lentsholongwane iHIV? (Which liquid of the body carries the HI-Virus? Does semen carry the HI-Virus?)
Ewe ☐ (yes)   Hayi ☐ (no)   Andiqinisekanga ☐ (not sure)

28c)
Yeyiphi incindi yomzimba enokuba nayo lentsholongwane iHIV? Ingaba iinyembezi zinayo lentsholongwane iHIV? (Which liquid of the body carries the HI-Virus? Do tears carry the HI-Virus?)
Ewe ☐ (yes)   Hayi ☐ (no)   Andiqinisekanga ☐ (not sure)

28d)
Yeyiphi incindi yomzimba enokuba nayo lentsholongwane iHIV?Ingaba igazi linayo lentsholongwane iHIV? (Which liquid of the body carries the HI-Virus? Does blood carry the HI-Virus?)
Ewe ☐ (yes)   Hayi ☐ (no)   Andiqinisekanga ☐ (not sure)

28e)
Yeyiphi incindi yomzimba enokuba nayo lentsholongwane iHIV? Ingaba umchamo unayo lentsholongwane iHIV? (Which liquid of the body carries the HI-Virus? Does urine carry the HI-Virus?)
Ewe ☐ (yes)   Hayi ☐ (no)   Andiqinisekanga ☐ (not sure)

28f)
Yeyiphi incindi yomzimba enokuba nayo lentsholongwane iHIV? Ingaba umbilo unayo lentsholongwane iHIV? (Which liquid of the body carries the HI-Virus? Does sweat carry the HI-Virus?)
Ewe ☐ (yes)   Hayi ☐ (no)   Andiqinisekanga ☐ (not sure)

28g)
Yeyiphi incindi yomzimba enokuba nayo lentsholongwane iHIV? Ingaba incindi yobumama inayo lentsholongwane iHIV? (Which liquid of the body carries the HI-Virus? Does secretion of the vagina carry the HI-Virus?)
Ewe ☐ (yes)   Hayi ☐ (no)   Andiqinisekanga ☐ (not sure)

29a)
Ingathatha ixesha elingakanani intsholongwane ukuphila ngaphandle komzimba? Ingaba lentsholongwane ingathatha imizuzu embalwa ukuphila ngaphandle komzimba? (How long can the HI-Virus survive outside of the body? Can the HI-Virus survive outside of the body for a few minutes?)
Ewe ☐ (yes) Hayi ☐ (no) Andiqinisekanga ☐ (not sure)
29b)
Ingathatha ixesha elingakanani intsholongwane ukuphila ngaphandle komzimba? Ingaba lentsholongwane ingathatha iiyure ezininzi ukuphila ngaphandle kozimba? (How long can the HI-Virus survive outside of the body? Can the HI-Virus survive outside of the body for some hours?)
Ewe ☐ (yes) Hayi ☐ (no) Andiqinisekanga ☐ (not sure)

30a)
Yintoni enokukhusela umntu kulentsholongwane iHIV? Ingaba xa nibukele umabonakude (TV) nomhlobo ningalali kungukukhusela ungasuleleki yinthsolongwane iHIV? (What protects you against the HI-Virus? Does watching TV with your friend without having sex with him or her protect you against the HI-Virus?)
Ewe ☐ (yes) Hayi ☐ (no) Andiqinisekanga ☐ (not sure)
30b)
Yintoni enokukhusela umntu kulentsholongwane? Ingaba ukusebenzisa ikhondomu xa nidibana ngesondo kungakukhusela na ekwasulelekeni yilentsholongwane? (What protects you against the HI-Virus? Does using condoms during sexual intercourse protect you against the HI-Virus?)
Ewe ☐ (yes) Hayi ☐ (no) Andiqinisekanga ☐ (not sure)

31a)
Kuthetha ntoni ukwabelana ngesondo okukhuselekileyo? Ingaba ukwabelana ngesondo okukhuselekileyo yindlela yokukhusela ukumitha? (What does "Safer Sex" mean? Is safer sex a method to prevent pregnancy?)
Ewe ☐ (yes) Hayi ☐ (no) Andiqinisekanga ☐ (not sure)
31b)
Kuthetha ntoni ukwabelana ngesondo okukhuselekileyo? Ingaba ukwabelana ngesondo okukhuselekileyo kukusebenzisa ikhondomu xa nisabelana ngesondo? (What does "Safer Sex" mean? Does safer sex mean using a condom during sexual intercourse (sex)?)
Ewe ☐ (yes) Hayi ☐ (no) Andiqinisekanga ☐ (not sure)
31c)
Kuthetha ntoni ukwabelana ngesondo okukhuselekileyo? Ingaba ukwabelana ngesondo okukhuselekileyo, kukuzigcina ungabelani ngesondo? (What does "Safer Sex" mean? Does safer sex mean practising abstinence from sex?)
Ewe ☐ (yes) Hayi ☐ (no) Andiqinisekanga ☐ (not sure)

32a)
Ngabaphi abantu abanokufumana lentsholongwane iHIV? Ingaba amapolisa angasuleleka yilentsholongwane iHIV? (Which people get an HIV infection? Can a policeman get an HIV infection?)
Ewe ☐ (yes)   Hayi ☐ (no)   Andiqinisekanga ☐ (not sure)

32b)
Ngabaphi abantu abanokufumana lentsholongwane iHIV? Ingaba abantu abathengisa ngomzimba bangasuleleka yintsholongwane (amahenyukazi) iHIV? (Which people get an HIV infection? Can people who sell their bodies get an HIV infection?)
Ewe ☐ (yes)   Hayi ☐ (no)   Andiqinisekanga ☐ (not sure)

32c)
Ngabaphi abantu abanokufumana lentsholongwane iHIV? Ingaba wonke umntu unokuwasuleleka yilentsholongwane iHIV? (Which people get an HIV infection? Can everybody get an HIV infection?)
Ewe ☐ (yes)   Hayi ☐ (no)   Andiqinisekanga ☐ (not sure)

32d)
Ngabaphi abantu abanokufumana lentsholongwane iHIV? Ingaba omama bangosuleleka yilentsholongwane iHIV? (Which people get an HIV infection? Can women get an HIV infection?)
Ewe ☐ (yes)   Hayi ☐ (no)   Andiqinisekanga ☐ (not sure)

32e)
Ngabaphi abantu abanokufumana lentsholongwane iHIV (f)? Ingaba amadoda anokwesuleleka yilentsholongwane iHIV? (Which people get an HIV infection? Can men get an HIV infection?)
Ewe ☐ (yes)   Hayi ☐ (no)   Andiqinisekanga ☐ (not sure)

33a)
Umntu unokulenza phi uvavanyo lwentsholongwane iHIV (f)? Ungalwenza na uvavanyo lwentsholongwane iHIV kwanompilo? (Where can one go to do a test for HIV? Can you do an HIV-test at an office of public health?)
Ewe ☐ (yes)   Hayi ☐ (no)   Andiqinisekanga ☐ (not sure)

33b)
Umntu unokulenza phi uvavanyo lwentsholongwane iHIV? Ungalwenza na uvavanyo lwentsholongwane iHIV kugqirha? (Where can one go to do a test for HIV? Can you do an HIV-test at a doctor?)
Ewe ☐ (yes)   Hayi ☐ (no)   Andiqinisekanga ☐ (not sure)

33c)
Umntu unokulenza phi uvavanyo lwentsholongwane iHIV? Ungalwenza na uvavanyo lwentsholongwane iHIV kwiklinikhi yendawo ohlala kuyo? (Where can one go to do a test for HIV? Can you do an HIV-test at a community clinic?)
Ewe ☐ (yes)   Hayi ☐ (no)   Andiqinisekanga ☐ (not sure)

Siyabulela kakhulu ngempendulo zakho ezinyanisekileyo!
(Thank you very much for your genuine answers!)

Appendix F
Commitments and Rules

⇒ We give everyone a chance to speak.

⇒ We listen to each other.

⇒ We must communicate.

⇒ We respect each other's opinion.

⇒ We must learn to be patient.

⇒ We do not laugh at people.

⇒ We learn to work together.

⇒ We do not use violence – here or outside the workshop – including hitting and being horrible to people.

⇒ Learners report problems to the facilitators.

⇒ Nobody's opinion is wrong!

⇒ We do not talk about what we have said outside the class!

Appendix G

Group Statistics (T-Test)

	Gender (female, male)	N	M	SD	SE mean
Pretest					
Self-esteem	female	39	2.6974	.48095	.07701
	male	40	2.5750	.44419	.07023
Self-efficacy	female	38	2.5296	.35288	.05724
	male	39	2.4038	.42386	.06787
Gender communication	female	39	2.0342	.53963	.08641
	male	40	2.2667	.46959	.07425
Social responsibility	female	38	2.7842	.26460	.04292
	male	40	2.6500	.44086	.06971
Knowledge on HIV/AIDS	female	39	.3147	.20156	.03228
	male	40	.3326	.13315	.02105
Posttest					
Self-esteem	female	63	2.6063	.47242	.05952
	male	58	2.4793	.48549	.06375
Self-efficacy	female	62	2.3387	.40004	.05081
	male	57	2.4189	.39774	.05268
Gender communication	female	63	1.8915	.44315	.05583
	male	58	2.2385	.44274	.05813
Social responsibility	female	62	2.7355	.28920	.03673
	male	57	2.5298	.48623	.06440
Knowledge on HIV/AIDS	female	63	.4281	.21589	.02720
	male	58	.4739	.18241	.02395
Follow-up 1					
Self-esteem	female	58	2.6379	.36410	.04781
	male	53	2.5057	.44481	.06110
Self-efficacy	female	59	2.2691	.35946	.04680
	male	52	2.3438	.35604	.04937
Gender communication	female	51	1.9150	.43764	.06128
	male	53	2.1667	.48481	.06659
Social responsibility	female	59	2.6983	.28131	.03662
	male	58	2.5655	.36923	.04848
Knowledge on HIV/AIDS	female	62	.3587	.15395	.01955
	male	58	.4101	.16936	.02224
Follow-up 2					
Self-esteem	female	49	2.6571	.42230	.06033
	male	55	2.5709	.42061	.05672
Self-efficacy	female	51	2.3873	.32332	.04527
	male	54	2.3750	.35188	.04789
Gender communication	female	47	2.0177	.44672	.06516
	male	52	2.1154	.41162	.05708
Social responsibility	female	52	2.7577	.34830	.04830
	male	55	2.5673	.37862	.05105
Knowledge on HIV/AIDS	female	51	.4130	.17855	.02500
	male	57	.4524	.15524	.02056

Note. M = Mean, SD = Std. deviation, SE mean = Std. Error Mean.

Appendix H

Correlation between Gender and the Evaluation Variables within the Intervention Group

Test phase		Levine's test for equality of variances		T-test for equality of means		
		F	Sign.	t	df	Sign. (2-tailed)
Pretest						
Self-esteem	Equal Variances assumed	.205	.652	1.176	77	.243
	Equal variances not assumed			1.175	76.162	.244
Self-efficacy	Equal variances assumed	.643	.425	1.413	75	.162
	Equal variances not assumed			1.416	73.233	.161
Gender communication	Equal variances assumed	.373	.543	-2.044	77	.044*
	Equal variances not assumed			-2.041	74.994	.045
Social responsibility	Equal variances assumed	6.212	.015	1.620	76	.109
	Equal variances not assumed			1.639	64.421	.106
Knowledge on HIV/AIDS	Equal variances assumed	5.742	.019	-.467	77	.642
	Equal variances not assumed			-.464	65.638	.644
Posttest						
Self-esteem	Equal variances assumed	1.079	.301	1.458	119	.147
	Equal variances not assumed			1.457	117.561	.148
Self-efficacy	Equal variances assumed	.115	.735	-1.095	117	.276
	Equal variances not assumed			-1.095	116.273	.276
Gender communication	Equal variances assumed	.531	.468	-4.305	119	.000*
	Equal variances not assumed			-4.305	118.196	.000
Social responsibility	Equal variances assumed	8.166	.005	2.831	117	.005*
	Equal variances not assumed			2.774	89.646	.007

Test phase		Levine's test for equality of variances		T-test for equality of means		
		F	Sign.	t	df	Sign. (2-tailed)
Posttest						
Knowledge on HIV/AIDS	Equal variances assumed	6.601	.011	-1.255	119	.212
	Equal variances not assumed			-1.263	118.155	.209
Follow-up 1						
Self-esteem	Equal variances assumed	5.774	.018	1.720	109	.088
	Equal variances not assumed			1.705	100.724	.091
Self-efficacy	Equal variances assumed	.054	.816	-1.097	109	.275
	Equal variances not assumed			-1.098	107.503	.275
Gender communication	Equal variances assumed	.133	.716	-2.775	102	.007*
	Equal variances not assumed			-2.781	101.592	.006
Social responsibility	Equal variances assumed	2.487	.118	2.190	115	.031*
	Equal variances not assumed			2.185	106.523	.031
Knowledge on HIV/AIDS	Equal variances assumed	.400	.528	-1.741	118	.084
	Equal variances not assumed			-1.735	114.981	.085

Test phase		Levine's test for equality of variances		T-test for equality of means		
		F	Sign.	t	df	Sign. (2-tailed)
Follow-up 2						
Self-esteem	Equal variances assumed	.364	.547	1.042	102	.300
	Equal variances not assumed			1.041	100.535	.300
Self-efficacy	Equal variances assumed	.646	.424	.186	103	.853
	Equal variances not assumed			.186	102.925	.853
Gender communication	Equal variances assumed	.765	.384	-1.132	97	.260
	Equal variances not assumed			-1.127	93.844	.262
Social responsibility	Equal variances assumed	.051	.821	2.703	105	.008*
	Equal variances not assumed			2.709	104.925	.008
Knowledge on HIV/AIDS	Equal variances assumed	2.528	.115	-1.229	106	.222
	Equal variances not assumed			-1.219	99.762	.226

Note. * = statistically significant ($p<0.05$).

Appendix I

Pearson Correlation Regarding Age of Samples –
Intervention Group

Test phase		Age of samples
Pretest		
Self-esteem	Pearson correlation	-.063
	Sig. (2-tailed)	.696
	N	41
Self-efficacy	Pearson correlation	.218
	Sig. (2-tailed)	.176
	N	40
Gender communication	Pearson correlation	.063
	Sig. (2-tailed)	.694
	N	41
Social responsibility	Pearson correlation	-.223
	Sig. (2-tailed)	.168
	N	40
Knowledge on HIV/AIDS	Pearson correlation	.139
	Sig. (2-tailed)	.387
	N	41
Posttest		
Self-esteem	Pearson correlation	-.077
	Sig. (2-tailed)	.633
	N	41
Self-efficacy	Pearson correlation	.156
	Sig. (2-tailed)	.336
	N	40
Gender communication	Pearson correlation	-.089
	Sig. (2-tailed)	.582
	N	41
Posttest Social responsibility	Pearson correlation	-.223
	Sig. (2-tailed)	.161
	N	41
Knowledge on HIV/AIDS	Pearson correlation	.277
	Sig. (2-tailed)	.080
	N	41
Follow-up 1		
Self-esteem	Pearson correlation	.043
	Sig. (2-tailed)	.800
	N	37
Self-efficacy	Pearson correlation	.248
	Sig. (2-tailed)	.145
	N	36
Gender communication	Pearson correlation	-.107
	Sig. (2-tailed)	.579
	N	29

Test phase		Age of samples
Follow-up 1		
Social responsibility	Pearson correlation	-.168
	Sig. (2-tailed)	.307
	N	39
Knowledge on HIV/AIDS	Pearson correlation	.231
	Sig. (2-tailed)	.146
	N	41
Follow-up 2		
Self-esteem	Pearson correlation	-.023
	Sig. (2-tailed)	.894
	N	37
Self-efficacy	Pearson correlation	.111
	Sig. (2-tailed)	.511
	N	37
Gender communication	Pearson correlation	.048
	Sig. (2-tailed)	.790
	N	33
Social responsibility	Pearson correlation	-.106
	Sig. (2-tailed)	.527
	N	38
Knowledge on HIV/AIDS	Pearson correlation	.447
	Sig. (2-tailed)	.005*
	N	38

Note. * = statistically significant ($p<0.05$).

Appendix J

Multiple Comparisons between Groups for Knowledge Scale 2 – Intervention Group

(I) Posttest (Age of samples)	(J) Posttest (Age of samples)	Mean Difference (I-J)	Std. Error	Sig.	95% Confidence Interval	
					Lower Bound	Upper Bound
9	10	.0210	.05296	.999	-.1608	.2029
	11	-.0616	.05945	.955	-.2658	.1425
	12	-.0644	.06907	.971	-.3016	.1728
	13	-.2727	.08615	.090	-.5686	.0231
	14	.0455	.11280	.999	-.3419	.4328
10	9	-.0210	.05296	.999	-.2029	.1608
	11	-.0826	.04580	.662	-.2399	.0746
	12	-.0854	.05775	.821	-.2837	.1129
	13	-.2937(*)	.07737	.021*	-.5594	-.0281
	14	.0244	.10624	1.000	-.3404	.3893
11	9	.0616	.05945	.955	-.1425	.2658
	10	.0826	.04580	.662	-.0746	.2399
	12	-.0028	.06375	1.000	-.2217	.2161
	13	-.2111	.08195	.264	-.4925	.0703
	14	.1071	.10962	.965	-.2694	.4835
12	9	.0644	.06907	.971	-.1728	.3016
	10	.0854	.05775	.821	-.1129	.2837
	11	.0028	.06375	1.000	-.2161	.2217
	13	-.2083	.08917	.374	-.5145	.0979
	14	.1098	.11512	.968	-.2855	.5052
13	9	.2727	.08615	.090	-.0231	.5686
	10	.2937(*)	.07737	.021*	.0281	.5594
	11	.2111	.08195	.264	-.0703	.4925
	12	.2083	.08917	.374	-.0979	.5145
	14	.3182	.12611	.286	-.1149	.7512
14	9	-.0455	.11280	.999	-.4328	.3419
	10	-.0244	.10624	1.000	-.3893	.3404
	11	-.1071	.10962	.965	-.4835	.2694
	12	-.1098	.11512	.968	-.5052	.2855
	13	-.3182	.12611	.286	-.7512	.1149

Note. * = a statistically significance (p<0.05).

Notes

Notes

Notes

Notes